Reboot Your Brain

Reboot Your Brain

Diet and Lifestyle Techniques to Improve
Your Memory and Ward Off Disease

Dr. Gary Null, PhD

Gary Null Publishing
an imprint of Skyhorse Publishing, Inc.

Gary Null Publishing books may be purchased in bulk at special discounts for sales promotion, corporate gifts, fund-raising, or educational purposes. Special editions can also be created to specifications. For details, contact the Special Sales Department, Gary Null Publishing, 307 West 36th Street, 11th Floor, New York, NY 10018 or info@skyhorsepublishing.com.

Gary Null Publishing is an imprint of Skyhorse Publishing, Inc.

Skyhorse® and Skyhorse Publishing® are registered trademarks of Skyhorse Publishing, Inc.®, a Delaware corporation.

Visit our website at www.skyhorsepublishing.com.

10 9 8 7 6 5 4 3 2 1

Library of Congress Cataloging-in-Publication Data is available on file.

Print ISBN: 978-1-63220-622-0
Ebook ISBN: 978-1-62873-531-4

Printed in the United States of America

Publisher's Note

Contents

An Important Note About Supplements and Multiple Conditions

This book is designed for individuals who have, or are specifically concerned about, only one of the conditions discussed on the following pages. To promote brain health and protect your brain, you should follow my protocol for optimal brain health in chapter 2.

In the chapters that follow, I'll recommend protocols for specific conditions. The vitamins, minerals, and supplements I recommend should be incorporated into the protocol from chapter 2. In some cases I will recommend increasing the dose of a particular vitamin or supplement to impact a specific condition. In these cases, you should increase the daily dosage from chapter 2 to the level recommended for that specific condition.

Do not combine the protocols in these chapters with each other. And do not add more than one additional protocol to the one given in chapter 2. If you are concerned about more than one of these brain conditions, consult with a health professional about how you can safely impact multiple conditions. If you are taking medications, or have any food restrictions, you should consult with your doctor before beginning any supplement program. Supplement overdoses are rare, but possible, and certain combinations may affect individuals adversely.

Reboot Your Brain

PART I

WHAT IT MEANS TO REBOOT YOUR BRAIN

Introduction

As of 2013, ninety-three million people over the age of forty-seven live in America. They make up the largest group of aging people in our country's history. Most of these individuals are overweight or obese and have poor diets. Many of them experience a high-stress lifestyle and turn to smoking, drinking, drugs, and prescription medications for short-lived "fixes." Our health care system makes matters worse through overtaxing and placing little to no emphasis on prevention. Given this state of affairs, the prognosis for America is a virtual pandemic of brain dysfunction, oxidative stress, and inflammation leading to dementia, Alzheimer's disease, Parkinson's disease, insomnia, multiple sclerosis, and amyotrophic lateral sclerosis (ALS). Current estimates by health care experts tell us that by 2050, two billion people worldwide will suffer from dementia, costing approximately one trillion dollars in medical expenses annually.[1] These projections may well become a reality *unless* we make some radical and fundamental changes.

This book is the culmination of thirty-five years of my own research into anti-aging sciences—thirty of them spent as a research fellow with the Institute of Applied Biology—as well as my clinical experience counseling more than ten thousand individuals as a nutritionist and dietitian. I have come to the conclusion that all the conditions mentioned above can be prevented and reversed with lifestyle modifications. It is my firm conviction that it is never too early or too late to change your behaviors to successfully maintain vigorous mental and physical health as you grow older. These claims are well-supported by thousands of studies published in peer-reviewed scientific literature.

Shifting the Paradigm of Aging

Science has told us we have approximately 65,100 trillion cells. We know that there are more than ten thousand gene alterations per cell per day. The reason our brains lose function as they age is that we damage them, rather than help them repair themselves. Coffee, cigarettes, white bread, hot dogs, hamburgers, pizza, french fries, milkshakes, cheesecakes, pretzels, bagels, grilled cheese sandwiches, white rice, colas, candies, and other junk foods allow for the biochemical reactions that cause oxidative stress, inflammation, free radical damage, and glycation that destroy, harm, or alter DNA. Such damage occurs all the time, and it will continue as long as we are doing nothing to change it.

A wealth of scientific evidence demonstrates that engaging in physical and mental exercise and adhering to a healthy, vegan diet rich in phytonutrients, vitamins, minerals, and antioxidants can effectively prevent DNA damage and help us maintain good health. In *Reboot Your Brain*, I gather knowledge from hundreds of the latest peer-reviewed studies from around the world showing that our lifestyle choices play a central role in keeping the brain fit and functional. In this book, we will review cutting-edge research showing that consuming a plant-based diet rich in nutrients, antioxidants, and omega-3 fatty acids can effectively protect against dementia and Alzheimer's disease. We will explore how modern science has identified the ancient practice of tai chi as a powerful treatment for individuals suffering from Parkinson's disease and depression. In addition, we will look at new evidence linking cognitive degeneration with a sedentary lifestyle and investigate the connection between staying mentally stimulated and maintaining a healthy brain.

This book is meant as a wake–up call, alerting you that everything in life is cause and effect. The concept of cause and effect has been explained by some truly brilliant minds: Hans Selye, who told us in the 1950s about the effects of stress; Lawrence LeShan, who taught us in the 1960s that what we think, we then become; as well as many others.

The concept is less theoretical than practical, in actuality. Throughout our lives, we have been conditioned to believe that disease exists and symptoms—be it heart attack, stroke, cancer—manifest suddenly, when the reality is every single choice we make in our lives contributes to the disease process or the wellness process. But that's hard to appreciate, as no one who eats a single hamburger has a heart attack and ends up in a hospital, and no one who smokes a cigarette ends up with lung disease, and no one who eats a slice of cheesecake ends up diabetic. Hence, we're lulled into a false pattern of behavior that reinforces no such things as cause and effect. All this occurs every day with every choice we make. Granted, you may not end up with a disease, but, in time, the quality of your life will be measured by the total cumulative impact of it all. We never think in terms of cumulative impact: the 3000th hamburger, or the 2000th drink of alcohol, the 170th pound of sugar every year! Then one day, we end up with symptoms represented by a healing crisis. Inflammation anywhere in the body is inflammation *everywhere* in the body. As blood courses through the body, hetracyclic amines in BBQ chicken or deep-fried french fries, or the brown crust of toast or the bagel or donut, all cause inflammatory agents in the blood. So every cell fed by blood is also impacted. But our monotheistic medical model consists of highly skilled specialists with highly specialized technology to determine specific damage to a specific part of the body, and they do not look beyond, they can't see the whole—not in the holistic way. We are looking at the whole process and the cumulative progression, whether positive or negative. In our culture, we don't often examine the problem until the breaking point—but look at the metaphor of the person who goes broke or gets divorced. It doesn't happen overnight.

Back when I was young, we infrequently had fast or junk food. We had family table dinners. We had backyard gardens where our fruits and vegetables were organic and pesticide-free. We'd store and date frozen foods. Our lives were in many ways less stressful. Today young people are living in a different world with considerable challenges: They don't have proper vitamin supplementation (vitamin deficiencies); they eat processed foods and have massive pro-inflammatory diets; they are surrounded by electromagnetic pollution; they get poor sleep; they consume caffeine and processed sugars and high fructose corn syrup and aspartame; they get excess calories from excess proteins and fats all of which have excess sodium; they experience mitochondrial destruction through chemical exposure; they battle allergies and therefore immune system over stimulation from diets high in gluten and dairy and yeast; they have high glycemic intake overtaxing the pancreas leading to pre-diabetes and metabolic syndromes; and they have high stress made worse only by a lack of exercise—all cause aging of the brain as they age the body.

So when I looked at former President Clinton, who had quadruple bypass surgery, I predicted he would be diagnosed with ALS or Parkinson's or dementia within ten to fifteen years, *unless* he made a radical change. And he did—he's been vegan for years and he's never seemed better. But the concept of radical change scares so many. And we have the concept backwards. We are extremely radical when it comes to consuming wrong things and very conservative with the right ones. Ask the average person to substitute coffee with green tea, even today, and they'll immediately think you're nuts.

We must remember diets are only part of this—our beliefs, the epigenetics of our family life, the understanding that everything that occurred emotionally from conception to adulthood impacts us. And we can't forget the significance of our environment—our water, the impact of stress, our responses to it, even reality TV—which is an escape, a way to say, "As bad as my problems are, I'm way better than these low-life degenerate idiots on TV!" And we champion the wrong people and attitudes—like the "food gladiator" at the heart of the recent reality TV show *Man v. Food* on the Travel Channel, who goes to popular restaurants around the country and eats several pounds of the worst foods imaginable. Our public cheers this behavior on. And what happens? Now we are faced with the first generation where parents will outlive their children.

So as we approach this puzzle, there is no one piece, but millions. Each element, regarded with discipline and mindfulness can connect the direction we have gone to the one we should go, and in time we can fix much of what we suffer and prevent worse from happening.

The time is ripe for a shift in the paradigm. The new fifty is thirty. The new sixty is forty. The new eighty is sixty. All biologically speaking, but for those who are doing it *right*. In that context, we are seeing a transition. We are seeing a whole new generation of people who are not willing to wake up one day and have Alzheimer's, dementia, Parkinson's, ALS, forgetfulness, wrinkles, and arthritic joints. They are finally willing to stop long enough to say, "Cause and effect. If it works in finance, if it works in raising a child, it certainly should work with my body."

This book is such a tool. It is specifically meant to help you understand what to do for your brain. In the end, this is not just about rejuvenating and protecting the brain as you age. It is about rejuvenating and protecting every cell of your body, with the brain as the primary focus. But everything you do for the brain will have a residual positive effect.

And so, I challenge you to examine your definitions of aging, to challenge a belief system that says you must accept a quiet decline, a gradual fading of mind, body, and spirit. I challenge you to remember that it is the quality of your own beliefs that ultimately determines the quality of your life and growth for your brain and your body, no matter what your age. If you're not convinced yet, maybe these testimonials will help.

MAUREEN MCGOVERN

I was a museum curator at the corporate level. But after my brain injury, when I went to the Met, I couldn't recognize the artwork. I could barely read and I could not write. I couldn't read *The New York Times*. After a while I couldn't bathe properly or take care of myself. I had a very hard time understanding where I was. I'd get confused at the grocery store and couldn't find the things I needed. When people helped me shop, I would swipe my credit card without knowing what I was paying. I would go home and I couldn't cook.

My brain injury was the result of an awful crime, in which I was the victim. At first, after the crime, I was just out of it and I figured that with a little time my mind would be back to normal. And then there was a medical accident that made things much worse. After that, I went to Gary. The doctors who diagnosed me with dementia, wanted to put me on Allon, which is for Alzheimer's, and a friend of mine luckily did some research and discovered that six people had died from Allon. When you have bad cognition, you're in a very vulnerable place, and it's easy to become a victim of someone's experimentation. But Gary's approach was different; he gave me a plan and he's given me a *life*.

Before I went to Gary, the doctors gave me a couple of things that really hurt me—permanently hurt me. They were doing AP04 studies on me, specifically for the Alzheimer's gene, and their experimentation left me with some permanent disabilities.

When I started following Gary's natural approach to healing, I made giant leaps forward with everything—you know, being able to talk, dress myself, walk. Now, I *can* read, I do my own paperwork, and I've begun working again. I still have a long way to go, but I'm making real progress.

I keep pushing and pushing. I've advanced in terms of my critical thinking, and my spirituality. I've gotten a lot of my life back. It's hard work, and I have to stick to it. I wake up at five, I pray, I organize my food, I juice, I lay out the plans for the day, I do the remediation, I get the injections, I do the trips— it's a tremendous amount of work. But the gift I get is life, and now the opportunity to help other people with similar problems.

Today my life is a happy one. I'm nourished physically, mentally, and spiritually. I am actually happier and healthier than I was before my brain injury. I thank Gary for my life.

KENNETH F. CIESLA

In 2008, I experienced the most severe MS symptoms. However, five years prior to that in 2003, every once in a while I would have phantom issues with my musculature. I would experience slurred speech, muscle weakness, dizziness, and vertigo. From time to time, I felt intense pressure on the top of my head, as though someone was pushing down on me with an almost angry force. That particular symptom would become more and more frequent. I thought they were all isolated issues, but looking back I see that they were certainly part of MS. It was progressing quite steadily. Sometimes I'd be okay walking, other times I would need assistance walking and doing activities.

The first person I went to was a general physician, because of the vertigo and pressure on my head. They checked me out and told me to go to a neurologist. The neurologist performed two MRIs and a spinal tap. They said it was probably MS because of the lesions on my brain, my symptoms, and the results from the spinal tap. The only thing that would have made it for sure is if I had lost mobility and had even worse symptoms. When my symptoms did get worse, I didn't go back to that doctor. He said if I was in worse shape, he would have given me the MS diagnosis. When they did get worse, I was already seeking alternative ways to handle it.

I got the probable diagnosis and was scheduled to go back to the doctor a week later. During that time I went to a reiki practitioner, whom I still visit to this day. She suggested I get a hair analysis heavy metal test and recommended a handful of different vitamins. A week or two later during my appointment with the neurologist, he prescribed me Avonex and gave me a number to an MS clinic in North Jersey where they were going to have to inject me—or I would inject myself—for the rest of my life. The funny thing is that even though I was a "probable" in terms of diagnosis, he was giving me MS drugs. I thought that sounded like a definite diagnosis to me. I never took the medications and I never went to the MS clinic in Jersey. I never went to my local Walgreens and never sent in the prescription.

At that time, I didn't listen to Gary. I kind of knew who he was, but never listened. My wife was a big listener and she heard him say he never turns down an opportunity to help someone heal and that all you needed to do was email him. I emailed him and he got back to me quickly.

I went into NYC and drove around until I found the East Side Vitamin Closet. Outside, I saw one of his employees and he had all these boxes. Before I know it, I'm helping him bring this entire load of inventory upstairs. So I go upstairs and I told him that I'll get some green supplements and red supplements. Harry mentioned that Gary has a health support group which gets a 50 percent discount. Then I called up and sent all my stuff in for the support group.

At the beginning of the support group, my symptoms were at their worst. I needed assistance coming up the stairs. But shortly thereafter, after all the vitamins and the diet change, my symptoms subsided.

Because I had such a resolve to take care of things, I dropped everything bad I was doing. I stopped going to McDonald's. I threw out the food in my refrigerator. I had two weeks of pretty severe withdrawal from the food changes. They were becoming less and less frequent as I maxed out on green supplements and red supplements. I was exercising and following the protocol.

The next person I went to see was a chelation therapist. The doctor gave me a test for heavy metals, which showed me that all the metals were off the charts. Everything was high. At the same time I was doing chelation, I went for ozone therapy three times a week. I was going for hydrocolonics to detox. I was going for acupuncture and getting my mercury fillings removed. Three months later, they tested for heavy metal again and all my heavy metal levels were either at below detectable or near below detectable. They all went down dramatically. At that point, my symptoms really began to subside. They were about 98 percent gone. About seven to eight months after the diagnosis I was symptom-free.

The reason why I am successful is because I made a simple choice. I chose to reverse my illness. And if that's what you choose; everything that you do has to be in line with that choice. You have to do all of it. It can be an expensive proposition. You can't be a victim. The biggest thing of all that I've learned out of this experience is to relax and have a tranquil mind.

If there's one thing in life that I've learned it's that if any disease creeps up on me in the future because of actions I've taken in the past, I can reverse it. Gary's protocols are spot on—you just have to follow them. If I hadn't, I wouldn't be walking around today. I'd be in a wheelchair taking injections every day. That's a lot to be grateful for.

Chapter 1

Your Aging Brain

"The brain is not, like the liver, heart, and other internal
organs, capable from the moment of birth of all the
functions which it ever discharges; for while in common
with them, it has certain duties for the exercise of which
it is especially intended, its high character in man, as the
organ of conscious life, the supreme instrument of
his relations with the rest of nature, is developed
only by a long and patient training."

—R. V. Pierce (*The People's Common Sense
Medical Advisor in Plain English*, 1917)

From the moment of conception, our brains are developing, growing, and changing, and scientists and researchers are constantly
discovering new information about how our brains develop
throughout our lives.

For instance, it had long been thought that the human brain
created crucial neural pathways in the early years of life and then,
over the course of a lifetime, worked to reinforce and strengthen
the most important of these connections, while pruning away those
that were underutilized. In other words, the brain was formed and

influenced in early years, remained largely unchanged in middle years, and declined in old age.

Throughout the last few decades, as scientific research techniques have become more sophisticated, our ability to learn about the complexities of the brain has accelerated. Now scientists are discovering that the growth of the brain is far more complicated and ongoing than previously supposed. Studies have shown that crucial development in the prefrontal cortex occurs after the teen years, and other researchers have discovered that brain cells can continue to develop well into old age.

It is amazing to consider how our brains—these three-pound organs that constantly grow and change throughout our lives—are charged with the oversight of our entire being. This mass of tissue and nerves drives our intelligence, interprets input from our senses, initiates the movement of our limbs, and regulates the social aspects of our behavior.

In this chapter, I will talk about the structure of the brain and how choices you make about your environment, lifestyle, nutrition, and other factors can impact the health of your brain as you age.

Understanding the Brain

To get the most out of the Reboot Your Brain program, you need to have some knowledge of the most basic structures and workings of the brain and to understand how external factors influence both the growth and decline of this amazing organ.

The Architecture of the Brain

Our brains sit under our scalps, within the bony safety of our skulls, floating in cerebrospinal fluid and covered by the meninges. The meninges consists of three layers: the dura mater, a thick membrane that can restrict the movement of the brain within the skull, preventing movements that may burst the blood vessels of the brain; the middle layer, or arachnoid; and the layer closest to the brain, the pia mater. Our brains are nourished by our circulatory systems, which convert the nutrients in our blood into fuel for the ongoing computations of the brain's billions of nerve cells. The brain is covered with a thin layer of tissue called the cerebral cortex. This coating is also called gray matter because the nerves in this area lack the insulation that makes other parts of the brain appear white. Most information processing takes place in the cortex.

The Forebrain

When you look at a picture of the brain, it is likely that the first part you notice is the cerebrum. This intricate, wrinkled area, along with its covering (the cortex) is the source of higher-level functions. It holds memories and allows you to plan, imagine, and create. This is the part of your brain you use in problem solving, abstract thinking, and making judgments. The cerebrum is split down the center by a deep fissure, creating two halves, each with very different functions. At the base of the split is a thick construct of nerve fibers called the corpus callosum, which keeps communication flowing between the halves of the brain. Signals from the brain cross over on their way to the body.

The right cerebral hemisphere controls primarily the left side of the body, and the left hemisphere controls primarily the right side of the body. In most people, the left hemisphere is dominant in controlling responses, as well as language production and understanding and cognitive functions. The right side of your brain controls temporal and spatial relations, pattern recognition, recognition of complex auditory tones, and communication of emotion.

Each of the cerebral hemispheres in the forebrain can be further divided into sections called lobes, which govern specific functions.

- The frontal lobes lie directly behind your forehead and control your ability to plan, reason, and imagine. They are also important in memory construction. The rear part of the frontal lobes has a motor area that controls voluntary movement. On the left frontal lobe, a section called Broca's area works to transform thoughts into words.

- The parietal lobes govern sensory combinations and comprehension of stimuli, such as touch, taste, temperature, and movement. The parietal lobes also function in reading and arithmetic.
- The temporal lobes are associated with music, memory, and sensation. These lobes also process emotion, including strong emotions such as fear. They are important in forming and retrieving memories.
- The occipital lobes process images from the eyes and link that information with images stored in memory.

The Midbrain

This area of the brain controls some reflex actions and is responsible for some voluntary movements.

The Hindbrain

The lowermost area of the brain is composed of the upper part of the spinal cord, the brain stem, and a wrinkled ball of tissue called the cerebellum. The hindbrain governs cardiac, respiratory, and vasomotor centers.

The Limbic System

Deep within the brain, hidden from view, lie the structures that make up the limbic system, the area of the brain that is responsible for our emotional states. These gatekeepers of the brain include:

- The hypothalamus, a structure the size of a pearl, which works as a regulator, returning your body's systems to a "set point." The hypothalamus controls hunger, thirst, response to pain, and sexual satisfaction, as well as our emotions, such as anger, unhappiness, joy, and excitement.

- The thalamus acts as a clearinghouse for information flow between the cerebrum and the spinal cord. Clusters of nerve cells called basalganglia surround the thalamus and are responsible for integrating movements.
- The hippocampus works as a memory indexer and is vital in the construction and reconstruction of memory.
- The amygdala regulates our stress responses to fear and anxiety.

Communication in the Brain

All the structures in the brain communicate with each other and the rest of the body by sending signals through cells called neurons. Information passes from one neuron to another at a junction called a synapse. Chemicals known as neurotransmitters are released by one neuron, cross the synapse, and attach to a receptor in a neighboring cell. There are at least one hundred known neurotransmitters, all with individual chemical reactions that occur constantly at the millions of synaptic junctions in our brains.

Key neurotransmitters, which help the brain function quickly and smoothly, include acetylcholine, serotonin, dopamine, glutamate, and gamma amino butyric acid (GABA). Maintaining the delicate balance of these neurotransmitters within the brain is crucial to brain health.

Aging and the Brain

Our brains begin to form just three weeks after conception and continue to develop, expand, and adapt throughout our lifetimes. Babies are born with more than one hundred billion neurons, roughly the same number they will always have. Throughout the next three years, trillions of synaptic connections form between these neurons. During this period of time, frequently stimulated synapses strengthen and proliferate, and rarely used synapses are discarded. Scientists use the term "plasticity" to define this period of adaptive growth.

Until rather recently, the prevailing theory had been that, from adolescence through adulthood and old age, the brain continues to simply discard neuronal connections. Doctors told elderly patients experiencing age-related conditions such as memory loss and mental fatigue that there was nothing they could do but accept the inevitable. "Old" neurons had died, and there were no new cells to replace them. A decline in mental sharpness was an inevitable by-product of aging.

But research has shown that our brain—this amazing organ that grows and learns through interacting with the world through both perception and action—can continually adapt and rewire itself. A Princeton research team discovered there is a natural regenerative mechanism in the mature brain that creates neurons that migrate to the cerebral cortex, where they "plug in" and become a new part of the brain's central circuitry.[1]

Think about the brain of an infant, which is constantly amassing new information and stimulation and enrichment for the neurons forming synaptic connections. Now consider your own perceptions about challenging your brain when you are middle-aged or during your elder years. Stimulation, mental activity, and challenge all are essential in brain growth and vitality. This new research brings new urgency to a key maxim for vigorous mental health at any age: "Use it or lose it!"

But clearly the issue of what weakens our brain function is not simply the act of aging. Despite what we have been told for decades, we need not accept the idea that our bodies, or our brains, simply and inevitably "wear out" as we grow older. Staying vital both mentally and physically as we age requires paying close attention to the mind–body connection and the effects outside factors such as environment, nutrition and diet, and stress and emotion bring to bear on our welfare.

Negative Factors and Brain Weakness

What does happen, as we grow older, is that we begin to experience the cumulative effects of negative lifestyle habits and outside influences. Mental health conditions that have been labeled "age-related" are more often the result of our neglect of our bodies and our brains. If we understand the negative factors and how they impact our mental vitality, we can make the changes necessary to ensure vigorous mental health throughout our lifetimes.

In the rest of this chapter, I discuss the key factors in your environment and lifestyle that can negatively impact your mental health as you age. In chapter 3, you will find out how you can protect yourself from these external hazards and rejuvenate your brain naturally.

Environment and the Brain

Pollution and poisons in our environment are especially harmful to our brains. Let's examine the substances of greatest concern.

Toxic Substances

Our daily environment can be hazardous to the health of our brains. It is shocking to realize that there are approximately one thousand substances that may cause brain toxicity and accelerate the decline of the brain. Of these one thousand substances, we are in danger of being exposed to several on a regular basis.

These substances cause brain damages in two main ways:

- Acute toxicity occurs when there is a single exposure to high levels of a substance, causing immediate neurological damage.
- Chronic toxicity results from continuous exposure to lower levels of a toxin and can result in long-term negative effects in the body.

Four general categories of substances may contribute to brain toxicity: heavy metals, solvents and fuels, pesticides, and carbon monoxide.

Heavy Metals

Heavy metals that are not metabolized by the body can accumulate in the soft tissue with toxic effect. Heavy metals enter our bodies through food, water, and air. They may also be absorbed through direct contact with our skin. Blood and urine tests can be used to assess levels of heavy metals in the body. According to Dr. Christopher Calapai, DO, "The biggest enemy of the brain is clearly heavy metals. Research going back thirty years has linked heavy metals with Parkinson's, ALS, MS, lupus, Alzheimer's, auto-immune disease—it runs the gamut. And as we pull metals out of the body with appropriate chelation therapy, and we get vitamins, minerals, glutathione back in the body, we start to see significant improvement."[1]

The list below contains four heavy metals that appear in the top ten substances on the 2003 Comprehensive Environmental Response, Compensation, and Liability Act (CERCLA) Priority List of Hazardous Substances, compiled by the Agency for Toxic Substances and Disease Registry (ATSDR).[2]

Arsenic. Arsenic is the most common cause of acute heavy metal poisoning in adults. Arsenic is released into the environment by certain manufacturing processes. It can be found in our soil, water, and air. The central nervous system, blood, kidneys, digestive system, and skin are the main targets of arsenic toxicity.

Lead. Children are particularly susceptible to lead toxicity because they are likely to ingest lead-containing substances, such as paint chips. (Paint manufactured prior to 1940 contains lead.) Lead exposure also occurs in the home as drinking water passes through pipes, drains, and soldering materials used on plumbing. Adverse effects of lead exposure occur in the brain, bones, blood, kidneys, and thyroid. A simple blood test can determine lead levels in your body.

Mercury. Mercury affects the cerebellum, the basal ganglia, and the visual centers of the occipital lobe. Among the many conditions linked to mercury in the body is short-term memory loss. Mercury is extremely toxic, and exposure can result in serious physical and neurological problems, and even in death. Mercury is used in thermometers, thermostats, and dental amalgams. Mining operations and paper industries are significant producers of mercury. Until 1990, mercury was added to paint as a fungicide. Mercury is also present in the medicines Mercurochrome and Merthiolate, as well as in some childhood vaccines.

Cadmium. Cadmium is a by-product of mining and the smelting of zinc and lead. Fertilizers with cadmium are used in agriculture and may leach into water supplies. Cigarettes also contain cadmium. Inhalation or ingestion of cadmium can result in damage to the brain, liver, kidneys, bones, and lungs.

Other Toxic Metals

While not considered heavy metals, two other metals pose serious dangers to the brain:

Aluminum. We are exposed to aluminum in abundance. It is found in food additives, antiperspirants, drinking water, automobile exhaust, tobacco smoke, foil, cookware, cans, and ceramics. Researchers have discovered significant amounts of aluminum in the brain tissues of patients with Alzheimer's disease. Although there is no conclusive evidence either for or against aluminum as a factor in Alzheimer's disease, research continues into the relationship between aluminum and such serious brain conditions as dementia and Alzheimer's.

Manganese. Manganese toxicity is a well-recognized hazard for those who may inhale manganese dust. Inhaled manganese is transported directly to the brain and may cause neurological symptoms similar to those of Parkinson's disease. The symptoms of manganese toxicity generally appear slowly, over a period of months or years. Used in gasoline as an antiknock additive, the manganese-containing compound methylcyclopentadienyl manganese tricarbonyl (MMT) was approved for use in the United States in 1995. Manganese may also be ingested by drinking contaminated water and may also cause neurological symptoms.

Solvents and Fuels

Paints, glues, and thinners contain substances that have been shown to cause neurological problems. The usual symptoms of people exposed to these toxins include fatigue, headache, and confusion.

Toluene. Toluene has been associated with long-term neurological problems, such as dementia, balancing and coordination problems, and brain atrophy. Toluene occurs naturally as a component of crude oil and is produced in petroleum refining and coke oven operations. It can also be found in gasoline. Do not be lulled into thinking you have escaped its ravaging effects once you are inside your home, however, because toluene can be found in household aerosols, nail polish, paints, and cleaning agents containing a solvent base.

Sniffing or "huffing" substances containing toluene on a continual basis causes permanent brain damage. Researchers have long studied how exposure to solvents has affected humans. Among the deleterious effects are a wide variety of brain conditions, such as cognition, attention, and memory problems. Depression and anxiety have also been associated with exposure to solvents.

Pesticides

In my research I have seen numerous varieties of pesticides that have neurotoxic effects on humans. When exposed to pesticides, a person may develop headaches and fuzzy vision and have difficulty speaking. In severe cases, the lungs or other organs may fail. The main ways in which a person is exposed to pesticides are through inhaling their gases or absorbing their chemicals through the skin.

Carbon Monoxide

Carbon monoxide is invisible, odorless, and tasteless and kills like a silent assassin. Unlike other toxic gases that emit noxious fumes, carbon monoxide is odorless, so people can unknowingly be exposed to its vapors and will become unconscious, and often die, because of a lack of oxygen to the brain. During the last decade, carbon monoxide poisoning has made big headlines in the United States. But until the deaths from carbon monoxide poisoning of high-profile individuals, such as tennis star Vitas Gerulaitis, the importance of carbon monoxide detectors was on the back burner. In many states, there are no laws mandating that each home be equipped with carbon monoxide detectors.

When carbon monoxide does not kill, it wreaks havoc on the brain, causing memory loss and other cognitive impairments. The hippocampus, a part of the brain vital for creating new memories, is especially vulnerable to the effects of carbon monoxide.

Electromagnetic Radiation

The popularity of wireless technology devices has skyrocketed over the past fifteen years. Millions of Americans cannot go a few waking hours without using their wireless phones or computers. Henry Lai, an expert in radiation at the University of Washington, has compiled more than four hundred studies that examine the possible connection between radiation generated by wireless devices and human health. In an interview with *The New York Times*, Lai stated that more than 67 percent of all independent studies into the subject showed that the use of wireless communication devices produces biological changes in the body.[2] Research has correlated exposure to radiation with an array of health conditions, including brain tumors and decreased cognitive function.[3, 4]

And it's not just wireless technology, but a wide variety of EMF sources that make up life in our world. As Dr. Ronald Klatz puts it, "There are significant adverse side effects from being engulfed in an environment of electro-frequency or radio-frequency pollution. Swiss researchers collected data on electrical towers and Alzheimer's risk. People who lived within 150 feet of the towers were 24 percent more likely to die of Alzheimer's than those who lived more than 2,000 feet away. The risk for Alzheimer's increased with the length of time people spent near electrical towers. This radio frequency pollution can have adverse side effects on your sleep cycle, on the release of melatonin (a natural hormone necessary for restorative sleep), the repair of DNA. So avoid electrical frequency pollution if for no other reason than to protect your cognitive function."[2]

Lifestyle and the Brain

Just as your external environment can influence the health and welfare of your brain, your internal environment—the way you react to events and emotions—has an equally powerful impact on your mental health. Our daily behaviors and habits, if unexamined and unchanged, can predispose us to suffer some of the serious health conditions associated with aging.

Stress

Much has been written about how stress affects the brain. For instance, according to the National Institute of Mental Health, stress and depression are closely linked. A recent study shows that stress can actually rewire the emotional circuits of the brain. Stress is not only psychological but physiological. As Dr. Hyla Cass puts it, "Our body chemistry actually changes as a result of stress—we actually use up the raw materials that we need to make the feel-good chemicals for our brain (serotonin, dopamine, etc.—the feel-good neurotransmitters that get used up in order to make adrenaline and cortisol, which are the stress hormones)."[3]

Specifically, constant stress produces disproportionate cortisol levels in the brain. Cortisol is a hormone that is released from the adrenal glands in response to a physical or psychological threat. When cortisol is continually produced, it will begin to impair the function of the hippocampus, the area of the brain that is related to memory. High cortisol levels from excessive stress result in atrophy and death of the neurons, destroying brain cells in the hippocampus and frequently affecting short-term memory.

In his book *Does Stress Damage the Brain? Understanding Trauma-Related Disorders from a Neurological Perspective*, J. Douglas Bremner, an Emory University professor of psychiatry and radiology, has used his more than ten years of research as a clinical psychiatrist to explain how changes in the brain that are the result of stress may be the cause of some psychiatric disorders, including, among others, depression and anxiety.

According to a report from Stanford University, intense stress may even cause brain damage that leads to major depression or eventual memory impairment. In an article written for the journal *Science*, Stanford researcher and professor Robert Sapolsky discusses what science has learned so far about how stress adversely impacts our bodies.

Sapolsky cites a number of studies: one that looked at the hippocampus (the part of the brain responsible for explicit, declarative memory) of people who had recovered from long-term, major depression; another that studied Vietnam veterans; and a third that measured the left hippocampus of adults who suffered from post-traumatic stress disorder because of childhood sexual abuse. In all of the studies, the hippocampus in these severely stressed individuals was smaller than those in the control groups.[5]

In his book *Why Zebras Don't Get Ulcers*, Sapolsky emphasizes how stress adversely affects our whole bodies. Once stress triggers the sympathetic nervous system, hormones are secreted, and a whole host of physiological changes occur that prepare the body for what it perceives to be impending danger.[6] This response is obviously beneficial to us when, for instance, we are being pursued by a tiger, but it also suppresses the immune system. Constant exposure to this type of stress and the resulting suppression of the immune system open the door to many diseases, both physical and mental.

Unhealthy Habits

There may be some daily habits that you indulge in that damage your brain. And remember that habits you recognize as being unhealthy for your body are just as damaging to your brain as those that you may indulge in without full knowledge of the risks.

Nicotine. Despite the well-advertised adverse effects of tobacco, nearly 25 percent of the world's population smokes cigarettes. While most people understand the link between smoking and cancer or heart disease, few are aware of the fact that the effects of nicotine on the brain are equally as dire. Cigarettes lower oxygen levels in the blood, and studies have shown that chronic smoking decreases blood flow to the brain. Nicotine prompts brain cells to grow nicotinic receptor cells that respond to the neurotransmitter acetylcholine. This rush of acetylcholine explains why smokers may feel energized and clearheaded.

But as acetylcholine production continues at an unnatural rate, the delicate balance of neurotransmitters in the brain is upset, and mental sharpness begins to suffer. This is particularly noticeable for anyone who has undergone the symptoms of nicotine withdrawal, which the American Psychiatric Association classifies as a mental disorder.[7]

Alcohol. The negative effects of alcohol on the body are generally obvious. Alcohol consumption hastens the breakdown of antioxidants, negatively impacts the central nervous system, inhibits vitamin absorption (leading to liver damage), and is toxic at a cellular level. The effects of alcohol on the functioning of the brain are also far-reaching, negatively influencing areas involved in emotion, processing sensory information, and regulating stress. Alcohol disrupts the balance of key neurotransmitters, including serotonin, endorphins, and acetylcholine. Evidence also suggests that alcohol can alter the activity in the hippocampus, a part of the brain that is vital in memory. Alcohol acts as a depressant, decreasing the activity of the nervous system.

Caffeine. Excess consumption of caffeine can wreak havoc with sleep patterns, deplete the body of critical B vitamins, and upset the stomach, as well as cause physical symptoms such as tremors and exacerbate anxiety. Withdrawal from this potent drug is associated with irritability, headaches, depression, and nervousness.

Inactivity and the Obesity Epidemic

Back in the day, people believed that as we age, we should slow down, take it easy, and accept that our bodies can no longer keep up with an active lifestyle. In the 1980s and 1990s, research emerged demonstrating that this prescription for physical inactivity is, in fact, the worst possible advice for both your body and your brain.

A sedentary physical lifestyle contributes to impaired cardiac and respiratory systems, diabetes, arthritis, obesity, high blood pressure, osteoporosis, and insomnia. A sedentary mental lifestyle can lead to anxiety, depression, memory loss, and loss of cognitive function. Dr. Klatz even cites recent research as linking obesity to major neuro-degenerative disease: "A recent Johns Hopkins Univerity report tells us that excess weight causes age-related cognitive decline. Having a BMI of 30 or higher increases a person's risk. Obesity was found to have a particularly high effect on Alzheimer's disease, increasing the risk of that disorder by as much as 80 percent."[4]

The mind-body connection is particularly clear when it comes to the connection between being both mentally and physically active. Muscle activity and chemical activity in the brain are closely related. In fact, bodywork practitioners find that deep muscle massage often triggers the release and awareness of powerful memories and emotions. Neurotransmitters such as acetylcholine and dopamine work to regulate muscle movement and fine motor skills, and, in return, muscle activity serves to stimulate and increase synaptic receptors.

The benefits of physical exercise on the brain are many: improved blood flow, increased oxygen, and the release of mood-regulating neurotransmitters. The benefits of mental exercise are equally impressive: stronger neural connections, stimulation of new neuron growth, balanced levels of neurotransmitters, and increased memory and cognitive functions.

There is no reason to let any of your muscles, including your mental muscles, atrophy simply because you are getting older. An active lifestyle with an active interest in stimulating and enriching activities is a key component in keeping our brains vital as we age.

Nutrition and the Brain

Poor nutrition and an inadequate diet are leading causes of many brain-related diseases and conditions that are often attributed solely to aging. Most Americans fuel their bodies and brains with fast food, refined carbohydrates, trans fats, and sugar. Those who think they are eating more healthfully don't consider the fact that they are consuming meats, fruits, and vegetables that have been genetically modified, irradiated, or raised in toxic environments where earth and water may be contaminated with pesticides and fertilizers.

While I have spent a great deal of time and effort working with people to educate them about the effects of poor nutrition on their bodies, I now feel that I have to speak out just as strongly about the damage their diets and ways of living are doing to their brains. According to Dr. Joel Fuhrman, who specializes in treating illness through nutrition and is the author of *Fasting and Eating for Health*, the frightening fact is that our American diet literally causes our brain to shrink by depriving it of necessary nutrients and oxygen over the course of our lives.[8]

In the next chapter, I talk about nutritional and lifestyle solutions that will protect your brain over a lifetime. But before you move on to reading about my Reboot Your Brain Nutritional Plan for Optimum Brain Health, you should fully understand the damage you are doing to your body, and thus your mind, by following the diet of the average American. When considering what you put into your body, you should know that your brain health is compromised by the consumption of sugar and fats and by a lack of vitamins and minerals.

Sugar

Sugar is high on my list of substances that should be completely banned from our diets. Sugar is nothing short of toxic to our bodies, yet Americans consume, on average, 140 to 160 pounds of sugar each year. Sucrose, or refined sugar, is quite different from glucose, the fuel that your brain needs to operate smoothly. Glucose is a simple sugar that is obtained from the metabolism of carbohydrates in foods and circulates through the bloodstream to provide the body with energy. Meanwhile, refined sugars challenge the immune system, causing diabetes, hypoglycemia, tooth decay, and obesity, to name only a few conditions. Sugar depletes B vitamins and calcium, and generates exceptionally high levels of cell-damaging free radicals, promoting inflammation throughout the body, especially in the brain. Overconsumption of sugar savagely attacks metabolism, causing a wide range of symptoms, including irritability, anxiety, confusion, nervousness, mood swings, lack of concentration, fatigue, depression, and headaches.

Fats

High-protein diets have been promoted, especially in recent years, as a quick way to lose weight. These diets preach what the average American wants to hear: You can consume lots of cholesterol and lots of saturated fats and lots of animal protein and still lose weight. Weigh these dietary tips against the fact that heart attacks and strokes kill about 50 percent of all Americans, and the connection is clear: The standard Western diet promotes cardiovascular disease.

As cholesterol and fats are transported through the bloodstream to the delicate tissues of the brain, the cells in the brain become coated with a waxy substance. This amyloidal protein buildup, or plaque, is found in the brains of individuals suffering from Alzheimer's disease. This amyloidal plaque has an inflammatory effect on the brain tissue. Inflammation is a prime cause of brain aging; I discuss it in more detail below.

There is no doubt that high-fat diets have an adverse effect on the entire circulatory system, but you may not recognize how this directly impacts the brain's health. As plaque buildup narrows arteries and tiny blood vessels (a process called arteriosclerosis), the flow of blood throughout the body and to the brain is slowed. Blood that does reach the brain is oxygen-poor and lacking in nutrients, literally causing brain cells to die and the very mass of the brain to shrink.

Even as fewer nutrients are reaching the brain as a result of a high-fat diet, there is still more damage being done. Saturated fatty acids interfere with glucose use in the brain, starving the brain of energy and impairing cognitive function.

Vitamin and Mineral Deficiencies

A diet that relies on refined carbohydrates, sugars, and animal proteins as its building blocks does not leave a lot of room for taking in important nutrients from plant products. The healthy brain needs B vitamins, especially B6 and B12, as well as folate, vitamins E and C, and zinc. Nearly all these important nutrients can be found in plant-based products. And few Americans are getting enough of them in their daily diets.

In recent years, much has been written about Vitamin D and the epidemic of Vitamin D deficiency for a sun-phobic public. According to a *New York Times* article citing the work of Dr. Michael Holick of Boston University, a leading expert on vitamin D and author of *The Vitamin D Solution,* everyone should ideally have 30 nanograms per milliliter. As Holick puts it, "currently in the United States, Caucasians average 18 to 22 nanograms and African Americans average 13 to 15 nanograms." The low levels could potentially be connected to the rise of everything from Type 1 diabetes to various cancers, Holick's research maintains. Dr. Klatz also notes, "An important study was published in 2010 that reports that Vitamin D reduces physiological brain changes that may trigger atrophy." It's clear that Vitamin D supplementation should be a key addition to our daily vitamin supplementation.

Special Risks

In addition to environmental, lifestyle, and diet factors, there are two other causes that play a significant role in brain aging.

Brain Inflammation

Inflammation is the body's response to stress, disease, and injury. One's environment and diet can bring on an inflammatory condition. It is the hallmark of every chronic disease. While the inflammatory response is a sign that the body's immune system is functioning and vital, when it is too strong or does not naturally suppress itself, it becomes damaging.

Inflammation of the brain plays a prominent role in Alzheimer's and dementia. The hippocampus, the region of the brain closely linked to memory, seems to be particularly vulnerable to neuroinflammation. Blood and urine tests can show whether markers of inflammation are elevated.

Hormone Imbalance

Hormones are natural chemicals produced in one location in the body and transported, via the bloodstream, to signal other organs or systems in the body. In short, they are responsible for the functioning of the trillions of cells in the human body. When any one hormone falls out of balance, the entire communication system in the body breaks down.

With aging, changes naturally occur in the level of hormones and the body's response to them. It is important to maintain a balance of hormones in the body to protect the brain against changes that may lead to depression, anxiety, or decreased cognitive functions.

Summary

Having read this chapter, you can see how important it is to practice a lifestyle that creates a healthy environment for your brain. When you ignore the health of your body, you are just as effectively ignoring the health of your brain. Just like your body, your brain doesn't have to become fragile or weak simply because it is growing older. The good news is that it is possible to make changes to create a healthy environment for your mind.

In the next chapter, I will show you a diet and supplement plan, as well as lifestyle practices, that will protect your brain and even reverse the impact that negative behaviors, habits, and environments have had up to this point.

In Part II of this book, I will discuss specific conditions and diseases of the brain, such as depression, mental fatigue, senile dementia, and Parkinson's disease, and show you how to naturally fight their debilitating symptoms.

It is never too late to implement these changes. The brain is a remarkable, adaptable, and regenerating organ. Given the right environment, the right nutrition, and proper stimulation, it will thrive, regardless of its chronological age. By making a concerted effort to make the positive changes I discuss in the next chapter, you can set the stage for optimal performance of both your mind and your body, and discard notions of inevitable and "age appropriate" mental and physical decline.

Chapter 2

Promoting and Protecting Brain Health

"For even the mind depends so much on the temperament and disposition of the bodily organs that if it is possible to find some means of making men in general wiser and more skillful than they have been up 'til now, I believe we must look for it in medicine. It is true that medicine as currently practiced does not contain much of any significant use; but without intending to disparage it, l am sure there is no one, even among its practitioners, who would not admit that all we know in medicine is almost nothing in comparison with what remains to be known, and that we might free ourselves from innumerable diseases, both of the body and of the mind, and perhaps even from the infirmity of old age, if we had sufficient knowledge of their causes and of all the remedies that nature has provided."

—René Descartes (*Discourse on Method*, 1637)

Aging successfully in both mind and body requires us to attend to all aspects of our lives: to embrace new challenges, to exercise limbs and cognition, to promote emotional health, and to provide our brains and bodies with the fuel that will allow them to grow healthily from infancy through old age.

In this chapter, I discuss the basic and fundamental strategies for maintaining brain health. Think of this chapter as the overview for having a healthy brain. Everyone needs to follow this advice. In later chapters in Part II, I'll discuss strategies tailored to specific disorders of the brain that only those of you with special concerns will want to follow.

But first, we all need to follow the advice in this chapter. I offer you ways to continue to stimulate your brain, ensuring that neuronal pathways remain strong and productive. I will touch on the role of exercise in keeping both the body and the mind healthy, and how nurturing healthy social and emotional relationships benefits our minds as we age. Finally, I will discuss optimal diet and nutritional habits and give you a plan of foods, vitamins, and supplements that will serve as your first line of defense against age-related mental decline.

Lifestyle Habits For A Healthy Brain

If I'd known I was gonna live this long, 100 years, I'd have taken better care of myself.

—Ubie Blake (1883–1983)

The way we choose to live can have a huge effect on brain health in the long and short term. Let's examine the crucial areas of our lives that can contribute.

Challenge Your Brain

Research has documented that the brain requires constant stimulation and challenge to develop to its fullest potential. From studies that stress the importance of stimulation in a child's first three years of life,[1] to those that show how using your five physical senses and your emotional sense in unexpected ways will strengthen, preserve, and grow brain cells, science has proven again and again that we must "use it or lose it." In an article published in the *St. Petersburg Times*, the Pittsburgh neurologist Paul Nussbaum, speaking at the joint meeting of the National Council on Aging and the American Society on Aging, stressed that specific training for the brain, such as learning sign language, can boost IQ and promote a lifetime of brain growth—which, if continued, can stave off dementia and other brain diseases as people age. Other brain-challenging activities include taking up a second language, learning to knit, practicing public speaking, or learning to play a musical instrument.[2]

Lawrence C. Katz, PhD, a professor of neurobiology at Duke University Medical Center and the coauthor of *Keep Your Brain Alive: 83 Neurobic Exercises*,[3] suggests a series of exercises that can easily be done on a daily basis and involve one or more senses in a novel way. This type of "cross training for your brain" can help keep your mind fit to meet any challenge.

Try some of the following ways to challenge your brain:

- Use your nondominant hand to go through your morning rituals of hair styling, tooth brushing, and makeup application.
- Shower with your eyes closed, using your tactile senses to adjust water temperature and flow and your sense of smell to locate shampoo and soap.
- With your eyes closed, locate your house keys and open the door to your home.
- Turn a photo album upside down and study the pictures.
- Shop at a new grocery store.
- Read part of the newspaper or a book upside down.
- Sleep on the other side of your bed.

The good news is that, young or old, we can continue to learn. The more complex the learning challenge, the more we stimulate our brains and the more vital they remain. Travel, reading, going to museums, and attending book group readings all contribute to an active brain life. So play Scrabble, or do crossword puzzles, or enjoy bingo, or learn a foreign language. Growing older does not mean that we should lose our sense of curiosity in the world around us or our desire to pursue new challenges.

Exercise Your Body

Most of us know that physical exertion is good for our bodies— but it is also essential for our brains. Exercise should be a natural part of your life, whatever your age. If you do not exercise on a regular basis, or feel that you are too old to embark on a physical fitness program, you can begin to build a stronger body and brain by the simple act of taking a walk. Studies show that senior citizens who walk regularly show significant improvement in memory skills compared to sedentary elderly people. Walking can also improve learning ability, concentration, and abstract reasoning.[4]

Another long-term study that tracked a group of older men and women with no signs of dementia over a seven-year period found that those with a high participation in leisure activities, including walking or participating in an exercise class, were 38 percent less likely than others in the study to develop dementia.[5]

In still another study on physical activity and its effects on brain health, researchers at the University of California in San Francisco measured the brain function of nearly six thousand women during an eight-year period. The results were then correlated with the women's normal activity levels. The study showed that no matter how much or how little the women did in terms of exercise, there was a direct correlation to cognitive performance. It wasn't simply a matter of all or nothing. For every extra mile walked per week, there was a 13 percent lower chance of cognitive decline.[6]

But walking is not your only choice. Citing a 2003 study published in the *New England Journal of Medicine* that showed that ballroom dancing at least twice a week made people less likely to develop dementia, the AARP (formerly the American Association of Retired Persons) recommends dancing as one of the best mind-body workouts.[7] Researchers speculate that the combination of learning and remembering specific steps and sequences specifically boosts brain power.

Looking for a sport that is easier on your muscles than dancing or walking? Advocates of the gentle, controlled movements of tai chi claim the significant benefits of stress reduction and improved balance and muscle tone. The memorization of specific movements and sequences is similar to learning new steps to a gentle and serene dance.

There is no doubt that even the most basic exercise offers our bodies and our brains long-term benefits. Dr. Kristine Yaffe, chief of geriatric psychiatry at the San Francisco Veterans Administration Medical Center, estimated the protective effects of regular activity against cognitive decline could be as high as 40 percent.[8]

Whether you choose to walk, dance, garden, or practice tai chi or yoga, the most important thing is to get your body moving. The effects of physical activity are beneficial in delaying the onset of dementia, preventing the development of Alzheimer's disease, and improving memory and reasoning skills. Exercise also acts as a powerful antidepressant. No matter how old you are, it is never too late to experience the powerful benefits of some kind of physical activity.

Begin slowly if you must, but attempt to work up to forty-five minutes of exercise at least five days per week.

Strengthen Your Spirit

As we grow older, we can experience a sense of isolation and perhaps feel like withdrawing from interaction in society. This type of shutting down of emotion, intellect, or spirit is as unhealthy for our brains as the more easily recognized damaging habits of poor diet or lack of exercise.

Numerous studies have shown that individuals who have a strong sense of purpose and meaning in their lives thrive in their later years. Frequent contact with family and friends, participating in one's community, and feeling satisfied with one's accomplishments are key in maintaining mental health.

A positive outlook and ongoing social and emotional involvement are essential in keeping our brains stimulated and vital as we age. Ursula Lehr, PhD, of the University of Heidelberg and the former secretary of health of the Federal Republic of Germany, states that many studies have found that people who are mentally active have a wider range of interests, farther-reaching perspectives, and a greater number of social contacts reach old age with greater feelings of psychophysical well-being.[9]

Practicing meditation may be valuable for brain health, as well. In a recent article published in the *Washington Post*'s online edition, Dr. Richard Davidson, a neuroscientist at the University of Wisconsin, discussed the findings of a study conducted over the past few years evaluating the effects of meditation on Tibetan monks. The results of the study demonstrate, according to Dr. Davidson, that "the brain is capable of being trained and physically modified in ways few people can imagine."[10]

When the monks' brains were measured by MRI, Davidson found that the ones who were the most accomplished practitioners of meditation had brain waves that were better organized and coordinated compared to those of novices who had not been practicing meditation for as long. The more years spent meditating, the higher the gamma wave activity. In previous studies, mental activities such as focus, memory, learning, and consciousness were associated with this kind of high level neural coordination.[11]

Research in this area is ongoing, but I have no doubt that meditation can be a powerful tool in promoting a healthy brain.

Nutrition for a Healthy Brain

In this section, I provide a nutritional plan that you can follow to ensure your brain is protected as you age. This basic plan provides the diet and supplements that our bodies need to fuel its cells, including those in the brain, for optimal performance and health.

This eating plan is simple, easy to follow, and nonrestrictive. I don't want you to think of this approach to healthy eating as a "diet." Diets can leave you feeling deprived and lacking in energy. Diets tend to focus on a goal of weight loss, rather than an overall enhancement of health. They can rob your body of essential nutrients and food groups and put you on the road to bad food habits. While you may lose weight when you follow my protocol for a healthy brain and body, what is more important is what you will gain: energy, focus, and mental vitality.

The supplements have been chosen specifically for their beneficial effect on brain function and health, but you will notice other health benefits, as well.

Of course, before you begin any new health program, you should get a comprehensive, full-body evaluation performed by a qualified health care practitioner. A proper health and medical evaluation should evaluate your blood chemistry to assess your blood markers, your metabolic rate, and your blood pressure for indicators of cardiovascular, hormonal, or other imbalances or danger signs. If you are taking medications of any sort, you need to inform your doctor of any supplements you are considering adding to your daily diet, as some may interact with prescription medications.

The Nutritional Plan

Let's start with a discussion of what to eat.

Complex Carbohydrates

Complex carbohydrates are the gold standard when it comes to brain foods. They are the starches and fibers in foods such as whole grains, nuts, tubers, beans, seeds, lentils, fresh fruit, and vegetables. Incorporate these foods into your diet in place of refined white rice, pasta, and bread.

To maximize the nutritional benefits of complex carbohydrates, you should eat them in whole-food form. For many years, I have recommended that you eat five or more servings of organic fruits and vegetables each day. You should especially choose dark green, leafy, and root vegetables, such as broccoli, watercress, carrots, sweet potatoes, Brussels sprouts, spinach, green beans, and peppers, either raw or lightly cooked. You should select fresh fruits, such as apples, berries, citrus fruit, pears, and melon.

In addition, you should consume at least four servings of whole-grain foods, such as oats, rice, rye, whole wheat, millet, corn, or quinoa, in cereal, breads, and pasta. Remember, when you can, to also include the skins of fruits and vegetables. Fruits and vegetables are excellent sources of fiber. You may wonder, "Gary, how can fiber help my brain?" Well, fiber helps lower cholesterol and blood pressure levels, which are linked to Alzheimer's disease, as well as other degenerative brain diseases.

A Note About Sugar. Carbohydrate sugar converts to glucose, and, as such, is indispensable to the health of our brains, but you should try to obtain it in as pure a form as possible. Eliminate all refined sugar from your diet. This is not quite as easy as it may sound, for sugar is a hidden ingredient, lurking in many processed foods. We all know sugar can be found in soda, candy, and cakes. But how many of us know that it is also in bread, breakfast cereals, condiments, cheeses, and canned foods? I am fully aware that eliminating sugar from your diet will not be easy. You need to read the nutritional labels on processed foods. It will be worth the effort.

Don't make the mistake of thinking that a quick candy bar is fueling your brain. Common table sugar has been processed to 99.9 percent sucrose, which is stripped of the vitamins and minerals found in sugar cane or sugar beets. The refined sucrose taxes the body's digestive system, depleting it of essential vitamins, minerals, and enzymes as the sugar is metabolized. For this and other reasons, white sugar is known as an empty food. Choose whole-grain carbohydrates as your body's source of glucose.

Fruits and Vegetables

Fruits and vegetables are packed with the essential vitamins and protective antioxidants that promote optimal brain function. Eating a wide variety of organic fruits and vegetables is crucial to a brain healthy diet.

Antioxidants. Free radicals (atoms with unpaired electrons that can cause damage, called oxidation) in the normal metabolic process, are an important factor in the aging process. Brain cells are particularly vulnerable to oxidation because of their high-energy production. They are constantly firing messages back and forth. As more energy is produced, a greater number of damaging free radicals occur. The destructive effects of the free radical process have been implicated in conditions such as Alzheimer's and Parkinson's disease.

But here's some good news: Two studies out of the University of South Florida Center for Aging and Brain Repair reinforce evidence that specific fruits and vegetables may guard against the brain being ravaged by free radicals as you age. "If these preclinical findings translate to humans, it suggests that eating a diet high in antioxidant rich fruits and vegetables may help reverse declines in learning and memory as you get older," said Paula Bickford, PhD, a professor at the University of South Florida Center for Aging and Brain Repair, and the lead author of the two studies.

The first study involved feeding older rats a diet with high amounts of spinach over a period of six weeks. The results showed a reversal in the normal loss of learning that occurs with age. As noted above, spinach is a great source of antioxidants.

The second study concerned the value of a diet high in fruits and vegetables. The results found that the benefit of such a diet depends on the amount of antioxidants contained in the fruits and vegetables. The researchers imply that the protective effects of antioxidants may be connected to their ability to reverse the havoc caused by inflammation in the brain. Dr. Bickford found the greatest benefit in richly colored fruits and vegetables, which have the highest antioxidant levels. She recommends having spinach salads for lunch and blueberries and strawberries for snacks.[12]

Antioxidants, which work to protect the cells against free radical damage, are naturally occurring in many fruits and vegetables. Eating these beneficial foods essentially detoxifies the brain, ridding it of free radicals. Antioxidants include vitamins E and C, alpha lipoic acid, grape seed extract, and coenzyme Q10. Antioxidants are specifically found in the following foods: apples, berries (including blueberries, raspberries, blackberries, cranberries, and strawberries), cherries, cooked kale, garlic, grapes, prunes, raisins, and raw spinach.

Organic Produce. All fruits and vegetables you eat should be organic, whenever possible, to avoid exposure to pesticides. Certain conventionally grown produce is especially risky to eat. According to the Environmental Working Group (EWG), a nonprofit environmental watchdog agency based in Washington, DC, eating the twelve most contaminated conventionally grown fruits and vegetables would expose a person to nearly twenty pesticides per day on average. These foods are as follows (and are also listed on the EWG's website, at www.foodnews.org/reportcard.php):

- apples
- celery
- lettuce
- grapes
- blueberries (domestic)
- cucumbers
- nectarines (imported)

- peaches
- potatoes
- spinach
- strawberries
- sweet bell peppers

The website also lists the fifteen least contaminated fruits and vegetables:

- asparagus
- avocado
- kiwi
- mango
- onion
- pineapple
- sweet corn
- cabbage
- sweet peas
- eggplant
- cantaloupe (domestic)
- sweet potatoes
- grapefruit
- watermelon
- mushrooms

To the list of most contaminated foods, I would add leafy greens—because we consume the part of the plant that is sprayed—and nuts and seeds, such as almonds, pumpkin seeds, walnuts, and sesame and sunflower seeds—because their oils can hold chemicals for longer periods of time.

Washing fresh produce may help reduce pesticide residues, but it does not eliminate them entirely. Peeling reduces exposure, but valuable nutrients are also lost along with the peel. If you cannot buy organic produce, choose foods from the least-contaminated list, and be sure to wash all fruits and vegetables thoroughly before eating them or using them in recipes.

Proteins

Most people are under the impression that you must have animal proteins to sustain life. This is a myth perpetuated by the meat industry. Consequently, we have given vegetables, grains, nuts, seeds, fruits, and herbs a nutritional backseat or relegated them to being an insignificant accompaniment or garnish to a meat-based or animal protein–based diet. This idea was the result of propaganda and marketing, but it was scientifically inaccurate.

In fact, my own original work with Dr. Hillard Fitsky and Dr. Victor Berman at the Institute of Applied Biology showed that virtually all foods contain all eight essential amino acids and that we have been led to believe that only animal foods contain these amino acids.

We must make sure that we are receiving high-quality amino acids—nine-tenths of a gram per kilogram of body weight, which is approximately 50 grams per day for women and 70 grams per day for men. (Pregnancy, lactation, recovery from various illnesses, surgery, and infection will cause a person to require more than this.)

The best foods for high-quality protein from fiber sources are grains (e.g., millet, buckwheat, brown rice, spelt, rye, quinoa, and oats), legumes, nuts, seeds, tofu, and tempeh. Good vegetable sources include yams, potatoes, sweet potatoes, gourds, squashes, and cruciferous vegetables (e.g., broccoli, cabbage, cauliflower, onions, asparagus, mustard sprouts, and sea vegetables), as well as soy and rice protein shakes.

Keep in mind that protein digestion is greatly improved by using the proper cooking techniques. By moderately heating most proteins, you increase their digestibility. This is especially true when dealing with beans, grains, and meat. Beans and other legumes contain several toxins that become nontoxic when cooked or sprouted.

Fats

Our bodies and brains need fat to function. But there are harmful fats and good fats. Making informed choices about the types of fat in the foods you eat is important in the proper feeding of your brain.

Most of us know that the saturated fats in fried foods and the trans fats in processed foods should be avoided. But let's talk about the good fats that we should be sure to include in our diets.

Eating nuts and seeds provides beneficial amounts of intelligent fat for your brain; the best choices are walnuts, almonds, pine nuts, pistachios, and pumpkin, sunflower, hemp, flax, sesame, and chia seeds. To increase the nutritional benefit from these seeds, you can grind them before using them in your meals.

Omega-3 fatty acids are known to benefit patients with chronic inflammatory diseases, including cardiovascular disease and arthritis.[13] Omega-3 fatty acids may help reverse brain damage resulting from chronic inflammation that is linked to aging and degenerative diseases. Another benefit of omega-3 fatty acids is that they prevent blood from clotting too rapidly, which could improve cerebral functioning by increasing cerebral blood flow.[14] According to a study from the Department of Veterans Affairs (VA) and the University of California at Los Angeles (UCLA), when given a diet high in docosahexaenoic acid (DHA)—an omega-3 fatty acid—mice exhibited a substantially slower progression of Alzheimer's disease.[15]

More benefits to omega-3 fats and other essential fatty acids (EFAs) called omega-6s exist. EFAs serve as building blocks for nerve cells and membranes. Our brains consist almost entirely of fatty acids. While both omega-3 and omega-6 fats are necessary for proper cell function, the Standard American Diet (SAD) provides an unhealthy omega-6 to omega-3 ratio of 10-20:1. The optimal ratio is 1:1 or at most 4:1. Without an adequate level of EFAs, dangerous saturated fats will take their place in cell membranes.

Foods high in omega-3 fatty acids include flax seeds, chia seeds, and walnuts.

Just as there are fats that are beneficial to your brain, there are fats that are clearly harmful to your brain. Saturated fats are very unhealthy. Excess saturated fat is linked to the increased likelihood of cardiovascular disease. Relative to all of the other fats, saturated fat is the most damaging. Saturated fats wreak havoc on blood vessels and interfere with blood circulation. They increase the production of LDL cholesterol (the "bad" cholesterol), which increases blood cholesterol levels, thereby increasing the risk of heart disease.

Saturated fats reduce membrane fluidity and efficiency, thereby contributing to premature aging and disease development. Deficiencies in fatty acids have been linked to chronic inflammatory conditions, such as arthritis, hypertension, memory loss, dementia, cardiovascular disease, and insulin resistance (leading to Type II diabetes).

You should avoid consuming foods that are high in saturated fats, which are commonly found in processed foods, such as salad dressings, french fries, pastries, and the majority of margarines, and hydrogenated vegetable oils found in processed foods, such as boxed cakes, microwave popcorn, and TV dinners.

Sixteen Rules of Nutrition

So far in this chapter, I have outlined the general principles of healthful nutrition to help protect your aging brain. This program is good for all of us, and the more closely you follow it, the more you will strengthen your brain. Even before you experience problems, you should follow these programs. They are preventive, too.

The more you incorporate these recommendations into your eating habits, the better off you will be. Some of us can only manage to follow a few of these guidelines. Others start with baby steps, and as they feel better, they want to do more.

For those of you who want to do everything you can to change your nutritional intake to strengthen your brain, I have included the following sixteen rules for best brain health. However, even if you can't follow all these guidelines, even choosing one or two will leave you better off than you would be if you took none of the advice in this chapter. But those of you who can keep to the sixteen rules all the time will have the best health of all.

1. Eat small amounts of nuts and nut butters, such as almond butter and walnuts, as well as sunflower seeds, pumpkin seeds, chia seeds, and sesame seeds.
2. Eat soybeans and soy products.
3. Eat whole grains, such as quinoa, amaranth, spelt, and teff. Include beans (of which there are more than seventy varieties commonly available, from black-eyed peas, navy beans, adzuki beans, lentils, split peas, and lima beans, to turtle beans).
4. Do not eat dairy, including milk, yogurt, cheese, butter, ice cream, or cream sauces. Replace them with rice milk, soy milk, almond milk, or oat milk. Do not use any non-dairy product with casein listed as one of the ingredients.
5. Do not eat animal meat, fish, or shellfish.
6. Do not use caffeine or alcohol. This means cutting out chocolate, coffee, tea, wines, hard liquor, and beer. Replace them with decaffeinated herbal teas and grain beverages, such as Postum, Cafix, Raja's Cup, or green tea (which has small amounts of caffeine but also has threonine, which neutralizes caffeine and has a very beneficial calming effect).
7. Do not eat sugar or artificial sweeteners. If you must use a sweetener beyond what naturally occurs in food, choose stevia root, raw unfiltered honey, molasses, brown rice syrup, or natural food sweeteners. You can also use chromium picolinate 200 mcg (micrograms) to curb sugar cravings.
8. Do not drink carbonated beverages, including sodas or seltzer. Replace them with spring water, distilled water, filtered water, or fresh-squeezed organic juices.

9. Do not eat processed bread or wheat products. Replace them with spelt bread, sprouted whole-grain bread, rice bread, or Essene bread. Make sure to read the labels to ensure that these products do not have refined flours, sugars, or trans fats.

10. Eat only certified organic produce. This applies to all vegetables, fruits, beans, grains, legumes, nuts, seeds, and potatoes.

11. Do not eat deep-fried or processed foods. Replace them with steam-fried, sautéed, steamed, stir-fried, or broiled meals.

12. Try to avoid using oils for cooking, or keep the amount extremely low. Every tablespoon of oil costs you 120 calories, and all oils damage the endothelium, the delicate lining of the arteries. If you must use oil, choose healthier oils for cooking, such as macadamia and safflower oils. For baking, use hazelnut, macadamia, coconut, or mustard seed oils. For salads, use walnut, flax seed, or extra virgin, cold-pressed olive oil.

13. Do not eat food additives, preservatives, coloring agents, flavorings, or MSG.

14. Do not eat bedtime snacks. Eat primarily during the day. Try to have your largest meal between 1:00 and 3:00 p.m. with a light breakfast and a very light dinner.

15. Avoid dehydration. Make sure you drink plenty of fluids throughout the day. It's important not to lose our liquid balance, because we will then upset our electrolyte balance, our lymphatic balance, and our cleansing and elimination program. Most people should drink a minimum of one gallon of water per day, but if you are sweating profusely or exercising vigorously, you may need more. It is best to have an impedance test, which will determine what percent of your body is water. Ideally it should be between 72 and 74 percent, because for each percentage under that, you will be losing your body energy and lessening the process

of cleansing and detoxification. Liquids can include purified water or juices, plus one or two cups of green tea daily, lemon juice to help alkalize the body, and digestive enzymes to help with the tea.

16. Do not make excuses. Keep a positive outlook and be sure to appreciate how your body and brain begin to feel and act younger after just a short time following this protocol. Commit to healthy living habits and maintain them for the sake of your long-term mental and physical health.

The Supplement Plan

In addition to choosing fresh, organic foods and using brain-healthy ways to prepare them, it is possible to further boost the health of our brains by supplementing our daily menu of foods with vitamins, minerals, and other supplements that specifically target and enrich the function of the brain.

In truth, it can be hard to get the optimal levels of the vitamins and minerals we need through diet alone. Although the nutrients we get from foods are more powerful, we should ensure we are getting adequate quantities by taking supplements as well to complement (not substitute for) our healthful eating habits.

Vitamins and Minerals

Vitamin B-Complex. The B vitamins play an important role in promoting brain health. One study reported that middle-aged men who had the highest amounts of vitamin B6 in their blood scored best on memory tasks, as compared to other middle-aged men who had B6 deficiencies.[16] Vitamin B6 is also thought to improve verbal memory and combat depression.

Vitamin B9, better known as folic acid or folate, is critical for brain health. Studies seem to indicate that up to 38 percent of adults who have been clinically diagnosed with depression are deficient in folic acid.[17] Additional research from the Universities of Oxford

(England) and Bergen (Norway) report that low folate and low vitamin B12 levels are connected to an increased risk of developing Alzheimer's disease. Both studies concluded that the risk for eventually getting Alzheimer's can be dramatically reduced through supplementation of folate and vitamin B12.[18]

I recommend that you take a vitamin B-complex that provides the daily amounts of all B vitamins as listed on the chart that appears toward the end of this chapter.

Vitamin C. A powerful antioxidant, vitamin C protects against inflammation within our bodies, working to protect our brains against the effects of poor blood flow associated with atherosclerosis. Because vitamin C is water soluble and rapidly excreted from the body, it is important that levels be replenished daily. I recommend that you take 1 to 3 grams every day.

Vitamin E. Vitamin E (tocopherol) is an antioxidant that helps protect tissue from unhealthy oxidative free radicals, which can cause damage and lead to premature aging and the development of chronic diseases, such as cancer, Alzheimer's, and cataract formation. There are a number of forms of vitamin E. The most common vitamin E supplement is alpha-tocopherol. Recent studies, however, suggest that gamma-tocopherol is the most effective form of vitamin E.

When choosing a vitamin E supplement, look for one containing compounds called tocotrienols, which synergistically combine with vitamin E to help protect our bodies against damaging processes. Tocotrienols also lower the levels of LDL (the dangerous form of cholesterol), which is an important risk factor for heart attack and stroke. (Remember, this directly affects the brain.)

I suggest that you choose a vitamin E supplement that has 268 milligrams of alpha-tocopherol, 200 milligrams of gamma-tocopherol, and 65 milligrams of tocotrienols.

Selenium. This vital mineral can be found in grains, garlic, and Brazil nuts. It is a powerful antioxidant that may protect against heart attack and stroke. Selenium appears to encourage a healthy cardiovascular system by increasing the ratio of good cholesterol (MDL) to bad cholesterol (LDL). A healthy cardiovascular system means a healthy flow of nutrient-rich blood to the brain. To promote brain health, I recommend taking 200 micrograms of selenium daily.

"Smart" Drugs and Nutrients

A revolution of sorts occurred in the 1970s, when reports began to surface that specific nutrients and drugs could improve concentration, learning, and memory in general, plus overall cognitive functions. Choline, phosphatidylcholine, ginkgo biloba, dimethylaminoethanol (DMAE), and phosphatidylserine were the nutrients heading the list. In the drug category, hydergine, piracetam, and centrophenoxine were at the forefront.

Acetyl-L-Carnitine (ACL). A form of the amino acid–like compound carnitine, acetyl-L-carnitine, or ACL, is produced naturally in the brain. Carnitine transports fatty acids to cells for conversion into energy used by the body's muscles, organs, and tissues. Carnitine deficiencies can place a strain on the heart muscles and create an energy drain on the body that may leave you feeling worn out. A simple urine test can determine if you have a carnitine deficiency.

Some studies show that acetyl-L-carnitine may boost memory and offer some protection against Alzheimer's disease, especially when taken in combination with alpha lipoic acid.[19] I recommend a supplement of 2,000 milligrams daily in two divided doses.

Alpha Lipoic Acid. This potent antioxidant dissolves in both water and fat, and is thus able to scavenge damaging free radicals more effectively than most antioxidants, which dissolve in either water or fat but not both. Because it dissolves in fat, alpha lipoic acid can reach tissues in the nervous system. Results from animal studies show that alpha lipoic acid may improve long-term memory and holds promise for protection against Alzheimer's disease, particularly when taken in combination with acetyl-L-carnitine.[20] I recommend taking a supplement of 300 milligrams daily in two divided doses.

Carnosine. This amino acid compound protects against damage by free radicals and is highly concentrated in the brain. Levels of this powerful antioxidant decline in the body as we age, and supplementing with carnosine may offer benefits in protecting against neurological degeneration. I recommend supplementing with 1,000 milligrams daily.

Coenzyme Q10 (coQ10). As we age, our body's natural production of coenzyme Q10 (coQ10) diminishes. Our older bodies produce only 50 percent of the coQ10 they did when we were younger. This makes coQ10 one of the most important nutrients for people over thirty. Because the cells of our body need coQ10 to produce energy and to combat mitochondrial free radical activity, a coQ10 deficiency can result in a greater incidence of many degenerative diseases associated with aging.

Though the heart is frequently affected by a coQ10 deficiency, scientific reports show that the brain is also likely to suffer adversely from an inadequate supply of coQ10.[21]

CoQ10 is a fat-soluble nutrient that goes into the mitochondria throughout the body. Once there, it governs the oxidation of fats and sugars into energy. When consumed in an oil-based capsule, the coQ10 can be absorbed through the lymphatic canals for better distribution throughout the entire body.

I recommend taking a supplement of 100 to 300 milligrams daily with meals for general brain health.

Dehydroepiandrosterone (DHEA). Youthful hormone balance is vital in maintaining health and preventing disease in individuals over the age of forty. One hormone that is deficient in virtually everyone who is over thirty-five is dehydroepiandrosterone (DHEA).

A large body of research indicates that DHEA is a critically important hormone that appears to protect the entire body against the ravages of aging. Studies on rats have shown that DHEA increases acetylcholine release in the hippocampus of the brain and has improved both short- and long-term memory in mice.[22, 23] Another study shows that DHEA can protect against early changes in the brain cells associated with Alzheimer's disease.

Not everyone, however, can take advantage of the multiple benefits of DHEA. Men and women with hormone-related cancers, for example, should not take DHEA. This supplement is available only by prescription from your doctor. But if your doctor says it's safe for you, I recommend taking a supplement of 25 to 50 milligrams daily.

Dimethylaminoethanol (DMAE). This nutrient, found in sardines, is a powerful brain stimulant that increases acetylcholine levels. Acetylcholine is a neurotransmitter associated with mood and energy levels. I recommend taking a supplement of 150 milligrams daily.

Glycerylphosphorylcholine (GPC). Choline and lecithin can reduce arterial plaque and lower blood pressure. They also enhance acetylcholine production, which plays an important role in memory and learning. One type of choline, called glycerylphosphorylcholine (GPC), has been shown to improve the condition of subjects with adult onset cognitive dysfunction, Alzheimer's disease, and stroke-related mental impairment. The therapeutic effects of GPC were noted as superior to either choline or lecithin alone. I recommend a dosage of 600 milligrams of GPC and 1 gram of lecithin daily.

Hydergine. Initially discovered in the 1940s, this drug was approved by the FDA for treatment of symptoms of dementia. Today it is used proactively to protect us against mental decline. Studies support my contention that hydergine protects the brain against age-related decline by enhancing glucose use;[25] increases intelligence, memory, learning, and recall;[26] and increases the blood and oxygen supply to the brain, enhancing metabolism in brain cells.[27] I recommend a daily supplement of 5 to 10 milligrams.

Phosphatidylcholine. Phosphatidylcholine is a phospholipid, a large molecule that covers the nerve cells that assist in transferring information between cells. A lack of phospholipids can result in abnormal brain activity and difficulties in the central nervous system. I recommend a supplement of 500 to 1,000 milligrams daily.

Phosphatidylserine (PS). PS helps the brain use fuel more efficiently. By boosting neuronal metabolism and stimulating production of acetylcholine, PS may be able to improve the condition of patients in cognitive decline. Studies have revealed that supplementing with phosphatidylserine slows down and even reverses declining memory and concentration, or age-related cognitive impairment, in middle-aged and elderly subjects.[28] An added benefit is its ability to reduce levels of the stress hormone cortisol.

Phosphatidylserine is a phospholipid found in all cells, but is most highly concentrated in the walls of brain cells (called membranes), making up about 70 percent of its nerve tissue mass. There it aids in the storage, release, and activity of many vital neurotransmitters and their receptors. Phosphatidylserine also aids in cell-to-cell communication. It also stimulates the release of dopamine (a mood regulator that also controls physical sensations and movement), increases the production of acetylcholine (necessary for learning and memory), enhances brain glucose metabolism (the fuel used for brain activity), reduces cortisol levels (a stress hormone), and boosts the activity of nerve growth factor (NGF), which oversees the health of cholinergic neurons.

As we grow older, aging slows the body's manufacturing of phosphatidylserine to levels that are detrimental to our functioning at our full mental capacity. This is where supplementation with phosphatidylserine comes into play. In one Belgian study that looked at the effects of phosphatidylserine, thirty-five senile demented patients, ages sixty-five to ninety-one, were hospitalized with mild to moderate memory problems. Seventeen patients were given, over the period of six weeks, phosphatidylserine at 300 milligrams per day. The other eighteen patients received a placebo. The study reported an improved quality of life for the patients who were given phosphatidylserine. Using three different evaluation methods, the researchers classified forty-nine functions—for example, getting dressed, eating, and control of bowel and bladder movements—into ten categories. The results were astonishing, as improvements in all ten categories were reported."[29]

I recommend taking a supplement of 300 milligrams daily.

Pregnenolone. A hormone produced by the adrenal glands, pregnenolone is abundant in the brain, where it facilitates communication between neurotransmitters. As we age, the amount of pregnenolone our bodies produce declines; levels can be determined by a basic urine test. I recommend a daily supplement of 50 milligrams.

Proanthocyanidins. Proanthocyanidins (chemical relatives of bioflavonoid) serve to benefit the brain in a twofold manner: They are antioxidants, and they protect collagen.

Brace yourself for what I am about to tell you. Research has shown that proanthocyanidins are fifty times more powerful antioxidants than vitamins C and E! Intricate tests prove that proanthocyanidins are great killers of the hydroxyl radical, the free radical that is responsible for the most damage and lipid peroxides (rancid fats).[30] This is extremely important because the brain is particularly vulnerable to free radical damage.

In protecting collagen, proanthocyanidins are, in essence, protecting the glue that holds the brain together. Enzymes can destroy the walls of blood vessels that are, essentially, made of collagen. Proanthocyanidins therefore protect the blood–brain barrier. Remember, the blood–brain barrier protects the brain from toxins and other potentially destructive substances. Thus, proanthocyanidins, as potent shields of the blood–brain barrier, are invaluable.

Although proanthocyanidins can be found in food, the levels are generally insufficient to provide the brain with the fortification it needs to ward off attack. Thus, the best way to obtain proanthocyanidins is through supplementation. In particular, the best two sources are grape seed extract and pine bark extract. I recommend supplementing with 80 milligrams daily.

Trimethylglycine (TMG). TMG is the most effective facilitator of youthful methylation metabolism. Research has shown that defective methylation is implicated in a variety of diseases, including cancer, neurological disorders, and birth defects.[31] Methylation produces S-adenosylmethionine (SAMe, pronounced "sammy"), which may have powerful anti-aging effects and has eased depression and improved Parkinson's symptoms in patients with the disease. TMG should be taken with vitamin B6 and folic acid to enhance the effectiveness of methylation. I recommend taking 200 to 300 milligrams per day.

Vinpocetine. Vinpocetine is an extract taken from the lesser periwinkle plant (Vinca minor). It is available by prescription in Europe and is used for mitigating stroke- and age-related decline in brain function. In the United States, it is available as an over-the-counter dietary supplement. Vinpocetine may provide protection against the types of cognitive decline associated with poor brain circulation, including memory loss and disorientation. It also enhances the brain's use of oxygen by boosting levels of adenosine triphosphate (ATP), an important brain fuel. I recommend a dose of 10 milligrams twice daily with meals.

Reboot Your Brain Chart of Daily Supplements for Best Brain Health

Supplemental vitamins and minerals, as well as smart nutrients and drugs, can be extremely beneficial to our brain health when used in combination with a healthful diet. But I know that keeping track of the proper dosages can be difficult. To help you reach that goal, I have provided the following chart, which summarizes the supplement program I recommend.

The plan that follows is intended to promote brain health and protect your brain. In Part II of this book, I discuss specific conditions and recommend vitamins and supplements that can be added to this basic plan to fight and impact brain conditions such as memory loss, Parkinson's disease, or headaches. When recommending protocols for specific conditions, I am assuming that you are already following the supplement program in the chart that follows.

Do not combine this protocol with more than one additional protocol from Part II of this book. If you are taking medications, or have any food restrictions, you should consult with your doctor before beginning this or any supplement program. Supplement overdoses are rare, but possible, and certain combinations may affect individuals adversely.

Vitamins and Nutrients	Daily Dose	Comments
acetyl-L-carnitine (ACL)	2,000 mg in two divided doses	
alpha lipoic acid	300 mg in two divided doses	
B-complex vitamins	• 75 mg thiamine (B1) • 50 mg riboflavin (B2) • 200 mg niacin (B3) • 500 mg pantothenic acid (B5) • 75 mg pyridoxine (B6) • 250 mg inositol (B8) • 800 mcg folic acid (B9) • 800 mcg vitamin B12 • 60 mcg biotin • 200–300 mg trimethylglycine (TMG) • 250 mg choline • 100 mg para-Aminobenzoic Acid	A B-complex vitamin should contain the dosages I recommend.
carnosine	1,000 mg	
coenzyme Q10 (coQ10)	100–300 mg with meals	

Continued

59

Vitamins and Nutrients	Daily Dose	Comments
dehydroepi-androsterone (DHEA)	25–50 mg	Must be prescribed by health practitioner. Individuals with hormone-related cancers should not take DHEA.
dimethylamino-ethanol (DMAE)	150 mg	May be overstimulating for some people. Headaches, muscle tension, and irritability may occur. Do not take if you have epilepsy, a history of convulsions, or bipolar disorder. If you have kidney or liver disease, consult your doctor before taking this supplement.
essential fatty acids (EFAs)	• 2,000 mg borage oil (equals 920 mg GLA) • 2,000 mg fish oil extract (equals 1,000 mg DHA) • 400 mg EFP	
glycerylphos-phoryl-choline (GPC)	600 mg	
hydergine	5–10 mg	
lecithin	1 g	This dose is about 1 heaping tablespoon of granules.
phosphatidy lcholine	500–1,000 mg	

Vitamins and Nutrients	Daily Dose	Comments
phosphatidylserine (PS)	300 mg	Do not use if you have a bipolar disorder; do not use if you suffer from depression.
pregnenolone	20 mg	Individuals with hormone-related cancers should not take pregnenolone.
proanthocyanidins	200 mg	These naturally occur in grape seed extract and pine bark extract.
selenium	200 mcg	
vinpocetine	10 mg two times daily with meals	
vitamin C	1–6 g	
vitamin E	268 mg 200 mg (gamma-tocopherol) 150 mg (palm oil–derived tocotrienols)	These are mixed tocopherols with an emphasis on gamma.

Summary

In this chapter, I have given you a plan for protecting brain health, no matter what your age. By following these nutritional guidelines and supplementing with essential vitamins, minerals, and smart drugs, you are taking an important step in safeguarding your brain against age-related decline. These measures are for us all. They are preventive at the very least.

In the chapters that follow in Part II, I address specific conditions that affect our brains and mental health. I offer a detailed protocol of diet, nutrition, supplements, and alternative therapies that can rejuvenate your brain and eliminate many of the symptoms and diseases that are associated with age-related mental decline. These individualized protocols should be followed in addition to the basic Reboot Your Brain plan in this chapter.

PART II

SPECIFIC BRAIN CONDITIONS AND TREATMENTS

The old repeat themselves, and the young have nothing to say. The boredom is mutual.

—Jacques Bainville

Chapter 3

Depression

"In addition to my other numerous acquaintances, I have one more intimate confidant. . . . My depression is the most faithful mistress I have known—no wonder, then, that I return the love."

—Søren Kierkegaard

The perceived link between aging and depression has been a real concern of mine for most of my career. As far as I'm concerned, the notion that suffering depression is an inherent risk of the aging process is absolutely false: Depression is absolutely not a by-product of aging. In my experience, many older people feel satisfied with their lives; they are vital, fulfilled, energetic individuals. It would not be considered normal for them to suffer from depression. In fact, there is nothing "normal" about depression at any age, and there is certainly no need to tolerate it simply because we are growing older.

Of course, anyone can feel sad or "down" at times, but these moods should pass. When these blue periods impact behavior, thinking, emotion, memory, energy levels, or physical health over an extended period of time, then a diagnosis of clinical depression must be considered. Unfortunately, the incidence of diagnosed depression is increasing in the aging population. Late-life depression affects about six million Americans age sixty-five and older. The National Institutes of Health has named late-life depression as a major public health problem.[1]

Depression is manifested both physically and emotionally. It affects the whole person: body, mind, and spirit. Any steps to overcome it must address all these areas. Depression is difficult to self-diagnose, and often equally difficult for medical professionals to pinpoint.

In this chapter, I start by discussing the different types of depression and their causes. Then I provide guidelines for determining whether you are suffering from depression. Once you know where you stand, I'll discuss the lifestyle and nutritional strategies you can use to fight depression naturally.

Understanding Depression

Your brain uses neurotransmitters to send information between nerve cells. When the neurotransmitter levels are low, messages cannot flow smoothly across the synaptic gaps. In essence, the communication in your brain becomes sluggish. When the delicate balance of these compounds is disrupted, depression may occur.

There are three main neurotransmitters directly related to depression:

Serotonin. Individuals with low serotonin levels are likely to be depressed or experience internal anger. When the brain creates serotonin, tension is eased.

Dopamine. An intermediate in the synthesis of epinephrine, dopamine is a compound that prepares the body to meet emergencies such as cold, fatigue, or shock. Low levels can affect sleep, appetite, mood, and sexual interest.

Norepinephrine. Related to the chemical epinephrine, norepinephrine is released in response to short-term stress. An excess release of norepinephrine can cause increased heart rate and blood pressure, an increase in glycogenolysis (the conversion of glycogen to glucose), and an increase in lipolysis (the conversion of fats to fatty acids) in fat tissues. Like dopamine, increased norepinephrine levels can have a positive effect on some of the symptoms of depression.

Let's start with a look at the different types of depression and how you can tell whether you are suffering from one of them.

Types of Depression

The cause of depression can generally be attributed to one of three broad categories: life events, a chemical imbalance induced by certain medications or environmental factors, or genetics and family history.

Dysthymia

Dysthymia is the most common type of depressive disorder. This type of reactive depression can occur at any time, triggered by an agonizing or anxiety-producing event. When afflicted with this disorder, an individual can function at a basic level, but may lose interest in formerly pleasurable activities.

Clinical Depression

Clinical depression is not related to an external event, but is brought on by an imbalance of chemicals in the brain. There are strong indications this may be a result of an individual having a genetic predisposition for this condition. More severe than reactive depression, clinical depression may cause an individual to experience an extreme loss of interest in practically everything. And, unlike reactive depression, it has the potential to adversely affect all aspects of everyday living.

Manic Depression

Manic depression is characterized by severe mood swings. A person with manic depression will fluctuate between periods of extreme energy and vivacity and those of complete hopelessness. The causes of manic depression are not fully known, although there are inherited components.[2] Chemical imbalances in the brain may play a role, and stressful or traumatic events may provide the trigger for an episode of mania or depression.

Heavy Metal Contamination

Dr. Lewis Harrison posits that depression may result from heavy metal contamination of the body.[4] Aluminum, lead, copper, and mercury are present in our cooking utensils, the wiring in our homes, our drinking water, the fish we eat, and even in the dental fillings in our teeth. Removing these metals from our bodies through a thorough detoxification program can be beneficial in preventing and impacting depression. To learn more about detoxification programs, visit my website: www.garynull.com.

Parasite Poisoning

Dr. Hazel Parcells has done extensive work on the connection between depression and parasitic infection. Natural remedies such as garlic, pumpkin seeds, grapefruit seed extract, and olive leaf extract have been found to be effective against a range of parasitic invaders.[5]

Diagnosing Depression

Many physicians today are inclined to use depression as a catch-all diagnosis for an array of symptoms that can't be traced to a physical cause. Below I list the most common symptoms of depression as they manifest in older people. Anyone experiencing these symptoms every day for more than two weeks should be evaluated by a health professional to see if they are suffering from depression.

Symptoms of Depression

The common symptoms of depression include a long list of behaviors:

- agitation
- anxiety
- persistent, vague physical complaints
- difficulty concentrating or remembering things
- lack of interest in social activities
- loss of appetite
- unexplained weight loss or weight gain
- sleep disturbances such as insomnia, oversleeping, or early morning waking
- irritability or overly demanding behavior
- lack of attention to personal care or hygiene
- confusion or delusion
- feelings of hopelessness
- sadness, excessive crying
- loss of interest in normally pleasurable activities, such as sex
- loss of self-worth
- prolonged grief after a loss
- low energy, fatigue, feeling of "slowing down"
- suicidal thoughts

As we age, we all experience an accumulation of negative life events. We may suffer from serious or chronic physical illnesses or impaired functioning. What makes age-related depression difficult to diagnose is that it shares symptoms with many other conditions, including Parkinson's, Alzheimer's, dementia, thyroid disorders, strokes, heart disease, and side effects of medications. Sleep disturbances, weight loss, and low energy can be symptoms of diabetes or heart disease. Poor concentration, apathy, and memory loss are found in Parkinson's and Alzheimer's diseases. Fatigue may be a side effect of certain medications. And general aches and pains may result from overexertion or inactivity. These common experiences of aging make the diagnosis of depression especially difficult for the elderly.

Geriatric Depression Scale

Because of the difficulties in obtaining a diagnosis of depression in older adults, the Geriatric Depression Scale (GDS)[6] was developed to gauge depression specifically in the elderly. This series of thirty questions can provide an indicator of whether an older person is suffering from depression.

Circle the answer that best represents how you felt this week:

1. Are you basically satisfied with your life? yes no
2. Have you dropped many of your activities and interests? yes no
3. Do you feel that your life is empty? yes no
4. Do you often get bored? yes no
5. Are you hopeful about the future? yes no
6. Are you bothered by thoughts you can't dismiss? yes no
7. Are you in good spirits most of the time? yes no
8. Are you afraid something bad is going to happen to you? yes no
9. Do you feel happy most of the time? yes no
10. Do you often feel helpless? yes no
11. Do you often get restless and fidgety? yes no
12. Do you prefer to stay home rather than go out and do things? yes no
13. Do you frequently worry about the future? yes no
14. Do you feel you have more problems with memory than most? yes no
15. Do you think it is wonderful to be alive now? yes no
16. Do you often feel downhearted and blue? yes no
17. Do you feel pretty worthless the way you are now? yes no
18. Do you worry a lot about the past? yes no
19. Do you find life very exciting? yes no
20. Is it hard for you to get started on new projects? yes no
21. Do you feel full of energy? yes no

22. Do you feel that your situation is hopeless? yes no
23. Do you think that most people are better off than you are? yes no
24. Do you frequently get upset over little things? yes no
25. Do you frequently feel like crying? yes no
26. Do you have trouble concentrating? yes no
27. Do you enjoy getting up in the morning? yes no
28. Do you avoid social gatherings? yes no
29. Is it easy for you to make decisions? yes no
30. Is your mind as clear as it used to be? yes no

Scoring Your Test

Calculate your score accordingly:

Give yourself 1 point for every "yes" answer to questions 2, 3, 4, 6, 8, 10, 11, 12, 13, 14, 16, 18, 20, 22, 23, 24, 25, 26, and 28.

Give yourself 1 point for every "no" answer to questions 1, 5, 7, 9, 15, 19, 21, 27, 29, and 30.

Total your points.

0–9 points = normal

10–19 points = mildly depressed

20–30 points = very depressed

Combating Depression Naturally

Now, if you were to take this test and become concerned about the state of your mental health, you might go to your doctor. You might complain about sleeping problems, low energy, poor concentration and memory loss, or even general aches and fatigue. And it is likely that your doctor will conclude you are suffering from depression. But rather than examining other factors, such as nutritional or hormone deficiencies that may be contributing to your depression, your doctor will probably suggest you begin taking antidepressant medication as a course of treatment.

What you must keep in mind is that while drug therapy with antidepressants, such as Prozac, can help people feel better, there are negative side effects to these drugs, and we do not know what the long-term effects are. What we do know is that, in general, depression must be viewed as a mind and body disorder, and the relationship between depression and environmental and physical factors is a complex one. Everyone's situation and needs are unique.

In the Reboot Your Brain protocol for impacting depression that follows, I recommend natural approaches that treat the body and mind gently. I will teach you not only how to impact the symptoms of depression, but also, perhaps more important, how to focus on overcoming the fundamental causes of the condition. You will learn how to use nutrition, supplements, and lifestyle changes to naturally prevent and control the symptoms of depression and to rejuvenate and protect your long-term physical and mental health.

Lifestyle

Life events and anxiety-provoking situations can trigger depression. By consciously making lifestyle choices that promote physical, mental, and emotional health, we create a mind–body balance that allows us to access vital tools for preventing and reversing depression.

Exercise

Exercise is an important factor in preventing depression, and equally important in overcoming the condition. The lasting effect of regular exercise is an increased energy level and a feeling of revitalization and accomplishment. Even the most moderate and mild type of exercise can be beneficial.

When you are depressed, your energy levels are low, and it can be hard to start any kind of activity. Begin with simple movements, such as going for a walk, or performing stretches while seated. Active hobbies, such as gardening or dancing, are pleasurable ways to introduce increased exercise into your life.

As you move more, you will experience a positive effect on both your mind and your body, and it will become easier to include exercise as a regular part of your daily activities.

Social Interactions

The nature of depression can interfere with a person's ability to seek assistance. Depression saps energy and self-esteem. Positive social encounters can make the difference between suffering and recovery.

Spending time with friends and family of all ages is important in remaining vital and connected. Emotional support can help us to weather a crisis of loss or grief. Humor lifts our moods and opens us to experiencing daily happiness. Volunteering to help others, learning new skills, and participating in engaging and pleasurable activities enhance feelings of worth at any age. Spiritual communities may offer comfort and promote positive feelings. Loving touch is a proven mood elevator: massage, hugs, and even stroking a pet can lift our mood.

Environment

Music, visual and dramatic arts, and even color can affect mood. There are therapists who specialize in using creative expression to help with mental health issues. Music, dance, and journaling help some individuals understand and process complex emotions. Our physical environment is a reflection of our emotional, spiritual, and intellectual state. Adjusting the elements in our environment can have a miraculous effect in fighting and overcoming depression.

Nutrition

What can be difficult in promoting proper nutrition as we age is the fact that our bodies may become less efficient in absorbing and utilizing key nutrients. Furthermore, someone suffering from depression may have little or no appetite or interest in food. Therefore, it is important that every bit of food you eat has the maximum positive impact on your mental health.

Foods and Depression

The first step in eating a brain-healthy diet is to eliminate fast foods, simple carbohydrates, alcohol, artificial sweeteners, white flour products, and caffeine. This change should improve the chemical balances in your brain.

To prevent and combat depression, your diet should contain lots of fruits and vegetables, with soybeans and soy products, brown rice, millet, legumes, and essential fatty acids. Placebo-controlled research conducted with medicated patients suggests that adding omega-3 fatty acids, particularly eicosapentaenoic acid, may ameliorate symptoms of major depressive disorder.[7]

At all costs, you must avoid meat or fried foods, such as hamburgers and french fries. These foods are high in saturated fats that block the arteries and small blood vessels, interfering with blood flow. Your blood cells become sticky and clump together, leading to poor cerebral circulation, accompanied by mental sluggishness and fatigue.

Depressed people are attracted to sugar because of the initial lift it provides. Sugar does stimulate serotonin levels, which in turn temporarily improves your mood. But this initial surge of energy disappears in a matter of minutes. The reason behind the initial boost is that sugar, regardless of which form you are talking about, does not have to be digested and passes directly into the bloodstream, where it dramatically raises the blood sugar level, and overstimulates the pancreas to produce too much insulin. The excess insulin then causes the sugar level to plummet. Within half an hour of consuming a sugary snack, your blood sugar level will drop to very low levels, allowing fatigue, irritability, and anxiety to creep in. With these feelings present, the person seeks another boost from sugar, resulting in repeating the same, vicious cycle.

The Latest Research

An increasingly large body of evidence shows that a junk food diet can exact a heavy toll on our emotional well-being. A long-term study appearing in the journal *Public Health Nutrition* in 2011 observed that people who commonly ate fast food and processed baked foods were 51 percent more likely to suffer from depression than those people who rarely or never indulged in these foods.[6] The study's data reflected a dose-dependent relationship, meaning that the more unhealthy staples one consumes, the more at risk one is of suffering from depression. These findings are consistent with a 2009 analysis by British researchers that produced a clear link between diet and depression. Published in the *British Journal of Psychiatry*, the study concluded that people who consumed a diet high in foods, such as fried food, processed meat, refined grains, and sweets were 58 percent more likely to experience depression compared to those who consumed a diet rich in fruits, vegetables, and fish.

The millennia-old practice of tai chi was shown to effectively combat major depression in seniors in a recent study by scientists at UCLA. The findings, which were published in the *American Journal of Geriatric Psychiatry*, indicate that elderly patients diagnosed with the condition saw remarkable improvements after practicing a Westernized version of the Chinese martial art. The study compared the outcomes of two groups of seniors receiving standard depression treatment. One group engaged in two hours of tai chi classes weekly over the course of ten weeks, while the other group spent the same amount of time attending a health education class. Both groups realized notable improvements, but the tai chi group experienced significantly better improvements in memory, cognition, and quality of life and had reduced levels of depression.[7] Speaking in an interview, the study's lead author, Dr. Helen Lavretsky, remarked, "With tai chi we may be able to treat these conditions without exposing [patients] to additional medications."[8]

Recipes

The recipes in Appendix II of this book are intended to help you get started on a healthy eating plan that will provide optimum mental health benefits. Each dish focuses on foods rich in vitamins and nutrients beneficial to our brains. Eating right does not have to involve a huge effort. Prepare healthy dishes in larger quantities and store them for use throughout the week. In the list below are my recommendations for easy-to-prepare meals full of nutrients proven to help prevent depression:

- Deep-Sea Juicing
- Everglades Punch
- Green Power Punch
- How Green Is Your Juice?
- Nuts and Seeds
- Pure Citrus Punch
- Four Bean Salad
- Mixed Sprout, Bean, and Nut Salad
- Cream of Sweet Potato Soup
- Blueberry Banana Pancakes
- Nutty Oatmeal
- Macaroni Marconi
- Original Broccoli Stir-Fry
- Pasta e Fagioli
- Sweet Kidney Bean Mash
- Heavenly Roasted Nuts

Supplements

Even with a diet rich in recommended vitamins and minerals, your body may not efficiently absorb and process these necessary nutrients. As you grow older, your appetite may decrease, and you may find that you are unable to consistently take in the recommended amounts of food nutrients. Furthermore, loss of appetite is a common symptom of depression. It may be that getting these nutrients in supplement form is the most efficient way for you to enhance your healthy diet. However, supplements are not intended to replace healthy food choices.

Of course, before you begin any new health program, you should get a comprehensive, full-body evaluation performed by a qualified health care practitioner. A proper health and medical evaluation should evaluate your blood chemistry to assess your blood markers, your metabolic rate, and your blood pressure for indicators of cardiovascular, hormonal, or other imbalances or danger signs. If you are taking medications of any sort, for depression or any other condition, you need to inform your doctor of any supplements you are considering adding to your daily diet, as some may interact with prescription medications and cause adverse effects. You should speak to your doctor before adding any of these supplements to your daily regimen.

Vitamins and Minerals

Certain vitamins and minerals are especially important in fighting depression.

Folic Acid. Folic acid levels are directly related to the severity of depression: The lower the level of folic acid in the blood, the more serious the level of depression. Low levels of folic acid have been linked to depression and bipolar disorder in a number of studies. Insufficient folic acid is one of the most common nutritional deficiencies, and one-third of all adults are low in this important vitamin.[8] I recommend that your daily B-complex vitamin contain at least 800 micrograms of folic acid. If you are taking folic acid as a separate supplement, always combine it with 1,000 micrograms of vitamin B12.

Vitamin B12. Vitamin B12 deficiency may also play a part in depression. As we age, it becomes increasingly difficult for our bodies to absorb sufficient amounts of B12 from what we eat. So even if you are consuming adequate quantities of foods rich in B12, your body is not getting the full benefit. I recommend that your daily B-complex vitamin contain at least 1,000 micrograms of vitamin B12.

Vitamin B6. Vitamin B6 converts tryptophan (an amino acid) into serotonin. While extreme deficiencies in B6 are rare, minor deficiencies (which occur frequently) can lead to depression. Heavy users of alcohol are likely to have a B6 deficiency, as are women who use oral contraceptives. I recommend that your daily B-complex vitamin contain at least 75 milligrams of vitamin B6.

Vitamin D3. Vitamin D3 is called the sunlight vitamin because the body produces it when the sun's ultraviolet B (UVB) rays strike the skin. It is the only vitamin the body manufactures naturally. Considered a mood elevator, vitamin D3 may be effective in dealing with seasonal depression. Ten to fifteen minutes of summer sun a few days per week generally supplies the body with sufficient amounts of vitamin D3. Our body's ability to produce vitamin D3 declines as we age, however, and those who are unable to spend time outside, or who suffer the effects of the lack of sun in winter climates, may want to supplement. For those suffering from depression, I recommend supplementing with 268 to 536 milligrams of vitamin D3 daily.

Inositol. Inositol, also known as B8, functions closely with lecithin and choline. It is a fundamental ingredient of cell membranes and is necessary for proper brain function. The neurotransmitter serotonin depends on inositol to function properly. I recommend increasing your daily inositol supplement from 250 to 1,250 milligrams. Do not exceed 1,250 milligrams daily.

Magnesium. Magnesium deficiency is also seen in people suffering from depression. When patients recover from depression, magnesium levels in the blood rise.[9] Magnesium supplements should be taken with calcium to lessen overreaction to stress and panic attacks. I recommend that women suffering from depression take a supplement of 320 milligrams daily; men should take a supplement of 420 milligrams daily.

Potassium. Potassium is one of the most abundant minerals in the human body. Most of the time, supplementation with potassium is unnecessary, because it is readily available in our diet in such foods as bananas, orange juice, and potatoes. Potassium is depleted from our bodies in times of stress, thus upsetting the delicate balance of neurotransmitter communication in our brains. For this reason, potassium supplements may be useful in impacting depression. Potassium can interact with some drugs, so if you are taking prescription medications, consult with your doctor before taking potassium supplements. If potassium is safe for you, I recommend a daily supplement of 300 milligrams.

Smart Drugs and Nutrients

A number of other naturally occurring nutrients may have beneficial impacts on depression.

5-Hydroxytryptophan (5-HTP). A derivative of the amino acid tryptophan, this mood-enhancing chemical is converted into the neurotransmitter serotonin. 5-HTP should be taken with carbidopa, a decarboxylase inhibitor that prevents 5-HTP from converting to serotonin before it reaches the brain. For depression, anxiety, and panic attacks, I recommend taking 50 to 100 milligrams three times daily.

Adapton (Garum Armoricum). This naturally occurring substance is taken from a deep-sea fish. It is widely used in Europe and Japan to help with stress, anxiety, and depression. It improves concentration, mood, and sleep. You should take four capsules as directed for fifteen days; stop for one week, then continue with a maintenance dose of two capsules daily.

Dehydroepiandrosterone (DHEA). Youthful hormone balance is vital in maintaining health and preventing disease in individuals over the age of forty. One hormone that is deficient in virtually everyone who is over thirty-five is DHEA. This building block for estrogen and testosterone enhances mood and a sense of well-being in menopausal women.

Not everyone, however, can take advantage of the multiple benefits of DHEA. Men and women with hormone-related cancers, for example, should not take DHEA. This supplement is available only by prescription from your doctor. If your doctor says it's safe for you, I recommend taking a supplementof 25 to 50 milligrams daily; if your doctor thinks DHEA will help in the treatment of your depression, he or she will prescribe an appropriate increase in your dosage.

DL-Phenylalaline (DLPA). DLPA contains two forms ("D" and "L") of the amino acid phenylalanine. The "L" form is naturally occurring and believed to bolster mood-elevating chemicals in the brain. The "D" form is a synthetic form of a substance that has a pain-relieving effect. In one clinical trial of individuals suffering from depression, twelve of twenty depressed men and women who took 200 milligrams of DLPA daily reported being free of depression after nearly three weeks of treatment, and four reported feeling somewhat better.[10]

You should not combine DLPA with prescription antidepressants or stimulants unless specifically directed to do so by your doctor. If you have high blood pressure, or are prone to panic attacks, DLPA may aggravate your condition. DLPA should also not be used if you are taking levodopa for treatment of Parkinson's disease. Women who are pregnant, or individuals with melanoma, should not take DLPA. People with PKU (a rare, inherited metabolism disorder) should avoid DLPA as well.

If you are able to take DLPA, I recommend a supplement of 1,000 to 1,500 milligrams daily.

Dimethylaminoethanol (DMAE). This nutrient, found in sardines, is a powerful brain stimulant that increases acetylcholine levels. Acetylcholine is a neurotransmitter associated with mood and energy levels. I recommend increasing your daily supplement from 150 milligrams to 650 to 1,650 milligrams daily. Do not exceed 1,650 milligrams per day.

Pregnenolone. A hormone produced by the adrenal glands, pregnenolone is abundant in the brain, where it facilitates communication between neurotransmitters. Low levels of pregnenolone have been linked to depression. As we age, the amount of pregnenolone we produce declines; levels can be tested by a basic urine test. To improve your ability to handle the stress brought on by depression, I recommend increasing your daily supplement from 50 milligrams to 100 to 250 milligrams daily. Do not exceed 250 milligrams daily.

S-Adenosylmethionine (SAMe). SAMe (pronounced "sammy") has long been prescribed by European doctors as a treatment for depression. SAMe promotes cell growth and repair, and maintains levels of glutathione, a major antioxidant that protects against free radicals and contributes to the formation of the mood-enhancing neurotransmitter serotonin. SAMe should not be taken if you are taking MAO inhibitor antidepressants. You should consult with your doctor before taking SAMe if you suffer from severe depression or bipolar disorder. If SAMe is safe for you to use, I recommend raising the dose gradually from 200 milligrams twice a day to 400 milligrams twice a day, to 400 milligrams three times a day, to 400 milligrams four times a day, over a period of twenty days.

Reboot Your Brain Chart of Additional Supplements for Impacting Depression

The following chart summarizes the supplements I recommend adding to the protocol for overall brain health from chapter 2. In some cases, I will recommend increasing the dose of a particular vitamin or supplement to specifically impact depression. In these cases, you should increase the daily dosage from chapter 2 to the level recommended for that specific condition.

This protocol is designed for individuals who suffer from, or are specifically concerned about, depression. If you are concerned about additional brain conditions discussed in other chapters, consult with a health professional about how you can safely impact multiple conditions.

If you are taking medications—whether prescription or over-the-counteror—that have any food restrictions, consult with your doctor before beginning any supplement program. Your health care provider should always be up-to-date on all vitamins, supplements, and herbal or homeopathic remedies you are taking. Supplement overdoses are rare, but possible, and certain combinations may affect individuals adversely.

Supplement	Dosage	Cautions
5-hydroxy tryptophan (5-HTP)	50–100 mg three times daily	If you are taking prescription medication for depression, you should consult with your doctor before taking 5-HTP. Excess levels of serotonin in the blood can be dangerous in cases of coronary artery disease.
adapton (garum armoricum)	Four capsules as directed daily for fifteen days; stop for one week, then continue with maintenance dose of two capsules daily.	
DHEA hormone	Follow doctor's directions for dosage.	Must be prescribed by your health practitioner. Individuals with hormone-related cancers should not take DHEA.

Supplement	Dosage	Cautions
DL-phenylalanine (DLPA)	1,000–1,500 mg	Do not combine DLPA with prescription antidepressants or stimulants unless specifically directed to do so by your doctor. Do not take DLPA if you have high blood pressure or are prone to panic attacks, are taking levodopa for treatment of Parkinson's disease, are pregnant, have melanoma, or have PKU (a rare, inherited metabolism disorder).
dimethylamino-ethanol (DMAE)	Increase daily dosage from 150 mg to 650–1,650 mg. Do not exceed a daily supplement of 1,650 mg.	May be overstimulating for some people. Headaches, muscle tension, and irritability may occur. Do not take if you have epilepsy, a history of convulsions, or bipolar disease. If you have kidney or liver disease, consult your doctor before taking this supplement.
Inositol	Increase daily dosage from 250 mg to 1,000 mg. Do not exceed a daily supplement of 1,000 mg. Take in two divided doses.	
Magnesium	320 mg (for women), 420 mg (for men)	May take six weeks or longer for effects to be felt.

Supplement	Dosage	Cautions
Potassium	300 mg	Do not take potassium supplements if you are taking medication for high blood pressure or heart disease or if you have a kidney disorder. Consuming foods rich in potassium is okay. Do not exceed a supplementary dose of 3.5 g daily without consulting with your doctor.
Pregnenolone	Increase daily dosage from 50 mg to 100–250 mg. Do not exceed a daily supplement of 250 mg.	Individuals with hormone-related cancers should not take pregnenolone.
S-adenosyl methionine (SAMe)	Dosage range of 400–1,600 mg	Raise the dose gradually from 200 mg twice a day to 400 mg twice a day, to 400 mg three times a day, to 400 mg four times a day, over a period of twenty days.
vitamin D	268 to 536 mg daily	Do not exceed 536 mg daily

Alternative Health Remedies

When suffering from a specific condition such as depression, we can also try some natural treatment options that are considered alternatives to traditional medicine. While a healthful lifestyle and the proper nutritional and supplement plan are vital to winning the battle against depression, there are some other targeted remedies that might help, too.

Herbal Remedies

Some herbal extracts and homeopathic treatments have properties similar to conventional medications, but are gentler and may lack the drugs' side effects. Always inform your medical practitioner of any herbal remedies you may be taking.

- **St. John's wort** (hypericum) is very popular in Europe, where double-blind, placebo-controlled studies exist to support its efficacy in alleviating depression.[11] Hypericum is taken by more than twenty million people in Germany to combat depression. In fact, it is covered by German health insurance as a prescription drug. I recommend taking 450 milligrams once daily.
- **Ginkgo biloba** is an extract of the ginkgo plant, is used in Europe to help fight dementia and Alzheimer's disease, and is a free-radical scavenger effective at eliminating free radicals. It increases blood circulation to the brain and protects nerve cells, and has shown promise in impacting mild depression. One study revealed that elderly people suffering from depression who showed no improvement on antidepressant drugs did respond when a ginkgo biloba extract was added.[12] Your daily supplement should be 300 milligrams in two divided doses.
- **Chinese schisandra berry** is an adaptogen, like ginseng. It redirects energy, calms nerves, and can act as a mild sedative. I recommend taking 100 milligrams twice daily.
- **Calamus root** can be used externally by adding it to a bath to induce a state of tranquility. It should be avoided during pregnancy.

Homeopathic Remedies

The following remedies may be used for both temporary and acute cases of depression. When dealing with a chronic condition, homeopathic remedies must be used in conjunction with other therapies, as prescribed by a qualified health professional. Consult with your health care provider before taking any homeopathic remedy, and follow your provider's recommendation for the appropriate dosage. Always inform your medical practitioner of any homeopathic remedies you may be taking.

- **Aurum metallicum** alleviates feelings of worthlessness, low self-esteem, and despair. It can help provide hope for a person with reactive depression and is said to be particularly beneficial to idealistic and goal-oriented individuals who have experienced life-altering events and feel they have somehow failed.
- **Natrun muriaticum** is used when depression results from an event generating profound bereavement and distress. It is prescribed for people who cannot show their feelings and who suffer in silence, believing they must appear strong and controlled.
- **Sepia** is used mainly for women experiencing depression associated with menopause. This type of depression can be characterized by irritability and indifference to others.
- **Pulsatilla** is used for people who show signs of manic depression.

Light Therapy

In his book *Beyond Prozac*,[3] Dr. Michael Norden states that light therapy has shown positive results in helping patients overcome the mild depression associated with seasonal affective disorder (SAD). The body chemistry of many individuals is thrown off by the decrease in the daylight hours during the winter season. But treatments that utilize bright light have shown promise in overcoming this type of depression. One such treatment is called dawn simulation and is a unique lighting system used in the bedroom that is manipulated to mimic sunrise. Using dawn stimulation therapy results in an increased energy level and ease of waking for some individuals.

Light therapy is administered by a 10,000-lux light box, which contains white fluorescent light tubes covered with a plastic screen that blocks ultraviolet rays. An individual sits in front of the box with his or her eyes open, but not looking directly into the light. Daily sessions of ten to fifteen minutes are gradually increased to thirty- to forty-five-minute sessions. Ninety minutes of exposure per day is often prescribed. This therapy can easily be practiced at home.

Aromatherapy

Essential oils can be used in baths or inhaled to provide rebalancing effects. Do not apply essential oils directly to the skin; they must be mixed with carrier oils. Experiment with various scents to see what you find most soothing or energizing. You can try the following:

- lavender
- basil
- jasmine
- rose
- bergamot
- sandalwood
- neroli (orange blossom oil)
- ylang ylang
- marjoram
- clary sage
- chamomile

Summary

With careful attention to our diets, our environment, and our physical and spiritual selves, we can enjoy lives rich in vitality, energy, and self-esteem at any age. The Reboot Your Brain program works to keep you in balance during stressful or anxious times, allowing you to weather life's experiences without falling victim to debilitating depression.

Chapter 4

Anxiety

"A crust eaten in peace is better than a banquet
partaken in anxiety."

—Aesop

Your first day at school, a first date, starting a new job, buying a house, facing a serious illness, and many rites of passage are marked by sweaty palms, rapid breathing, and a stomach full of butterflies. Our bodies switch into high gear: We feel alert, ready to react, poised for any possibility. Anxiety is a typical and appropriate reaction to many types of stress. When experienced at an optimum level, anxiety keeps you sharp and allows you to foresee things that need attention.

We experience anxiety throughout our lives; it is part of our genetic makeup. We wouldn't be alive today if our ancestors had lacked the ability to anticipate dangers and threats. A low level of anxiety is as natural a part of our existence as breathing, eating, and sleeping. Dr. Richard Restak, a clinical professor of neurology at George Washington University School of Medicine and Health Sciences in Washington, DC, describes anxiety as a biological function with a preservative aspect: the ability to use the frontal lobe of our brain to imagine future possibilities. These future possibilities sometimes include events that induce a reaction of anxiety and provoke a particular biochemical reaction in the brain.[1]

When an anxious moment changes from a short-lived period of stimulation to an uncontrollable period of worry and accompanying stress, however, and feelings of restless foreboding become excessive, what is supposed to be a helpful biological reaction becomes a dysfunctional state. Clinical anxiety disorders are marked by an ongoing and pervasive sense of threat and vulnerability. Given our day-to-day living environment, in which we are bombarded by constant news of global terrorism and local crime, it may not surprise you to find out that more than nineteen million Americans suffer from some sort of acute anxiety.[2]

Until recently, anxiety disorders were thought to be most prevalent in the younger population. Experts are now beginning to recognize that anxiety disorders are common in the elderly population, however, especially in older people who suffer from depression. In fact, conditions generally associated with aging, such as chronic physical problems, cognitive difficulties, and significant emotional losses, may be triggers for anxiety disorders.

Because anxiety disorders spring from many—often interrelated—causes, the treatment modality varies from person to person. Increased age should not mean increased anxiety. By addressing both the physical and emotional components of anxiety, we can alleviate suffering and restore quality of life. In this chapter we'll look at just what causes anxiety and talk about natural ways to combat it.

Understanding Anxiety

There are several theories on the causes of anxiety disorders. In fact, many experts believe that both physical and environmental components combine to trigger anxiety disorders. Heredity, brain chemistry, personality, and life experiences may all be interrelated in causing anxiety. Particularly among older adults, anxiety disorders are closely associated with depression.

Some experts believe that a biochemical imbalance in our brains may lead to anxiety disorders. This certainly makes sense when you consider the strong relationship between anxiety and stress and between anxiety and depression. But what these experts have yet to determine is the root cause of this imbalance. Does the chemical imbalance in the neurotransmitters of our brain cause the anxiety disorder? Or is the disorder present first, with the subsequent stress reaction of our bodies causing the brain's chemical imbalance?

Individuals who suffer from anxiety disorders may have a brain chemistry imbalance resulting from a depletion of serotonin, as well as an excess of dopamine and adrenaline compounds.

Serotonin is an important chemical in the brain that regulates mental well-being and other brain functions, such as learning and sleep. Individuals with low serotonin levels are also likely to suffer from depression. When the brain creates serotonin, tension and anxiety are eased.

Dopamine is an intermediate in the synthesis of epinephrine, a compound that prepares the body to meet emergencies such as facing cold, fatigue, or shock. When the brain is creating dopamine, we may feel alert and think and act more quickly. Unregulated production of dopamine may produce symptoms of anxiety.

Adrenaline systems regulate important body functions such as blood pressure and wakefulness. An excess of adrenaline production and release can take a toll on the nervous system. Extended states of hyperarousal and the accompanying release of stress hormones, such as cortisol, can wreak havoc on an individual's physical and emotional health.

While some doctors believe this imbalance in brain chemistry can be corrected through prescribing medications that regulate the transmission of these compounds in the brain, it is clear to me that the treatment of an anxiety disorder is more complex than simply prescribing medications.

Let's begin by looking at the types of anxiety and how you can tell whether you are suffering from one of them.

Types of Anxiety

There are several types of anxiety disorders, each with its particular manifestation of symptoms. A single situation or event does not cause an anxiety disorder to appear. A combination of physical and environmental triggers can provoke any of the following anxiety disorders.

Generalized Anxiety Disorder

This is the most common anxiety disorder in older adults. Generalized anxiety disorder (GAD) is characterized by uncontrollable worry about one or more issues for a six-month period or longer. Chronic tension or excessive worries about health, money, family, or anticipated disasters are hallmarks of GAD. Women are more susceptible to GAD than men, and it is often linked to depression in the elderly. Physical symptoms may include trembling or twitching, muscle tension, headaches, irritability, sweating, nausea, hot flashes, lightheadedness, and difficulty breathing.

Panic Disorder

Marked by intense fear and dread, this anxiety disorder is often accompanied by specific physical symptoms, such as chest pains, dizziness, nausea, flushes or chills, racing heartbeat, or tingling or numbness in the hands. People who suffer from panic disorder feel emotionally and physically less healthy than average and may suffer from alcohol or drug abuse.[3] If left untreated, panic disorder can cause a person to avoid certain situations or events that make him or her feel anxious, leading to the development of phobic behavior. Panic attacks are more prevalent in late adolescence and adulthood and usually recede with age.[4]

Phobias

Phobias are fears that have become extreme and irrational. People with phobias experience an overwhelming desire to avoid the source of these fears. This dread interferes with their ability to interact normally in family, work, or social situations. Physical symptoms of phobias are similar to those associated with severe stress: rapid heartbeat, shortness of breath, trembling, and an overwhelming flight response.

Obsessive Compulsive Disorder (OCD)

People who suffer from OCD have an uncontrollable urge to repeat simple actions, check things repeatedly, or have ceaseless unwanted thoughts. These obsessive thoughts intrude persistently throughout the course of a normal day, causing great anxiety and stress. Compulsions are acts that are performed over and over again in an attempt to alleviate feelings of discomfort or anxiety. OCD is common in the elderly, and women are more likely than men to experience this anxiety disorder.

Post-traumatic Stress Disorder (PTSD)

This anxiety disorder is triggered by traumatic events that fall outside the range of what might be considered normal human experience. Survivors of war, sexual abuse, violent accidents, or near-death experiences may continue to experience the resulting stress of these traumas throughout their lifetimes. Someone who suffers from PTSD may re-experience feelings of intense fear, helplessness, or horror associated with the event. They may suffer from nightmares or flashbacks. They may feel emotionally numb and withdraw socially. Problems with concentration, insomnia, and mood swings may also be persistent.

Diagnosing Anxiety Disorders

Late-life anxiety disorders can be difficult to diagnose for a number of reasons. Traditionally, medical professionals considered anxiety disorders to be less prevalent in the elderly than in younger adults. In fact, until recently, anxiety disorders were thought to decline with age. Research now shows that anxiety disorders in the elderly are indeed real and treatable. Data on panic disorders, OCD, phobias, and GAD indicate that anxiety disorders are clinically significant in the aging population.[5] Like depression, anxiety disorders impact women at a disproportionate rate: nearly twice that of their male counterparts.[6]

Diagnosing anxiety disorders in older adults is complicated, however, by several factors. As we age, we may experience certain medical conditions that may increase our worry about physical problems, and thus increase our anxiety.

Medical problems can mimic the symptoms of anxiety, or even trigger it. An irregular heartbeat can cause palpitations and short-ness of breath. A clot in the lung (pulmonary embolism) may cause sudden, unexplained feelings of anxiety. Epilepsy and brain disor-ders may have anxiety as a symptom. Anemia, diabetes, thyroid disease, and adrenal problems all may cause symptoms of anxiety. Even when caused by medical problems, anxiety may not always be relieved by the treatment of the underlying disease.

Depression and anxiety disorders are closely linked, particularly in the elderly. Commonly prescribed medications used by many doc-tors as a first course of action to treat complaints they associate with aging may produce increased anxiety as a side effect. Prescription and some over-the-counter drugs can also cause anxiety symptoms. Cold medicines, diet pills, antispasmodic medications, stimulants, digitalis, thyroid supplements, and, ironically, antidepressants may all cause anxiety. Withdrawing from certain medications, including certain blood pressure medicines, can also trigger anxiety.

Individuals suffering from the early symptoms of dementia, such as memory loss and other cognitive impairments, may suffer from generalized anxiety, which can blossom into panic attacks. In this case, the panic attacks and anxiety may mask the true diagnosis of dementia.

Thus, to diagnose and impact anxiety in older adults, we must consider the complex relationships between anxiety and other disorders and take a comprehensive approach that addresses the special physical, emotional, and social needs of this particular population.

Symptoms of Anxiety Disorder

In generalized anxiety disorder (one of the most common disorders in the elderly), the pervasive feeling of anxiety is associated with at least three of the following symptoms:

- restlessness or edginess
- fatigue
- lack of concentration
- irritability
- muscle tension
- disturbed sleep cycles

Individuals who suffer from anxiety disorders of varying types also report a combination of the following symptoms:

- unrealistic worries
- excessive fear
- exaggerated reactions to startling events
- flashbacks to past trauma
- ritualistic behaviors as a way to deal with anxieties
- shakiness or trembling
- muscle aches
- sweating
- cold or clammy hands
- dizziness
- tension
- dry mouth
- racing or pounding heartbeat
- upset stomach
- increased pulse or respirations

Acute anxiety disorders, such as panic attacks, may also manifest physical symptoms, including:

- hot or cold flashes
- choking or smothering sensations
- chest discomfort
- faintness
- tingling
- unsteadiness
- nausea

Identifying Anxiety Disorders[7]

Whether we are suffering from stress or anxiety, or caring for someone who may be suffering from an anxiety disorder, it is helpful to assess both the level of worry and the impact such worries are having on daily life. The questions below have been adapted from the Anxiety Disorders Association of America's website and may help you separate feelings of anxiety from physical symptoms and determine whether you should seek help in treating a disorder that can become incapacitating, no matter your age.

Circle the answer that best represents how you've felt over the last week:

1. Have you been constantly concerned or worried over a number of things? yes no
2. Is there anything in your life that is causing you ongoing concern? yes no
3. Do you have a hard time putting worries out of your mind? yes no
4. Do your worries keep you from thinking clearly about other things? yes no
5. Do you avoid previously routine activities? yes no
6. Do you avoid social situations you used to enjoy? yes no

7. Do your worries seem out of proportion to reality? yes no
8. Have you experienced frequent weepiness, apathy, or unexplained weight loss or gain? (These symptoms can indicate depression, which is often accompanied by anxiety.) yes no
9. Were you exerting yourself physically when you noticed the chest pain? yes no
10. Were you exerting yourself physically when your heart started to race? yes no
11. Have you changed, or begun taking new, medication? yes no
12. Have you increased or changed your medication without supervision? yes no

Scoring Your Test

Give yourself 1 point for every "yes" answer to questions 1, 2, 3, 4, 5, 6, 7, and 8.

Give yourself 1 point for every "no" answer to questions 9, 10, 11, and 12.

If your score is higher than 4, you may want to talk to your health care provider about whether you are suffering from anxiety.

Combating Anxiety Naturally

Success in treating anxiety in the older person depends on a partnership that includes the patient, the patient's support network, and the patient's primary care provider. Everyone must recognize and agree on the nature of the problem and make a commitment to stick to a treatment plan that addresses not just the immediate symptoms but also necessary lifestyle changes that will help the individual return to normal functioning.

Many doctors, once they have concluded that a patient suffers from an anxiety disorder, will probably prescribe a course of therapy that includes both counseling and drug therapy. Both of these approaches may offer relief from crippling anxiety disorders, but there are other treatment options that may offer the same results. For instance, in a Swedish study, a simple exercise program was nearly as effective in reducing panic attacks as any antidepressant.[8] If you are taking prescribed medications, even in combination with psychotherapy, you may find that your anxiety is not alleviated. According to Dr. Jeremy Coplan, a researcher at Columbia University Medical College, "Drugs don't work in a quarter to a third of cases." He further notes that this is "exactly the same criticism directed at talk therapy."[9]

But when therapy and medications don't work to regulate the stress that can trigger more severe conditions, what can we do to protect our mental health? In the Reboot Your Brain protocol for impacting anxiety that follows, I recommend natural techniques for reducing stress and impacting anxiety. Changes in lifestyle, diet, attention to our emotional status, vitamin and mineral supplementation, and simple alternative treatments can prevent everyday stress from turning into crippling anxiety and control the symptoms of anxiety disorders.

Lifestyle

Stressful life events can trigger an anxiety reaction. Left unchecked, free-floating generalized anxiety can bloom into a severe and function-impairing disorder. By consciously making lifestyle choices that promote physical, mental, and emotional good health, we create a mind/body balance that allows us to access vital tools for preventing and reversing anxiety.

Exercise

Studies have shown that moderate exercise can release endorphins and natural cortisol, which act to elevate mood and reduce stress. Bodily pain and discomfort can increase anxiety in older adults, and gentle exercises, such as stretching, yoga, or even walking, can reduce discomfort while releasing stress. Exercise is also beneficial in normalizing sleep patterns and enhancing self-confidence. Choose a pleasurable activity and stick with it. It will not take long before you experience a positive effect.

Meditation

Meditation acts to calm the mind and relieve stress. Twenty minutes, twice a day, of mindfulness meditation is recommended to prevent and reduce anxiety. Engaging in breathing exercises and being generally aware of your breathing patterns throughout the day can be beneficial in eliminating anxiety. Focusing on the positive aspects of life and nurturing an optimistic outlook will reduce the effects of stress on the body and aid in coping with anxiety.

Cognitive Behavioral Therapy

For individuals suffering from anxiety disorders, cognitive behavioral therapy can help teach them to both change behavior resulting from anxiety and revamp their thought processes to prevent symptoms from worsening or developing. This type of therapy is short term, lasting perhaps eight to twelve weeks. Goals of cognitive behavioral therapy include learning to identify behavior patterns and interrupt them with physical activities, such as tapping, learning breathing and other relaxation techniques to prevent some of the symptoms of anxiety from gaining hold, and gradually becoming less sensitive to situations and thoughts that provoke stress and anxiety. It is important that a participant in this type of therapy be motivated to understand his or her behavior and work to change it.

Foods and Anxiety

Studies indicate that a poor diet may be a significant factor in producing anxiety. To prevent and impact anxiety disorders, I recommend some very specific dietary guidelines.

One of the most important steps is the elimination of caffeine from your diet. Caffeine and caffeine-like substances found in coffee, tea, and many soft drinks can induce symptoms of anxiety, such as nervousness, fear, heart palpitations, nausea, restlessness, and tremors. Caffeine overstimulates the adrenal system and can deplete your body of important B-complex and C vitamins. The effect of caffeine has been specifically studied in patients with agoraphobia and panic disorders. An astounding 71 percent of the study subjects who consumed caffeine reported that the effects were extremely comparable to the symptoms they experienced during a panic attack.[10] A separate investigation showed that patients with anxiety experienced a degree of anxiety that directly correlated with their consumption of caffeine. Even more astonishing, this report suggested that the persons most at risk from suffering from anxiety effects have a heightened sensitivity to the effects of just one cup of coffee.[11]

Hypoglycemia (lowered blood glucose levels) is also directly correlated to anxiety and its related symptoms. Anxiety, sweating, tremors, and palpitations are some of the physiological warning signs that indicate our autonomic nervous system is sensing lowered blood glucose levels. Maintaining proper blood sugar levels by avoiding refined carbohydrates is essential to controlling anxiety.

Drawing upon the recommendations of Dr. Paul Epstein, a naturopathic physician practicing in Norwalk, Connecticut, and an advocate of a dietary approach to banishing hypoglycemic reactions, I have created the ABC approach to managing anxiety through diet:

- **Avoid.** Eliminate alcohol, caffeine, and nicotine from your lifestyle.
  Analyze your current diet and learn to recognize foods that cause distress. Eliminate these foods from your diet and replace them with foods that provide the body with optimal nutrients and support.

- **Banish** simple sugars from your diet. Sugar, fructose, glucose, corn syrup, corn sweeteners, fruit sugar, and brown sugar are the most obvious forms of simple sugars. Alcoholic beverages and many canned, packaged, or frozen foods are also high in simple sugars. If you do experience a hypoglycemic attack and must take a simple sugar in the form of fruit juice, for instance, be sure to couple the sugar with a source of protein (e.g., beans, brown rice, nuts, or seeds) to slow down your system's absorption of the glucose and prevent rapid changes in blood sugar levels.

- **Choose complex carbohydrates.** Unrefined carbohydrates deliver the required energy more rapidly and efficiently than protein. Vegetable proteins provide time-released energy, as opposed to animal-based proteins, which do not.

The Latest Research

A recent study published in the *Nutrition Journal* by French scientists suggests that anxiety sufferers may benefit significantly from introducing more antioxidant nutrients into their diets. Lead author Marie-Anne Milesi and her team found that individuals given a supplement derived from melon juice and high in the antioxidant superoxide dismutase experienced significant reductions in perceived stress after four weeks compared to a group given a placebo.[9] The findings confirm the connection between psychological stress and oxidative stress in the body.

The role of magnesium in reducing anxiety and stress was examined in a 2011 study by researchers at Center for Learning and Memory, School of Medicine, at the University of Texas in Austin. Published in the *Journal of Neuroscience,* the study found that elevating levels of magnesium enhanced synaptic plasticity in the brain, which in turn, altered learned fear responses.[10] The results indicate that magnesium can help lessen anxiety by enhancing the brain's neural network. The study's authors also point out that higher levels of magnesium boost the production of brain-derived neurotrophic factor (BDNF), a protein that supports brain cell development and is necessary for long-term memory.

Recipes

In the list below are my recommendations for easy-to-prepare meals full of nutrients proven to help prevent anxiety. The recipes can be found in Appendix II.

- Everglades Punch
- Green Power Punch
- Nuts and Seeds
- Relax Your Mind
- Sleep Insurer
- Velvety Pecan Milk
- Mixed Beans Vinaigrette
- Mixed Sprout, Bean, and Nut Salad
- Cream of Sweet Potato Soup
- Nutty Banana Breakfast
- Nutty Oatmeal
- Indonesian Kale
- Original Broccoli Stir-Fry
- Pasta e Fagioli
- Sweet Kidney Bean Mash
- Heavenly Roasted Nuts

Supplements

Vitamins and Minerals

Certain vitamins and minerals are especially important in fighting anxiety.

Vitamin B6. Vitamin B6 is an important coenzyme in the synthesis of gamma-aminobutyric acid (GABA), dopamine, and serotonin neurotransmitters that impact anxiety and depression. Research suggests that vitamin B6 protects against neurological damage from hypoglycemia.[12] I recommend that your daily B-complex vitamin contain at least 75 milligrams of vitamin B6.

Vitamin B3 (Niacin). Nicotinamide (a type of the B vitamin niacin) has an effect on the brain similar to that of the class of drug known as benzodiazepines (tranquilizers and sleeping pills). Nicotinamide activates specific neurons in the brain, resulting in a calming effect, and can be beneficial in regulating anxiety disorders.[13] I recommend that your daily B-complex vitamin contain at least 200 milligrams of niacin.

Vitamin B8 (Inositol). Derived primarily from cereals and legumes, inositol has been proven effective in treating panic attack and OCD.[14] I recommend increasing your daily inositol supplement from 250 milligrams to 1,000 milligrams. Do not exceed 1,000 milligrams per day.

Magnesium. Magnesium is well known for its calming properties in people with anxiety symptoms, but proper amounts of magnesium are generally lacking in the average American diet. Individuals who use oral contraceptives or diuretics, and who overuse laxatives, are at risk of magnesium deficiency. I recommend that women suffering from anxiety take a supplement of 320 milligrams daily; men should take a supplement of 420 milligrams daily.

Smart Drugs and Nutrients

A number of other naturally occurring nutrients may have beneficial impacts on anxiety.

Adapton (Garum Armoricum). This naturally occurring substance is taken from a deep-sea fish. It is widely used in Europe and Japan to deal with stress, anxiety, and depression. It improves concentration, mood, and sleep. I recommend taking four capsules as directed for fifteen days; stop for one week, then continue with a maintenance dose of two capsules daily.

Melatonin. Melatonin is a hormone manufactured by the pineal gland in the brain. It is released into the bloodstream and is involved in synchronizing the body's hormone secretions and setting daily biorhythms. I recommend supplementing with 300 micrograms to 1 milligram taken nightly a half hour before bed.

Theanine. Theanine is an amino acid found in the leaves of green tea. It increases levels of neurotransmitter chemicals, including dopamine, which may explain its mood-regulating properties. In Japan, theanine is added to soft drinks and chewing gums for the purpose of inducing relaxation. I recommend taking 200 milligrams daily.

Reboot Your Brain Chart of Additional Supplements for Impacting Anxiety

The following chart summarizes the supplements I recommend adding to the protocol for overall brain health from chapter 2. In some cases, I recommend increasing the dosage of a particular vitamin or supplement to specifically impact anxiety. In these cases, you should increase the daily dosage from chapter 2 to the level recommended for this specific condition.

This protocol is designed for individuals who suffer from, or are specifically concerned about, anxiety. If you are concerned about additional brain conditions discussed in other chapters, consult with a health professional about how you can safely impact multiple conditions.

If you are taking medications, whether prescription or over-the-counter, or have any food restrictions, consult with your doctor before beginning any supplement program. Your health care provider should always be up-to-date on all vitamins, supplements, and herbal or homeopathic remedies you are taking. Supplement overdoses are rare, but possible, and certain combinations may affect individuals adversely.

Supplement	Dosage	Cautions
adapton (garumarmoricum)	Four capsules as directed daily for fifteen days; stop for one week, then continue with maintenance dose of two capsules daily.	

Supplement	Dosage	Cautions
inositol (vitamin B8)	Increase daily dosage from 250 mg to 1,000 mg. Do not exceed a daily supplement of 1,000 mg. Take in two divided doses.	
magnesium	320 mg (for women), 420 mg (for men)	May take six weeks or more for effects to be felt.
melatonin	300 mcg to 1 mg at night a half hour before bed	
theanine	200 mg	

Alternative Health Remedies

When suffering from a specific condition such as anxiety, we can also try some natural treatment options that are considered alternatives to traditional medicine. While a healthful lifestyle and the proper nutritional and supplement plan are vital to winning the battle against anxiety, some other targeted remedies might help, too.

Herbal Remedies

Some herbal extracts and homeopathic treatments have properties similar to conventional medications, but are gentler and may lack the drugs' side effects. Always inform your medical practitioner of any herbal remedies you may be taking.

- **Ashwagandha** has antistress properties. I recommend taking 450 milligrams twice daily.
- **Chamomile** is a gentle yet effective remedy for anxiety and the digestive disturbances that may accompany it. I recommend taking 650 milligrams daily, preferably with food. Chamomile may also be used as a tea and is best taken in the hours before bed.

- **Ginseng** is an adaptogen that may help protect and strengthen the body against the damaging effects of chronic stress reactions. Do not take ginseng if you have uncontrolled blood pressure. If ginseng is safe for you to use, I recommend a dose of 200 milligrams per day.

- **Ginkgo biloba** increases blood circulation to the brain, protects nerve cells, and has shown promise in ameliorating mild depression and accompanying anxiety. Ginkgo can act as an anti-coagulant, and individuals taking antithrombotic drugs such as ASA, anti-inflammatories, and warfarin or Coumadin should consult with their doctors before taking ginkgo. Your daily supplement should be 300 milligrams daily, in equally divided doses.

- **Indian snakeroot (Rauwolfia)** is a plant that grows wild in India and Africa and is used in impacting various conditions of the nervous system, including anxiety. Do not take Rauwolfia if you are suffering from depression. This herb is most effective when the whole herb is taken and used over an extended period of time. I recommend a dosage of 600 milligrams daily.

- **Skullcap** acts as a gentle sedative for the central nervous system. Consult with your doctor if you are taking any other medications, including over-the-counter drugs such as antihistamines. If skullcap is safe for you to use, I recommend taking 350 milligrams three times daily. Skullcap is often combined with other mildly sedative herbs, including valerian, passionflower, hops, and lemon balm. If you are taking such a preparation, follow the manufacturer's instructions.

- **St. John's wort** is very popular in Europe, where double-blind, placebo-controlled studies support its efficacy in alleviating depression. It has a calming and mildly sedative effect on the nervous system. I recommend taking 450 milligrams twice a day.

- **Valerian** is effective for people who experience anxiety-related insomnia. I recommend taking 400 to 450 milligrams daily. Do not take valerian for more than two consecutive weeks. Valerian is often combined with other mildly sedative herbs, including skullcap, passionflower, hops, and lemon balm. If you are taking such a preparation, follow the manufacturer's instructions.

Homeopathic Remedies

The following remedies may be used for both temporary and acute cases of anxiety. When dealing with a chronic condition, homeopathic remedies must be used in conjunction with other therapies, as prescribed by a qualified health professional. Consult with your health care provider before taking any homeopathic remedy, and follow your provider's recommendation for the appropriate dosage. Always inform your medical practitioner of any homeopathic remedies you may be taking.

- **Arsenicum album** is a remedy for exhaustion accompanied by anxiety.
- **Kali phosphoricum** is considered useful for anxiety and fear.

Acupuncture

By examining a patient's symptoms, appearance, and pulse, acupuncturists can diagnose and impact anxiety.

Acupuncture releases tension in the muscles. It causes a relaxation response in the body, resulting in lowered blood pressure and heart rate. Acupuncture increases the flow of blood, lymph, and nerve impulses to affected areas and decreases stress while promoting feelings of energy and well-being. Acupuncture also is effective in relieving the physical symptoms associated with stress-related and anxiety disorders.

Therapeutic Touch

A variety of treatments involve the transfer of energy from the practitioner to the patient, which can help relieve pain and anxiety.

In one study, massage reduced anxiety and lowered saliva cortisol levels (a key measurement of stress).[16]

Reiki. Pronounced "ray-kee," this method employs a powerful, hands-on healing technique in which the universal life force energy is channeled through the practitioner and transferred to the patient. Chronic stress and anxiety can deplete the energy in our bodies. Reiki is used to support the body's natural ability to heal itself. It releases spiritual and emotional blocks and brings a feeling of harmony and vitality.

Massage. This popular technique can enhance general relaxation and provide an outlet for stress and tension. Massage therapy can reduce feelings of anxiety, promote better sleep patterns, and increase feelings of well-being.

Shiatsu. This form of physical therapy combines traditional Chinese medical theory and various Japanese massage techniques. The therapist uses direct pressure with hands and fingers to redirect the flow of energy throughout the body. Shiatsu treatment is deeply relaxing and can be beneficial in both chronic and acute conditions.

Thought Field Therapy

According to Stephanie Marohn, a writer and editor of books on psychospirituality and alternative thought, Dr. Roger Callahan has pioneered a kind of energy therapy known as Thought Field Therapy (TFT).[17] TFT uses acupuncture points on the body to break up energy patterns that produce anxiety. By tapping on these acupuncture points, the energy is redirected, and the pattern contributing to anxiety is broken. TFT is a self-practiced therapy that gives the individual immediate control in reducing anxiety in particular situations.

Aromatherapy

Essential oils can be used in baths or inhaled to provide rebalancing effects. Do not apply essential oils directly to the skin; they must be mixed with carrier oils. Experiment with some of the scents below to see what you find soothing:

- bergamot
- cypress
- frankincense
- jasmine
- lavender
- lemon balm
- lime
- neroli
- patchouli
- rose

Summary

The Reboot Your Brain program in this chapter stresses the importance of nutrition and lifestyle modification, both in preventing and impacting anxiety disorders. Remember, anything that impacts this disorder can be used to prevent it from occurring. Anxiety has many causes, and the appropriate treatment will vary from person to person. What is important is to promote good physical health and a higher standard for one's spiritual and emotional life to combat the daily stresses that can contribute to more severe anxiety.

Chapter 5

Memory Loss

"The advantage of a bad memory is that one enjoys several times the same good things for the first time."

—Friedrich Nietzsche

People may joke about "senior moments"—those times when their memory suddenly fails, and they are unable to come up with the name of their boss or the time they are supposed to meet for dinner. The truth is that throughout our lives there are always times when our memory fails us. But because we have been taught that memory decline is a natural consequence of aging, and because we fear the onset of serious mental conditions often related to advancing age, such as dementia or Alzheimer's disease, lapses in short-term memory as we age can result in ongoing stress or worry.

Ironically, stress and worry are two factors that contribute to continued lapses in memory. The fact is, bouts of forgetfulness are usually unrelated to Alzheimer's disease, and there are simple ways to prevent and impact memory loss and even maximize your memory as you age.

For decades, scientists believed that the health of the brain and our mental functions deteriorated as we advanced beyond our middle years. They told us that our alertness and decision-making abilities naturally decline as we move into the later phases of our lives. The accepted thinking was that the brain cells and connections begin to die off as we age, and that this deterioration was inevitable and irreversible. We now know that this is not, and does not have to be, the case. Significant data shows there can be an ongoing regeneration and birth of brain cells throughout our lifespans, well into our elder years.

This news should not come as a surprise. Goethe completed his great work *Faust* at age eighty-three. Michelangelo designed the dome of St. Peter's cathedral when he was nearly seventy. Winston Churchill, widely recognized as one of the greatest political leaders of the twentieth century, became prime minister of Great Britain at the age of sixty-five. The bottom line is this: The majority of people who live their lives engaged in vigorous and diverse mental activities remain neurologically robust, even at advanced ages. In this chapter, I tell you how to strengthen your memory, protecting and maximizing its potential even as you grow older.

Understanding Memory Loss

Let's begin by taking a look at how our brains collect memories.

How Memories are Acquired

The roots of memory have been studied and debated for centuries, yet many questions remain as to how the brain performs this basic function. What is known is that memories are constructed through a series of interactive steps triggered by exposure to new information.

Paul Scheele, the founder of Learning Strategies Corporation—a company involved in providing self-empowerment, educational, and health programs—points out that memory is not something that is retained in a particular part of your brain.[1] Unlike a computer, which can store information on a hard drive and return to access that specific information, your brain constructs memory from input from the entire neural network in your body. Memory is nonlocal. Each time you remember something, your brain is literally rebuilding an original construction. In other words, you can't remember something you don't already know.

The practice of construction and reconstruction is critical to memory. Scheele refers to this ongoing process as "mental hygiene."[2] Dr. Dharma Singh Khalsa, president and medical director of the Alzheimer's Prevention Foundation International in Tucson, Arizona, stresses the same thing when he talks about how important it is to "maintain the brain."[3]

Remembering something, whether it's the name of your mother-in-law's poodle or how to dance the cha-cha, is a process that involves much of your brain. The two primary types of memory are: declarative and procedural.

The brain's medial temporal lobes, particularly the hippocampus, and the prefrontal cortex are responsible for maintaining declarative memory. Sometimes called explicit memories, these include facts, people, places, and things that we encounter frequently.

The capacity to learn skills or procedures, including new motor skills, is governed by our nondeclarative, or implicit, memory. This memory function is governed by brain structures outside the medial temporal lobes, including the amygdala, cerebellum, and motor cortex.

How Memories are Lost

Scientists are unclear as to the specific reasons for age-related memory loss. It may be that our brain becomes less agile as it ages, or that imbalances in the system of neurotransmitters that communicate within the brain cause memory loss, or that other types of chemical imbalances in our bodies, such as changing hormone levels, impact our ability to remember things. What is known is that it is normal for anyone at any age to have lapses of memory, but that older individuals may face a higher incidence of memory loss.

Difficulty Learning

Studies suggest that the reason we have trouble remembering things as we age is that it becomes more difficult to learn new information in the first place. Memory studies have shown that about one-third of otherwise healthy older adults have difficulty with declarative memory. However, a substantial number of eighty-year-olds perform as well as people in their twenties on difficult memory tests. Furthermore, all age groups retain newly learned information equally well, although it may take the older group longer to learn the information.[4]

Brain Circuitry

Brain researchers are not sure what exactly causes memory to be affected by aging, but for years they have speculated that changes may result from the subtly changing environment in the brain as it ages. Particular focus has been on the loss of brain cells and physical deterioration of the brain itself. But the role of an imbalance in the delicate systems of neurotransmitters that conduct all communication in the brain has been an area of recent study in relation to memory loss and brain function in aging.

A study in the September 2000 issue of the *Journal of Neuroscience* asserts that defective brain circuits could be more responsible for memory problems than the loss of brain cells.[5] Researchers at the Mount Sinai School of Medicine conducted a study that examined the synapses in the brains of rats and discovered that the ability of neurons to carry a signal was lessened in older rats whose learning ability was impaired. This reduced neuron activity was not correlated to age, but rather related to each rat's degree of learning impairment.

The Blood–Brain Barrier

It is important to understand the importance of the entire body's circulatory system in relation to the health of the brain. Blood carries nutrients to every part of the body, but the delicate tissues of the brain require a specialized security system. This tightly woven net of endothelial cells is called the blood–brain barrier (BBB) and acts as a filter, permitting only certain substances to travel from the blood to the brain. The BBB is responsible for providing neurons with glucose and other nutrients and also maintaining proper neurotransmitter balance.

The function of the blood–brain barrier is crucial, as it protects the brain from foreign substances in the blood that may be toxic to the brain, maintains a constant environment for the brain, and protects the brain from hormones and neurotransmitters in the rest of the brain.

The blood–brain barrier can be weakened in several ways, including high blood pressure; hyperosmolality (or high concentration of a particular substance in the blood); microwave exposure; radiation exposure; infection or exposure to infectious agents; as well as trauma, ischemia, inflammation, pressure, or injury to the brain.

Age-Related Alterations in the Blood–Brain Barrier

Studies have shown age-related alterations in the blood–brain barrier transport function, including a decrease in choline transport and a decrease in brain glucose influx.[6] Choline, one of the B vitamins, is critical in the manufacture of the neurotransmitter acetylcholine. Glucose is the primary fuel for the brain and supports many of the cognitive functions of the brain.

It is important, therefore, that the blood circulating throughout your body and brain is nutrient-rich and full of antioxidants, such as NADH or N-acetylcysteine, and amino acids, such as acetylcholine.

As Dr. James LaValle says,[7] "When you restrict blood flow you restrict oxygen delivery to a very vital area in the brain." Problems with our circulatory system start to surface when we have a deficit of blood and nutrients going to the brain because the arteries are clogged, due often to eating foods that are not promoting proper circulation or not exercising enough which also promotes proper circulation. According to Dr. Martin Feldman, "The improvement of circulation to the brain can actually make the brain more efficient and even reverse some of the potential problems we associate with aging of the brain."[6]

The Role of Hormones

Though memory loss affects both genders, it can be particularly devastating to women during and around menopause. In the book *Female and Forgetful: A Six-Step Program to Help Restore Your Memory and Sharpen Your Mind,* authors Elisa Lottor, PhD, ND, and Nancy Bruning explore the uncharted waters that link memory loss to menopause.[8] Estrogen has a powerful influence on the brain, playing an important role in functions such as memory, language skills, moods, and attention. The authors describe case studies of women who, in the beginning of menopause, suddenly cannot remember simple things, such as their social security or phone numbers. The authors posit that the sharp decline in hormonal levels during menopause wreak havoc on memory. Fortunately, as the reported incidences of menopause-linked memory loss increase in scientific literature, so do the reported efficacies of treatment.

Diagnosing Memory Loss

It is difficult to know exactly when memory failure is a simple lapse on the part of your brain in processing known information, and when it is indicative of a more serious condition, such as dementia (chapter 13) or Alzheimer's disease (chapter 8). It is this uncertainty, perhaps, that makes these episodes of forgetfulness so stressful to the older population.

Let's start with the important distinction doctors make between normal, age-associated mental impairment and conditions such as dementia that signal a disease process. Not all memory difficulties or cognitive complaints indicate the presence of Alzheimer's disease or other mental disorders. Many changes in memory or cognitive function in older adults are temporary and are linked to environmental factors, such as stress or poor nutrition, rather than to physiological processes.

A doctor evaluating a patient who complains of memory loss will have to consider underlying factors, such as illness or medications, head injury or trauma, the possibility of stroke or heart disease, or drug or alcohol abuse. These factors can make it unclear whether their patient is suffering the "inevitable" memory decline associated with aging, or experiencing symptoms that indicate the onset of a serious condition such as dementia or Alzheimer's disease.

Your doctor should also consider:

- essential fatty acid deficiencies
- chronic inflammation of the brain, which can damage cerebral blood vessels or neurons
- nutrient deficiencies
- hormone imbalances, especially decreased levels of DHEA, thyroid, and testosterone
- poor health habits, such as smoking, or drug or alcohol use, which can shortchange the amount of oxygen the brain receives
- atherosclerosis or heart disease, which can affect the amount of oxygen the brain receives
- brain neurotransmitter levels
- adverse side effects of prescription medications

Generally speaking, a memory problem is serious when it affects your daily functioning. If you sometimes forget names, you should not be worried, and there is much you can do to correct this tendency. In fact, researchers suggest that people who are aware of their memory loss probably do not have a serious problem.

If you have trouble remembering how to do things you have done many times before, or a place you visit often, or difficulty in understanding the order in which to do things (e.g., following a recipe), your doctor should be notified.

Combating Memory Loss Naturally

The good news is that the birth of new nerve cells in the brain is an ongoing process throughout our lifespans. Rejuvenating your memory or preventing decline in cognitive functions in the first place requires a holistic approach to a healthy lifestyle that considers proper nutrition and beneficial supplementation, mental and physical exercise, and stress management.

We must reject the notion that memory decline is a natural consequence of aging. A person's memory should function at optimal levels well into old age. Simple memory deficits, if not addressed, can worsen over time. We must act now to keep our minds sharp.

Mental maintenance is a "use it or lose it" proposition. You must make a commitment to continually learn new information, to undertake new physical challenges, and to endeavor to remain open to new experiences. In the Reboot Your Brain program for preventing memory loss that follows, you will find the most important nutrients for your brain, the best ways to challenge your mental muscles, and the most effective ways to reduce the stress that can adversely affect your memory.

Lifestyle

As I said earlier in this chapter, we cannot underestimate the importance of the mind–body connection in maintaining mental sharpness. We need nourishment in all areas of our lives—physical, spiritual, and emotional—to prevent or reverse impairments of the mind. By concentrating on therapies and behaviors that improve circulation to the brain, rejuvenate brain cell metabolism, suppress free radical damage, and strengthen our mental muscles, we can boost neurological function and expect to maintain robust memory even as we age.

Exercise

The brain is nourished by blood, so it should come as no surprise that physical activity that promotes circulation is beneficial in preventing memory loss and mental fogginess. Changes in the body can adversely affect the brain, as one study involving male twins demonstrated. Tests showed that high blood pressure in men during midlife was a clear marker for increased brain aging, and led to an elevated chance of stroke later in life. The male twins with high blood pressure, when assessed twenty-five years later, had smaller brain volumes and increased strokes when compared to their twin brothers with normal blood pressure.

The hippocampus section of the brain is vital for acquiring new memories. It is one of the select few areas in the adult mammalian brain that can grow new nerve cells. One study demonstrated that voluntary exercise increases neurogenesis in the hippocampus.[10] This was the first study indicating that neurogenesis can occur without learning enhancement.

Aerobic exercise, such as walking, gardening, swimming, tai chi, or dancing, has also been shown to sharpen memory skills.

Stress

Chronic stress—those day-to-day, irritating occurrences that continue to build up in our bodies—causes the body to release cortisol into the bloodstream. Cortisol then travels through the circulatory system to the brain, where it begins wreaking havoc on the hippocampus.

As we age, our bodies find it more difficult to signal to the adrenal gland that it should stop producing cortisol. Prolonged exposure to stress then leads to the loss of brain cells in the memory center. Dr. Sonia Lupien at McGill University has shown that the higher our cortisol levels are as we age, the higher the incidence of severe memory loss we suffer.[11]

Music

Exposure to certain types of music, especially classical music, produces transient increases in cognitive performance. One report examined a group of healthy elderly people and Alzheimer's disease patients to determine the effects of listening to an excerpt of Vivaldi's *The Four Seasons*. The results of the study showed that listening to music enhanced the patients' ability to pay attention.[12]

Mental Exercise

The best way to keep your memory skills strong is to use them. Memorizing dates, lists, and even telephone numbers can help keep your mind sharp as you age. The practice of construction and reconstruction of knowledge is critical to memory, so learning new skills stimulates your brain, too. A study in the January 2004 issue of *Nature* followed twenty-three healthy people (average age: twenty-two) who learned how to juggle. After three months, MRI scans showed enlargement of the gray matter—the part that drives higher mental functions—in their brains. Learning a new skill had actually made their brains grow. When the study participants stopped juggling, their brains shrank again.[13]

Keep your brain entertained and engaged by practicing crossword or jigsaw puzzles, doing word search and brainteaser puzzles, or playing board games or card games. Learn a second language, take up a musical instrument, or take a college course online.

Providing your brain with a healthy body, good nutrients, and a stress-free environment is important. Challenging your memory and continuing the lifelong process of learning is critical to prevent short-term memory loss as you age.

Learning and storing new information may help prevent memory decline. Practice memory skills to enhance learning and improve your recall.

- **Relax:** Tension and stress cause short-term memory failure.
- **Concentrate:** Pay attention as you are receiving new information; you'll be surprised at how much more you retain.
- **Focus:** Reduce distractions when you are involved in new undertakings that require concentration.
- **Slow down:** It doesn't matter how long it takes you to learn something; it's the acquisition of new information, not the speed with which you acquire it, that's important.
- **Follow a routine:** Put important items, such as keys, in the same place each time.
- **Organize:** Knowing where important information is can reduce stress; storing vital information in a visible place may be enough to trigger your memory without even having to look.
- **Write it down:** Write down important things; keep lists.
- **Repeat:** Repetition improves recall; use it, especially when learning names.
- **Visualize:** A strong link to a visual clue can improve memory; use landmarks to help you find places.

Foods and Memory Loss

The nutrients present in the food you eat are the building blocks for neurotransmitters, the main network of communication in your brain. It's an easy correlation to make: If you don't nourish your brain with the proper foods, the health of the neurotransmitters will be compromised. When your mind suddenly goes blank, it may be that your lack of attention to diet has negatively impacted your brain's ability to do its job. It's a classic case of the domino effect, a perfect illustration of cause and effect.

A good maxim to remember is "What works for the heart, works for the head." When planning a brain-healthy diet, remember that, like your heart, your brain needs oxygen, it needs to be blood-rich in antioxidants and vital nutrients, and it needs glucose for energy. Processed sugars, simple carbohydrates, fast foods, alcohol, and artery-clogging saturated fats are as bad for your mind as they are for your body.

Foods rich in the omega-3 fatty acids found in green leafy vegetables, walnuts, chia seeds, and flax seeds, as well as unrefined complex carbohydrates, high-quality proteins, and fruits rich in antioxidants, such as blueberries, blackberries, and prunes, are the basic ingredients for a diet that promotes a healthy body and a healthy mind.

The Latest Research

Research presented at the American Academy of Neurology's 64th Annual Meeting in April 2012 by scientists at Mayo Clinic Study of Aging illuminated the association between overeating and memory loss. Measuring mild cognitive impairment among 1,233 seniors ages seventy and above, the researchers discovered that those seniors who consumed between 2,143 and 6,000 calories per day more than doubled their risk of suffering from memory loss and other manifestations of mild cognitive impairment compared to those who consumed 600 to 1,526 calories daily.[12]

Sugar intake and brain function were the subject of a recent study by scientists at UCLA. The researchers found that rats given a diet high in fructose performed poorly in tests using mazes that were designed to assess memory and learning.[13] In addition to being fed a fructose-enriched diet, some rats were fed omega-3 fatty acids in the form of flaxseed oil and docosahexaenoic acid (DHA); this group completed the tests much more quickly than did the rats not given omega-3s, suggesting that healthy fats may counteract the harmful effects of sugar on brain health.

In an article published in the *Journal of Applied Physiology* in 2011, researchers from the University of Iowa reviewed more than one hundred studies that investigated how aerobic and resistance training exercise influences brain fitness. The group found that aerobic exercise corresponds with improved ability to multitask and maintaining concentration over extended periods of time, while resistance exercise is associated with greater ability to focus in the face of distractions.[14] Discussing her team's findings in an interview with the *Los Angeles Times,* lead researcher Michelle Voss stated that the hippocampus, a part of the brain crucial to memory formation, tends to shrink by 1 percent or 2 percent annually once we reach age sixty, but in the case of seniors who are physically active, it increases in size by approximately 1 percent or 2 percent.[15]

In an article appearing in the journal *Biological Psychiatry* in 2011, scientists at the University of New South Wales in Sydney, Australia, gathered compelling evidence demonstrating that leading a mentally active lifestyle may slow or prevent dementia and its symptoms, which include memory loss, in previously unidentified ways. In addition to showing that mental activity helps preserve the integrity of brain circuits, the team discovered that cognitive stimulation also improves our mental health through preserving blood flow to the brain and increasing neuron density.[16]

The relationship between a mentally active lifestyle and cognitive decline were the focus of a review published by the prestigious *Cochrane Collaboration* in early 2012. Analyzing the results of fifteen studies involving more than seven hundred patients with mild to moderate dementia, the authors found that those patients who participated in cognitive stimulation intervention programs performed significantly better on thinking and memory tests than did the individuals who did not undergo treatment.[17] The benefits of the programs were observed to last at least one to three months after treatment ended. The patients evaluated in the review engaged in a variety of mentally stimulating activities, including discussion of past and present events, word games, puzzles, music, baking, and indoor gardening.

Recipes

In the list below are my recommendations for easy-to-prepare meals full of nutrients proven to help prevent and restore memory loss; the recipes can be found in Appendix II:

- Antioxidant Punch
- Brain Juice
- Brain Power
- Cranberry Cooler
- Enzyme Enhancer
- Fountain of Youth
- Melon Boost
- Ruby Red
- Four-Bean Salad
- Nature's Total Salad
- Black Bean Soup
- Cold Strawberry Soup
- Blueberry Breakfast Treat
- Rice and Strawberries
- Brazilian Rice
- Chickpea Hummus with Toasted Pita
- Tantalizing Tempeh Dinner
- Tex-Mex Tofu Scramble
- Carob Power Brownies

Supplements

Vitamins and Minerals

Certain vitamins and minerals may provide protection against memory loss.

Vitamin E. In one study, researchers examined the possibility that vitamin E and other antioxidants could protect against neurodegenerative diseases.[14] The longitudinal study was conducted on 2,889 community residents, between the ages of 65 and 102 years.

Those monitored had their cognitive function measured by being told a long and detailed story and then being asked to recall items that were paired together. Those in the survey who had taken the highest amounts of vitamin E performed best on the cognitive tests. Based on the results of specific tests given the study's participants, the report concluded that vitamin E intake from foods or supplements is associated with less cognitive decline with age. I recommend increasing your daily vitamin E supplement from 268 milligrams to 536 milligrams. Do not exceed 536 milligrams daily.

Vitamin C. A powerful antioxidant, vitamin C plays a key role in maintaining healthy nerve cells in the brain. Vitamin C can reduce and reverse oxidative damage to tissues caused by free radicals, and vitamin C's immune system–enhancing capabilities are also well known. It has the ability to regenerate oxidized levels of vitamin E in the body, thus enhancing the potency of that vitamin. I recommend a daily dosage of 1,000 to 5,000 milligrams, taken twice daily.

Folate (Vitamin B9). A recent nationwide health and nutrition survey reported that grain products fortified with the B vitamin folate could help reduce memory loss in the over-sixty age group. A study linking the level of homocysteine (an amino acid found in the blood) with the level of B vitamin intake demonstrated that older adults with low vitamin B intake (in particular, folate) showed elevated blood homocysteine levels and suffered from a greater degree of memory loss than those with sufficient vitamin B intake. In fact, the participants in the study who had proper folate levels appeared to be immune to memory loss, even when their homocysteine levels were elevated.[15]

In another study, researchers at the Jean Mayer USDA Human Nutrition Research Center on Aging at Tufts University in Boston looked at the correlation between high homocysteine levels and memory loss. The subjects whose blood folate levels were highest seemed immune to memory loss, even though their homocysteine levels were elevated. The report suggested that consuming grain products fortified with folate may reduce memory loss in people over sixty,[16] although it makes more sense to consume large amounts of vegetables, which naturally contain abundant amounts of folate.

I recommend that your daily B-complex vitamin contain at least 800 micrograms of folic acid.

Lecithin and Choline. Lecithin is manufactured in the body and found in many animal- and plant-based foods, such as eggs, liver, peanuts, soybeans, wheat germ, and brewer's yeast. It is often found as an additive in processed foods, such as ice cream and salad dressing.

Lecithin is a precursor to the neurotransmitter acetylcholine and has a positive effect on cerebral and memory functions. Double-blind, placebo-controlled studies have shown that patients with mild cognitive disorders showed clear improvement when lecithin was given to them.[17]

A key component of lecithin, phosphatidylcholine, is broken down in the body and becomes choline, a building block of acetylcholine, a key neurotransmitter that plays an important role in memory. Levels of acetylcholine are known to decline with age, and studies have shown that supplementation with choline—which can also be found in liver, egg yolks, peanuts, cauliflower, soybeans, cabbage, and grape juice—can improve memory and learning. I recommend increasing your daily lecithin supplement from 1 gram to 2.5 grams for men and 2 grams for women. Take in two divided doses, and do not exceed a daily supplement of 2.5 grams for men or 2 grams for women.

Iron. Studies have shown that iron deficiency may be linked to problems with short-term memory. Iron is crucial in building brain neurotransmitter activity, and can be found in foods and supplements. Iron should be taken with vitamin C to improve absorption. Consult with your doctor about adding iron supplements to your daily regimen.

Smart Drugs and Nutrients

A number of other naturally occurring nutrients may have beneficial impacts on memory loss.

DMAE (Dimethylaminoethanol). This nutrient, found in sardines, is a powerful stimulant that increases acetylcholine levels. Acetylcholine is an important neurotransmitter in the brain. It plays a role in memory, concentration, and focus. I recommend increasing your daily

DMAE supplement from 150 milligrams to 300 milligrams. Consult your physician before taking heavy doses of DMAE.

N-acetylcysteine (NAC). This amino acid protects the brain from damaging free radicals by boosting quantities of glutathione, one of the body's most powerful antioxidants. I recommend a supplement of 500 milligrams taken three times daily.

Nicotinamide Adenine Dinucleotide (NADH). An enzyme that helps improve neurotransmitter function, NADH is present in all living cells and plays a critical role in energy production. It helps prevent cellular degeneration and may increase concentration and memory capacity. I recommend a supplement of 2.5 milligrams taken twice a day for two or three days of the week.

Phosphatidylserine (PS). PS helps the brain use fuel more efficiently. By boosting neuronal metabolism and stimulating production of acetylcholine, PS may be able to improve the condition of patients in cognitive decline. Studies have revealed that supplementing with phosphatidylserine slows down and even reverses declining memory and concentration, or age-related cognitive impairment, in middle-aged and elderly subjects.[18]

As we grow older, aging slows the body's manufacturing of phosphatidylserine to levels that are detrimental to our functioning at our full mental capacity. For impact on memory loss, I recommend increasing your daily PS supplement from 300 milligrams to 400 milligrams. Do not exceed a daily supplement of 400 milligrams.

Reboot Your Brain Chart of Additional Supplements for Impacting Memory Loss

The following chart summarizes the supplements I recommend adding to the protocol for overall brain health from chapter 2. In some cases, I recommend increasing the dose of a vitamin or supplement from chapter 2 to impact a specific condition.

This protocol is designed for individuals who suffer from, or are specifically concerned about, memory loss. If you are concerned about additional brain conditions discussed in other chapters, consult with a health professional about how you can safely impact multiple conditions.

If you are taking medications, whether prescription or over-the-counter, or have any food restrictions, consult with your doctor before beginning any supplement program. Your health care provider should always be up-to-date on all vitamins, supplements, and herbal or homeopathic remedies you are taking. Supplement overdoses are rare, but possible, and certain combinations may affect individuals adversely.

Supplement	Dosage	Cautions
B9 (folate)	800 mcg of folic acid	
dimethylaminoetha-nol (DMAE)	Increase from 150 to 300 mg.	Tension and irritability may occur. Do not take if you have epilepsy, a history of convulsions, or bipolar disorder. If you have kidney or liver disease, consult your doctor before taking this supplement.
iron	Consult your doctor.	Have a blood test to determine true iron deficiency, as iron overload can cause health problems. Iron can interfere with a number of drugs, including thyroid hormone drugs, antibiotics, and drugs used to treat Parkinson's disease. Tannins found in coffee and tea can inhibit iron absorption.
lecithin and choline (combine):	2.5 grams for men, 2 grams for women.	Take in two divided doses and do not exceed those amounts.

Supplement	Dosage	Cautions
N-acetylcysteine (NAC)	500 mg, three times daily	Regular supplementation of NAC increases urinary output of copper. If supplementing with NAC for an extended period, add 2 mg of copper and 30 mg of zinc to your daily supplement regimen.
nicotinamide adenine dinucleotide (NADH, also called coenzyme Qi)	2.5 mg twice daily, two or three times per week	High doses (10 mg per day or more) may cause nervousness, anxiety, and insomnia.
Vitamin E	400 IU to 800 IU daily. Do not exceed 800 IU.	
Vitamin C	Increase daily dosage of 500-1000 mg to 1000 mg taken up to twice daily.	

Alternative Health Remedies

When suffering from a specific condition such as memory loss, we can also try some natural treatment options that are considered alternatives to traditional medicine. While a healthful lifestyle and the proper nutritional and supplement plan are vital to winning the battle against memory loss, there are some other targeted remedies that might help, too.

Herbal Remedies

Some herbal extracts and homeopathic treatments have properties similar to conventional medications, but are gentler and may lack the drugs' side effects. Always inform your medical practitioner of any herbal remedies you may be taking.

- **Butcher's broom** promotes healthy circulation to the brain, resulting in enhanced memory and clearer focus. I recommend two to four 425 milligrams capsules daily.

- **Chamomile** is widely recognized for its ability to reduce stress and anxiety, resulting in increased focus and concentration. I recommend two 325 milligrams capsules three times per day, preferably with food.

- **Eye bright** is excellent for impacting inflammation; its cooling and detoxifying properties may help with memory loss. Take two 430 milligrams capsules three times per day, preferably with food.

- **Garlic** cleans clogged arteries and increases blood flow to the brain. Add to your diet or take prepared capsules as directed by the manufacturer.

- **Ginkgo biloba** enhances cerebral circulation, improves brain function and memory, and scavenges free radicals. Ginkgo can act as an anticoagulant, and individuals taking anticoagulant and antithrombotic drugs such as ASA, anti-inflammatories, and warfarin or Coumadin should consult with their doctors before taking ginkgo. If ginkgo is safe for you to use, I recommend taking 40 to 60 milligrams ginkgo biloba extract three times a day.

- **Ginseng** boosts energy and concentration and may help protect and strengthen the body against the damaging effects of chronic stress. Ginseng can interact with many medications. Talk to your health care provider before supplementing with ginseng, and follow your provider's instructions for use.

- **Gotu kola** improves memory and mental alertness. Elephants, animals known for their excellent memories, love gotu kola. Do not use gotu kola if you take medication for diabetes or to control cholesterol. If gotu kola is safe for you to take, I recommend 200 milligrams taken three times daily.

- **Huperzine A** sharpens the mind, wards off memory decline, and improves cognitive and behavioral functions. I recommend 50 micrograms per day with meals.
- **St. John's wort (hypericum)** is very popular in Europe, so much so that it is actually covered by German health insurance as a prescription drug. The recommended dose for combating memory impairment is 300 milligrams twice a day.
- **Vinpocetine** is a derivative of an extract taken from the periwinkle shrub. It enhances circulation to the brain and may improve mild, age-related cognitive impairment. I recommend taking 10 milligrams twice daily with meals.

Homeopathic Remedies

The following remedies may be of use for mild cases of short-term memory loss. When dealing with a chronic condition, homeopathic remedies must be utilized in conjunction with other therapies, as prescribed by a qualified health professional. Consult with your health care provider before taking any homeopathic remedy, and follow your provider's recommendation for the appropriate dosage. Always inform your medical practitioner of any homeopathic remedies you may be taking.

- **Barytci carbonica** is for memory loss of recent events and general difficulty comprehending.
- **Lycopodium** is for loss of memory due to anxiety.
- **Argentum nitricum** can help a generally weak memory.
- **Anacardium** is for impaired memory that seems worse after a hot bath and better after eating.

Stress-Reduction Techniques

Practicing stress-reducing techniques may aid in enhancing memory and focus.

Relaxation Response. One should begin each morning in a positive way, with some form of stress reduction technique. Dr. Dharma Singh Khalsa calls it "Wake Up to Wellness." Simply put, instead of starting your day with coffee, turning on the news, or reading the paper, you should start your day off in a positive manner. Find a quiet place so that you can practice some form of relaxation meditation technique, which lowers cortisol levels, which in turn improves memory.

Meditation. Quiet contemplation allows your body to relax completely. Meditation can be done at any time, in nearly any place. Simply sit comfortably with your spine straight. Let your gaze drop downward, allowing your eyes to rest comfortably while remaining open but unfocused. Allow your breathing to become rhythmic. If your attention drifts, or your eyes close, this is normal. Simply redirect your attention back to your relaxed, downward gaze.

Deep Breathing. After taking several normal breaths, begin to breathe deeper with longer inhalations and exhalations. Breathe from your diaphragm—your chest will rise, your ribs will expand, and your belly will rise in sequence as you breathe. Breathe deeply and slowly, paying attention to each breath as you imagine tension draining from your body with each exhalation.

Visualization. Use your imagination to recall successful or positive life events and link the feelings of those events to your present state.

Prayer. A way of getting in touch with our spiritual selves, prayer can take the form of silent meditation, affirmations, chanting, or traditional words. Repeat calmly, quietly, and in harmony with your breath.

Aromatherapy

Essential oils can be used in baths, or inhaled, or mixed with a carrier oil, such as massage oil, and rubbed on the skin. Experiment with some of the following scents to see which are stimulating to you:

- rosemary
- peppermint
- frankincense
- rosemary
- sage
- geranium

Summary

Diet, exercise, and stress reduction are all equally crucial in preventing declines in cognitive functions as we age. The Reboot Your Brain program recognizes that our brains are flesh-and-blood organs, depending on proper blood flow, nutrients, and mental gymnastics to keep them in peak condition. We are never too old to learn, and constructing an ongoing knowledge base is vital to reconstructing important memories. Living life fully, both physically and mentally, is the key to staying mentally sharp as we age.

Chapter 6

Mental Fatigue

"I've got a great ambition to die of exhaustion rather than boredom."

—Thomas Carlyle

If at times it feels as though the wind has gone out of your mental sails after you have worked too hard, in all likelihood it has. Imagine the activity of the billions of nerve cells in your brain as a steady breeze that propels your mental and physical boat. Sometimes, when the wind stops blowing, you can still move forward using the momentum you have already built up. In most instances, the wind will start up again before your boat stops.

When a neuron is stimulated, it emits an electrical message, and then it needs time to recover. While it is resting, a phase that lasts about ten seconds, other active neurons continue to transmit messages so that there is always a steady breeze of information flowing. Usually, the resting neurons are not missed because other neurons have picked up the slack. For a variety of reasons, however, sometimes too many nerve cells use too much energy too rapidly, enabling the brain to notice the gaps.

In this chapter, I start by discussing types of mental fatigue and their causes. Then I tell you how you can implement healthful lifestyle and nutritional strategies to combat mental fatigue.

Understanding Mental Fatigue

Mental fatigue, also called mental burnout or brain fog, is characterized by symptoms ranging from forgetfulness to confusion, lack of focus, and inability to think clearly. Unfortunately, people often suffer from these symptoms for such an extended period of time that they come to believe that having these symptoms is normal.

Mental fatigue can exist over extended periods of time or merely be a passing phase. Both your physical and mental condition can contribute to a case of mental fatigue.

Types of Mental Fatigue

Your brain can become fatigued for a variety of reasons. When you have overworked your mental capacities, or when your body is physically stressed, your mental sharpness can decline.

Mental Causes

Just as muscles become exhausted after grueling exercise, the brain cells, too, can become tired when they are overworked.

Hyperfocus. Unrelenting mental activity that is focused on one particular matter can exhaust neurons. Acute mental fatigue is fairly common among mathematicians and accountants after prolonged periods of working with dull facts or figures. Writers frequently encounter this conundrum, referring to it as writer's block.

Intense Stress. Essentially, whenever the mind goes into overdrive, mental fatigue looms on the horizon. A particular worry or stressful event can exhaust your brain and impair clear thinking.

Misuse. Investing mental energy in something that is against your nature can also trigger mental fatigue. For instance, if you are an honest person and you find yourself in a position that requires you to lie and, in general, become dishonest, you are misusing your mind, and that can cause mental fatigue.

Underuse. Mental fatigue can set in when a task is repetitious and monotonous, requiring only rote memory to complete it. This form of mental fatigue is more closely related to physical fatigue.

Physical Causes

Imbalances in your body chemistry can influence your brain as much as your body. Several physical conditions can directly impact your brain's energy levels and ability to function optimally over time.

Hypoglycemia (Low Blood Sugar). Hypoglycemia arises when there is an unusually low level of glucose (sugar) in the blood. When the glucose level is dangerously low in the blood, it is precariously low in the brain, as well. Hypoglycemia can lead to a lack of proper fuel reaching the brain.

Candidiasis. Mental fatigue symptoms can occur because of candidiasis (also known as a yeast infection or thrush), an infection caused by a parasitic yeast-like fungus called *Candida ulbicans* that is found in the intestines, mouth, esophagus, and throat. Normally this fungus is kept from overgrowth by naturally occurring bacteria (acidophilus) that are present in our bodies. An overgrowth of the bacteria causes a white discharge that can be itchy or painful. The overgrowth of the fungus can be controlled through diet changes, or medications can be taken to clear up the infection. Sometimes, mental fatigue may be the result of dying yeast. As yeast die, they have been known to release toxins that provoke temporary symptoms of mental fatigue.

Chronic fatigue syndrome (CFS) (also known as myalgic encephalomyelitis, chronic mononucleosis-like syndrome, chronic EBV syndrome, and post-viral syndrome) is a condition with complex, chronic, and debilitating disorders that has a multiplicity of symptoms. The cause of CFS is unknown, and there is no single diagnostic test. Some specialists link CFS to the Epstein Barr virus (EBV), which is in the herpes family. Some authorities list possible causes of CFS as hypoglycemia, Candida, and intestinal parasites.

Food Allergies. A food allergy occurs when the body responds improperly to a food or beverage that is not generally damaging to the body. Food allergies may affect your body and brain's energy production, leading to mental fatigue.

Nutritional Deficiencies. A diet lacking in necessary nutrients directly impacts the amount of energy available to the neurons. When your body is not receiving proper nutrition, your brain cannot function optimally.

Viral And Bacterial Causes. Epstein Virus, Cytomeglo Virus, Human Herpes 6, Mycoplasma Bacteria, plus other viruses and bacteria are commonly found in the blood of people suffering from mental and physical fatigue.

Diagnosing Mental Fatigue

We have all experienced some form of fatigue. It is not hard to understand how running a race, playing basketball, or engaging in other aerobic activity can leave us physically exhausted. But identifying the causative factors involved in mental fatigue poses a different problem altogether.

Symptoms of Mental Fatigue

Mental fatigue, or mental burnout, is formally defined as physical, emotional, and mental exhaustion caused by long-term involvement in situations that are emotionally demanding. Mental fatigue is closely related to, and often interlinked with, emotional fatigue. They are both psychogenic conditions, that is, states that are mental or emotional rather than physiological in origin.

Mental fatigue does not suddenly occur. It is a gradual process that takes place over a period of time. As the chronic pressures of everyday life mount, the body is placed under continual stress. We all know how damaging stress can be to our physical and emotional health. Scientific literature is replete with reports demonstrating how stress causes impotence, irregular menstrual cycles, heart disease, and even cancer.

Common symptoms of mental fatigue include:

- insomnia
- inappropriate drowsiness
- feelings of anxiousness
- feelings of stress
- loss of appetite
- inappropriate emotional reactions

Testing for Mental Fatigue

An indication as to whether you may be a candidate for mental fatigue is how you respond to the following questions:

1. Do you continue to do more, even when your resources are low or exhausted? yes no
2. Has your level of frustration risen so high that you do not see a way out? yes no
3. Has someone imposed or have you imposed on yourself unreasonable expectations that, because they are unattainable, have caused you to become sick and quick to anger at work or in your personal life? yes no
4. Do you feel stress shadowing you when you walk down the street, or do you see it staring back at you when you look in the mirror? yes no

Scoring Your Test

If you answered "yes" to any or all of these questions, you may be a candidate for mental fatigue or burnout.

Combating Mental Fatigue Naturally

Once you have arrived at a diagnosis of mental fatigue, you cannot simply take an aspirin or a multivitamin or a nap and wake up relieved of your malady. Mental fatigue and burnout are not something you can get rid of quickly, as you did not acquire them quickly. And because mental fatigue is so closely linked to disruptions in emotional and physical symptoms, you must take a holistic approach to restoring your brain's vitality.

In addition to examining the emotional and psychological stresses in your life, you must also look closely at your diet and nutritional habits. A hair mineral test can pinpoint nutritional deficiencies, metal poisonings, or other imbalances.

Mental fatigue affects millions of people. It causes accidents, crime, and problems in school and on the job, and interferes with relationships. That is the bad news. The good news is that there are corrective measures that can be taken to alleviate the problems associated with the condition.

In the following Reboot Your Brain protocol for impacting mental fatigue, I recommend natural, gentle treatments that will help rebalance the delicate chemical structure of your brain and revitalize your mental energies.

Lifestyle

Being aware of certain aspects of your lifestyle may help to prevent the symptoms of mental fatigue. Keeping your body and spirit refreshed will help your brain function optimally and prevent mental fatigue.

Environment

Psychology professor Stephen Kaplan of the University of Michigan has extensively researched mental fatigue. He asserts that the most powerful cure for mental fatigue is the natural environment. One does not have to go to the suburbs to gain the benefits of nature.

According to Kaplan, simply looking out the window and seeing a natural setting with trees and grass can reap rewards.[1]

A consistent body of research has documented the restorative value of nature in a wide range of illnesses, from recovering from cancer to keeping prisoners healthy, to helping AIDS caregivers with burnout. Researchers examining the biophilia hypothesis (*biophilia* literally means "the love of living things") believe that humankind's relationship with nature covers a period of about one million years.[2] If these researchers are correct, they are explaining why so many people thrive in a natural environment, but are ill at ease in large cities.

Exercise

Exercise improves your ability to think. Why? Even though the brain accounts for less than 5 percent of your entire body weight, it uses 30 percent of the oxygen in the body—and probably the same amount of glucose (which is the energy that runs your body). Quite simply, the more oxygen there is in your body, the more oxygen there is for your brain to use.

One recent study has shown that exercise may increase an individual's brain power. After placing twenty men and women between the ages of eighteen and twenty-four on a treadmill for thirty minutes of moderate to heavy running, the researchers measured the subjects' thinking capacity. When the subjects' heart rates returned to their normal resting rates, they were then connected to an electroencephalogram (EEG), an instrument that measures brain waves. They were then given two computer tests that were markedly different in their degree of difficulty. The results of these tests were measured against their previous tests, taken when they had not exercised in advance. The results were remarkable. They showed that when it came to decision making, not only did exercise increase brain wave measurements but, in fact, cerebral activity began thirty-five milliseconds (a millisecond is one-thousandth of a second) faster after the patients had exercised than when they had not exercised.[3]

Any kind of exercise you are able to do will benefit your brain. Walking, gardening, dancing, swimming, yoga, and tai chi are all excellent ways to promote both physical and mental health.

Foods and Mental Fatigue

A good starting point for improving mental energy is improving your diet. Organic fruits and vegetables should be incorporated into your diet, while foods that cause allergies should be eliminated. While you're at it, get rid of junk food and too much sugar. Drink at least eight 8-ounce glasses of fresh, organic, raw vegetable juice every day. These juices should have celery, cucumber, wheatgrass, broccoli sprouts, kale, watercress, red and yellow peppers, ginger, apple, lemon, and whole leaf aloe vera concentrate. Anyone with mental fatigue should not consume wheat and dairy. Foods that contain gluten rye, oats, and barley are also responsible for allergic reactions that may affect the brain. Certain vitamins and minerals can also help your body fight the signs of mental fatigue.

To remain energized and functioning at optimal levels, the brain needs a full spectrum of nutrients, including vitamins, minerals, essential fatty acids, antioxidants, and amino acids. Deficiencies in any of these nutrients can upset the delicate chemical balance of the neurotransmitters and contribute to conditions such as metal fatigue.

Recipes

In the list below are my recommendations for easy-to-prepare meals full of nutrients proven to help prevent mental fatigue. The recipes can be found in Appendix II of this book:

- Antioxidant Supreme
- The Big Cleanse
- Brain Power
- Chilling Relaxer

- Chlorophyll Boost
- Delicious Detox
- Detox Tonic
- Flax Cruncher
- Head Cleaner
- Wisdom Drink
- Fabulous Wild Rice Salad
- Herbed Tomato Salad
- Mixed Sprout, Bean, and Nut Salad
- Pasta Salad
- Chilled Cantaloupe Soup
- Blueberry Breakfast Treat
- Cream of Barley
- Gary's Vegetable Pan
- Good Shepherd's Pie
- Original Broccoli Stir-Fry
- Cherry Grape Kanten

Supplements
Vitamins and Minerals

Certain vitamins and minerals are especially important in fighting mental fatigue.

Calcium. Your body stores calcium in the bones and teeth, which is what keeps them strong. It helps muscles relax, lowers blood pressure, reduces stress, and improves the quality of sleep. It helps nerve cells communicate normally and promotes blood clotting. To perform these essential functions, the body simply takes as much calcium as it needs, leaching it from the bones. If there is too little calcium in your diet to replenish this supply, your bones will eventually become porous, weak, and prone to breaking. To safeguard your bones and prevent mental fatigue, I recommend a supplement of 500 milligrams taken twice daily with food.

Magnesium. Magnesium plays a variety of roles in the body. Not only is it critical for energy production and proper nerve function; it also promotes muscle relaxation and helps preserve the health of the nervous system. Magnesium deficiency may play a role in mental fatigue. Magnesium is also a building block for serotonin, an important mood-enhancing neurotransmitter that plays a role in reducing mental fatigue. I recommend a supplement of 320 milligrams daily for women and 420 milligrams daily for men.

Potassium. Potassium aids in converting blood sugar, or glucose—the brain's (and body's) foremost fuel—into glycogen, a form of energy that can be stored in the muscles and liver and released as needed. Inadequate stores of glycogen lead to physical and mental fatigue. Potassium is depleted from our bodies in times of stress, thus upsetting the delicate balance of neurotransmitter communication in our brains. Potassium can interact with some drugs, so if you are taking prescription medication, consult with your doctor before taking potassium supplements. If potassium is safe for you to take, I recommend supplementing with 300 milligrams daily.

Smart Drugs and Nutrients

A number of other naturally occurring nutrients may have beneficial impacts on mental fatigue.

Creatine. Creatine was recently in the news because of its use by both professional and amateur athletes in bodybuilding, and evidence of its beneficial effects seems to increase daily. Scientists from the University of Tokyo reported that creatine supplementation (8 grams per day for five days) reduced mental fatigue when the test subjects repeatedly performed a simple mathematical calculation. Specifically, after taking the creatine supplement, those in the test group showed a task prompted increase in the brain's utilization of oxygen.[4] Because creatine is naturally found abundantly in the brain and is an energy source for ATP synthesis, it makes sense that it should be effective in preventing mental fatigue. I recommend supplementing with 8 grams per day for five days. If mental fatigue persists, repeat the five-day dose as needed.

L-Glutamine. Glutamine is one of the most abundant nonessential amino acids in the bloodstream. It is produced in the muscles and is able to pass freely through the blood–brain barrier. Once in the brain, it is converted into glutamic acid and increases GABA, a neurotransmitter essential for proper mental function. The two types of glutamine supplements are: D-glutamine and L-glutamine. L-glutamine is the form that more closely mimics the glutamine in the body. For mental sharpness, I recommend supplementing with 500 milligrams, taken three times daily for not more than one month.

Rebooting the Brain Chart of Supplements for Impacting Mental Fatigue

The following chart summarizes the supplements I recommend adding to the protocol for overall brain health from chapter 2. In some cases, I recommend increasing the dose of a particular vitamin or supplement to specifically impact mental fatigue. In these cases, you should increase the daily dosage from chapter 2 to the level recommended for this specific condition.

This protocol is designed for individuals who suffer from, or are specifically concerned about, mental fatigue. If you are concerned about additional brain conditions discussed in other chapters, consult with a health professional about how you can safely impact multiple conditions.

If you are taking medications, whether prescription or over-the-counter, or have any food restrictions, consult with your doctor before beginning any supplement program. Your health care provider should always be up-to-date on all vitamins, supplements, and herbal or homeopathic remedies you are taking. Supplement overdoses are rare, but possible, and certain combinations may affect individuals adversely.

Supplement	Dosage	Cautions
calcium	500 mg twice a day	Take with food to increase absorption.
creatine	8 g per day for five days. Repeat as needed.	
L-glutamine	500 mg three times daily	Take while symptoms persist, but not for more than one month.
magnesium	320 mg daily for women, 420 mg daily for men	May take six weeks or more for effects to be felt.
potassium	300 mg daily	Do not take potassium supplements if you are taking medication for high blood pressure or heart disease, or if you have a kidney disorder. Consuming foods rich in potassium is okay. Do not exceed a supplementary dose of 3.5 g daily without consulting your doctor.

Alternative Health Remedies

When suffering from a specific condition such as mental fatigue, we can also try some natural treatment options that are considered "alternatives" to traditional medicine. While a healthful lifestyle and the proper nutritional and supplement plan are vital to winning the battle against mental fatigue, there are some other targeted remedies that might help, too.

Herbal Remedies

Some herbal extracts and homeopathic treatments have properties similar to conventional medications, but are gentler and may lack the drugs' side effects. Always inform your medical practitioner of any herbal remedies you may be taking.

- **Rhodiola (Rhodiola rosea)** is a plant that has been used throughout the world, particularly in colder regions, for hundreds of years. Rhodiola's an adaptogen, which means it bolsters a person's ability to combat stressors. According to a study in *Phytomedicine,* a placebo-controlled, double-blind study in Armenia of fifty-six nightshift physicians who used 170 milligrams of Rhodiolaper each day for two consecutive weeks had 50 percent less mental fatigue than did those who took the placebo.[5] For mental fatigue, I recommend a dosage of 500 milligrams taken twice daily while symptoms last.

- **Ginseng** is considered a rejuvenation herb. Research shows that ginseng is an antioxidant that slows the free radical damage of aging. It can promote better focus and boost energy levels. Ginseng can interact with many medications. Talk to your health care provider before supplementing with ginseng, and follow your provider's instructions for use.

Homeopathic Remedies

The following remedies may be used for relief from the symptoms of mental fatigue. When dealing with a chronic condition, homeopathic remedies must be used in conjunction with other therapies, as prescribed by a qualified health professional. Consult with your health care provider before taking any homeopathic remedy, and follow your provider's recommendation for the appropriate dosage. Always inform your medical practitioner of any homeopathic remedies you may be taking.

- **Calcarea phosphorica** relieves feelings of mental fatigue and forgetfulness.
- **Alumina** can help restore mental clarity.
- **Kali phosphoricum** is useful for nervous exhaustion and relieves mental fatigue.

Detoxification

Because the brain needs a substantial amount of blood, it is one of the first organs adversely impacted by the toxins residing in the blood. Metal and general body toxicity can contribute to mental fatigue. Toxic metals such as mercury can be found in our water, vaccines, dental fillings, food, soil, herbicides, and pesticides. Our bodies absorb these dangerous metals, and our brains feel the effect.

When debris from the colon is not properly eliminated, the body absorbs these toxins, which causes the body to become poisoned. Brain fog, depression, and mental fatigue are some of the symptoms of body toxicity. The colon is not the only part of the body that is responsible for eliminating waste, however; the liver and kidneys also play a vital role. When these organs are malfunctioning, a host of toxic substances are allowed to remain in the blood.

Many people choose to detoxify their systems by following the cleansing plan below:

- Follow a two-week diet consisting of only raw, organic foods. Drink ten 8-ounce glasses of water per day.
- Avoid dairy products. Use fiber, such as psyllium, each day.
- Use bentonite, a claylike substance that is used in a drink, which draws out toxins from the colon.
- Utilize colon therapy.

Breathing Exercises

Reduced oxygen to the brain is another common cause of mental fatigue. Shallow or interrupted breathing can be caused by anxiety, stress, or illnesses such as asthma, bronchitis, or emphysema. Simple breathing techniques can help relieve stress and tension. Long, deep breathing can increase oxygen flow to your brain and body. Alternate nostril breathing focuses your thoughts and concentration, improves circulation, and energizes the mind. Try both of the following breathing exercises to fight the onset of mental fatigue.

Long, Deep Breathing. Sit comfortably with shoulders and chest relaxed. Inhale, relaxing your abdomen as you push your belly muscles forward, and fill your middle with air. Exhale, allowing your abdomen to shrink back in, tightening your belly muscles as you squeeze the air back out. Place one hand on your abdomen to feel your belly moving with your breath. Breathe in even lengths, breathing out for the same amount of time as you breathe in.

Alternate Nostril Breathing. Close your eyes. Press your right nostril closed with the thumb of your right hand. Draw in a deep breath through the left nostril. After taking a full breath, close the left nostril with the middle, ring, and little fingers of your right hand, taking the thumb away from the right nostril, and slowly let the air out. Expel your breath fully. Inhale through your right nostril. After a full inhalation, close your right nostril with your right thumb and release your left nostril and breathe out fully. This completes one round. Begin with three rounds of alternate breathing and gradually increase. Stop if you feel dizzy or faint.

Correcting Structural Imbalances

Believe it or not, the spinal column being misaligned, or any encroachment on the cervical, cranial, or other nerves, can result in mental fatigue. Something as simple as an improper sleeping position can cause a pinched nerve that affects the brain, causing mental fatigue. Chiropractic and osteopathic treatment and craniosacral therapy have proven effective in correcting structural imbalances.

Yoga and Meditation

Many have discovered the joy of yoga and meditation in helping clear the mind of thoughts that fatigue it. Brief periods of meditation throughout the day can help refocus the mind and reinvigorate mental energy. The practice of walking meditation is particularly useful for clearing mental fatigue, as it combines both meditation and simple exercise.

To practice walking meditation, focus your attention on each foot as it contacts the ground. When the mind wanders away from your feet or legs, or the feeling of your body walking, refocus your attention. To deepen your concentration, don't look around, but keep your gaze forward and soft.

Aromatherapy

Essential oils can be used in baths or inhaled to provide an energizing effect. Do not apply essential oils directly to the skin; they must be mixed with carrier oils. Experiment with various scents to see which are most effective at clearing away your mental fog. You can try any of the following:

- basil
- cardamom
- celery seed
- hyacinth
- lavender
- peppermint
- rosemary
- thyme

Summary

Mental fatigue can be largely avoided, provided we pay careful attention to the amount of stress in our lives and strive to maintain a balance between work and relaxation. The importance of the mind–body balance is especially significant in overcoming the effects of mental fatigue. Proper diet and nutrition, as well as appropriate supplementation, can ensure that episodes of mental fatigue are brief and generally nondisruptive. By consciously seeking to keep our minds engaged but tranquil, we allow our brains to function optimally at any stage of our lives.

Chapter 7

Parkinson's Disease

"Your nervous system in fact is a circulating nervous system. It thinks. It's conscious."

—Deepak Chopra

After Alzheimer's disease, Parkinson's is the second most frequent adult neurodegenerative disease. Dr. James Parkinson, a British physician, was the first to officially describe the condition in *An Essay on the Shaking Palsy*, which was published in 1817. In all likelihood, however, the disease has existed for thousands of years.

A slowly progressive disorder affecting the central nervous system, Parkinson's is caused by the loss of the brain cells that produce the neurotransmitter dopamine. Without this vital brain chemical, the information transmitted on neural pathways in the midbrain becomes garbled and distorted, resulting in the breakdown of communication to the body's muscles.

What is amazing to me is that, for hundreds of years, doctors have taken notice of the initial signs of Parkinson's disease—a small tremor in the hands or a slight dragging of one foot—symptoms that are exacerbated when an individual is fatigued or under stress; they have learned that the absence of the neurotransmitter dopamine in the brain causes the physical symptoms of Parkinson's; but, tragically, after more than 150 years of desperately trying, traditional medicine has been unable to pinpoint an underlying cause or find a cure for this disease.

In this chapter, I talk about the symptoms and progression of Parkinson's, as well as what modern medicine knows about this condition. I tell you what type of lifestyle and nutritional changes you can implement to help prevent the onset of Parkinson's. I'll also discuss supplements and alternative treatments that may help with symptoms of Parkinson's.

Understanding Parkinson's

Parkinson's affects about 1 in 100 persons over the age of sixty—that's approximately one million Americans. Researchers estimate that this number will continue to rise—by fifty thousand or more each year—as the average age of the population increases. While certain symptoms of Parkinson's—lack of coordination, muscle tremors, and stiffness—are clearly physical, it must also be noted that more than 40 percent of individuals with Parkinson's also experience serious mental decline.[1]

Although Parkinson's disease usually starts in later years—the average age of onset is sixty—younger individuals are not immune to the disease. When the disorder appears before the age of forty, it is called early-onset Parkinson's. In younger people who are afflicted, the onset usually occurs following an inflammation of the brain, as in encephalitis, or from poisoning by carbon monoxide, metals, or certain drugs.

You probably don't think much about the cause and effect of bodily movements as you go about your daily routine. It just happens. You want a drink of water, so you get up and walk over to the sink. To understand how the disruption of the delicate chemical balance in your brain results in the symptoms of Parkinson's disease, however, it is necessary to grasp some of the nuances involved in the functional relationship between your mind and your body.

For you to get up from your chair and walk over to the sink, your brain first has to go through a series of calculations that would be the envy of the most complex computer. These calculations involve accumulating all of the necessary information relative to the position of your body—the location of your hands and your feet, whether you are you sitting down or standing up, and so on. Once your brain has this information, it then assesses as much information as it can about where you are headed (the sink). The brain triggers all of the senses in gathering such information. The eyes relay information to the brain about whether it is day or night, whether it is raining or snowing, and how far it appears you must travel. Your skin, along with other parts of the body, assesses the temperature. Your feet ascertain whether the terrain is hilly or flat.

Let's go back to the scenario in which you decided to get a drink of water. When you initially thought about getting that drink of water, your nervous system used the neurotransmitters to send messages to the muscles to enable you to do so. The role of neurotransmitters cannot be overemphasized. In essence, they are enablers; they enable thought to be transferred into motion.

As I hope the explanation above makes clear, dopamine is crucial in bodily movement. But there is another component to movement: fluid movement. Another neurotransmitter, acetylcholine, is invaluable in allowing the body to move fluidly. For the body to move smoothly, it is imperative to maintain the proper balance between dopamine and acetylcholine.

When a person is afflicted with Parkinson's disease, the number of nerve cells in the substantia nigra declines. This leads directly to less dopamine being available in the brain. When this occurs, the delicate balance between dopamine and acetylcholine is thrown out of kilter. This interference causes a lack of coordination in bodily movement that manifests as tremors, muscle stiffness, and/or difficult movements.

Causes of Parkinson's Disease

While the symptoms of Parkinson's are generally clear, and the damage to crucial neurotransmitters eventually becomes apparent, there remain differing theories for the underlying cause, or causes, that may act as a trigger for the development of Parkinson's.

Dopamine Deficiency

Although there has been no conclusive underlying cause confirmed for Parkinson's disease, there is widespread belief that Parkinson's is caused at least partially by a deficiency of dopamine. In actuality, Parkinsonian symptoms are ascribed to a loss of cells in the substantia nigra region of the brain, which are responsible for producing this extremely important neurotransmitter. The parts of the brain damaged by this deficiency of dopamine are the parts that help regulate the nervous system and body.

A logical conclusion would seem to be that if one were to monitor the loss of dopamine, the first sign of it diminishing would be an indicator of the possibility of Parkinson's. Unfortunately, Parkinson's doesn't develop until 80 percent of the substantia nigra cells that manufacture dopamine are lost. Consequently, doctors remain unable to identify people in the early stages of the disease. Perhaps one day a test will be developed that detects the decline of the brain's dopamine levels earlier.

Free Radical Damage

Free radical damage is also suspected of causing Parkinson's disease.[2] (A free radical is an atom or group of atoms that has at least one unpaired electron, and thus is unstable and highly reactive. In animals, free radicals damage cells and are thought to hasten the development of cancer, cardiovascular disease, and age-related diseases.) Many believe that other causes such as viruses or bacteria are the principal threats to health. They are not. Free radicals are the principal threat to your good health, and controlling them may very well save your life.

Strokes

Interestingly enough, a person who suffers a series of small strokes can consequently develop Parkinson's. The symptoms in these patients are more likely to manifest as problems in walking than any of the other traditional signs of Parkinson's. In fact, the difficulties are more probable in the lower tremor and are more likely to have symptoms that are worse in the feet and the legs than in the arms. Traditional medicine treats this condition as if it were Parkinson's disease.

Chemical Toxicity

Pesticides and herbicides used on farms have been the subjects of studies to investigate a possible link between Parkinson's disease and long-term exposure to chemicals. Individuals who use pesticides in their homes are twice as likely to develop Parkinson's as those who are not exposed to pesticides.[3] Our food and water contain countless combinations of low-level toxic residues, and it is not fully known how these toxins impact the health of our bodies and brains.

A recent study in the *Journal of Neuroscience* demonstrated that the pesticide rotenone caused Parkinson's symptoms when given to rats.[4] The study indicated that the pesticide might cause the mitochondria to produce free radicals, and the destruction caused by the free radicals would subsequently lead to Parkinson's disease.

Metals Toxicity

High levels of aluminum, mercury, cadmium, lead, iron, and copper may also play a role in the development of Parkinson's disease.

- Aluminum is ingested from sources such as food additives, cooking utensils, antacids, buffered aspirin, nasal sprays, antiperspirants, automobile exhaust, soda cans, ceramics, and tobacco smoke. This metal is even found in some municipal water supplies.

- Mercury, cadmium, and lead are three heavy metals that can accumulate in the body with toxic effects. Mercury is a neurotoxin known to destroy nerve cells and cause tremors.
- Iron excess can intensify the symptoms of Parkinson's. Potential sources of iron include iron supplements, drinking water, iron plumbing pipes, and cookware.
- Copper levels can become high as a result of chronic inflammation, such as that caused by autoimmune or undetected allergy reactions. High copper levels, in combination with antioxidant deficiencies, can result in increased free radical damage to cells.

Bacteria Overgrowth

Certain bacteria produce toxic poisons called endotoxins. These toxins are released when cells die and cell walls become compromised. Bacterial endotoxins may flourish in the body as a result of the liver's inability to detoxify the system. When endotoxins reach the brain, they act as neurotoxins, producing acute psychotic symptoms in younger individuals and chronic nerve and brain degeneration in elderly individuals.

Diagnosing Parkinson's Disease

There is no known test that definitively identifies Parkinson's. It cannot be diagnosed through blood tests, MRIs, or X-rays, although these tests may be performed by your doctor to rule out other conditions. If you are concerned that you have symptoms of Parkinson's disease, you should immediately consult a trained neurologist, as there are many causes other than Parkinson's that are responsible for tremors.

While scientists have ascertained quite a bit about the symptoms of Parkinson's, relatively little has been learned about its cause and cure, and there remains little known about the risk factors for Parkinson's. Parkinson's disease affects both men and women equally. It knows no social, ethnic, economic, or geographic boundaries.[5]

Even today, doctors cannot recognize the beginning stages of Parkinson's, and there is a large degree of uncertainty in the diagnostic process that determines whether a patient, in fact, has Parkinson's.

For instance, side effects of prescription and nonprescriptive drugs (pain medications and selective serotonin reuptake inhibitors, or SSRIs, a class of antidepressant drugs effective in blocking the reabsorption of serotonin following the transmission of a nerve impulse across a synapse) can cause symptoms similar to those of Parkinson's disease, making a misdiagnosis possible.[6] These types of drugs may cause a condition called Parkinsonism, a nervous system disorder caused by damage to nerves in the brain. The symptoms closely mimic those of Parkinson's disease. If you find this hard to believe, consider that a study of autopsied bodies showed that 25 percent of patients who had been diagnosed with Parkinson's did not actually have the disease!

But there is no doubt as to what occurs in the brains of those who have the disease: the death and destruction of brain cells. An autopsy is sometimes the only definitive way to confirm the presence of Parkinson's. Lewy bodies (microscopic brain structures that may be observed in an autopsy) are an extremely strong indicator of Parkinson's disease.

Symptoms of Parkinson's Disease

Signs and symptoms of Parkinson's include:

- shaking (tremors)
- stiffness and rigid limbs (generally asymmetric)
- extremely slow movement (bradykinesia)
- impaired postural reflexes (extended arm tremor or trouble with handwriting)

When two of these symptoms are present, it is probable that the patient is suffering from Parkinson's. When three or more symptoms are evident, the patient is positively considered to have Parkinson's disease.[8]

Other, related symptoms may include:

- poor balance
- walking problems
- involuntary eye closure
- memory loss
- constipation
- sleep disturbances
- dementia
- speech, breathing, or swallowing problems
- stooped posture

Frequently, tremor (trembling or shaking) of a hand or a leg, particularly when the person is resting, is the first indication of Parkinson's disease. The tremor often begins on one side of the body (asymmetric), oftentimes in one hand. Eventually, a person's voluntary movements become increasingly difficult. For example, a once-simple task such as walking becomes stiffer and slower. This is followed by speech difficulties (speaking in a hushed tone). Then the face becomes expressionless because of increased muscular rigidity. Because the person cannot control his or her facial muscles, there is often drooling. There may also be numbing of the hands and feet. Also, the person's handwriting becomes small (known as micrographia) and is illegible. (If you have ever seen Muhammad Ali's handwriting, the first thing that strikes you is how small it is.) Although the person's thinking processes remain normal, they are stuck inside a debilitated body. For this reason, as symptoms worsen, a great depression may set in and lead to a shortened lifespan.

Combating Parkinson's Disease Naturally

As of now, we do not have a way to prevent the loss of nerve cells that produce dopamine or to restore those that have already been lost. Thus, effective treatment of Parkinson's would seem to rest on the ability to halt the damage to, and death of, the nerve cells that manufacture dopamine.

In fact, many individuals suffering from Parkinson's are prescribed the drug levodopa (L dopa), which can be converted into dopamine in the brain. Levodopa is often used in combination with other drugs that appear to have protective effects on brain cells. Treatment with these drugs, however, does not completely alleviate the symptoms of Parkinson's, although the disease may progress slower. Long-term treatment with these drugs may result in neurotic or psychotic symptoms.[9]

Research is ongoing on the effects of other drugs and methods of treating Parkinson's, including a new generation of drugs that work to mimic levodopa and inhibit the enzymes that break down levodopa in the brain. Research is also progressing on surgical options, including a brain "pacemaker" that blocks brain signals that cause tremors. In late stages of the disease, some patients are treated with a surgical option called pallidotomy, in which a small section of the globus pallidus is destroyed. Some patients also undergo thalatomy, another surgical procedure that destroys a specific group of cells in the thalamus (the brain's communication center). Neurotrophic proteins and neuroprotective agents are also being studied, along with neural tissue transplants and genetic engineering.

Obviously, Parkinson's is a serious condition, and professional medical management and prescription drugs are crucial in staving off the progression of the disease and maintaining quality of life.

Recent advances in molecular science, however, are beginning to alter the diagnostic approach to Parkinson's and the ways in which we approach treatment of the condition. Prior to these recent developments, the chief focus—and rightfully so—was on oxidative damage. Now, other causes—mitochondrial damage, excitotoxicity, and inflammatory cytokines—are being examined for the part they play in the death of brain cells.[10] At some point in the future, the chief cause of Parkinson's may be determined to have come from this group. But, as of now, any of these can lead directly to Parkinson's. Hence, the treatment modality should be multifaceted.

In the Reboot Your Brain protocol for impacting Parkinson's disease that follows, I discuss natural treatments that support the body and brain and are generally protective and supportive of good physical and mental health. Following this protocol may help protect you from the onset of Parkinson's disease or help reduce the severity of symptoms if you have been diagnosed with this condition.

Lifestyle

Although full-blown Parkinson's can be crippling or disabling, early symptoms of the disease may be so subtle and gradual that patients attribute them to other causes. Even if your doctor is fairly certain you are suffering from Parkinson's, there is much you can do in the early stages that may help to slow the progression of the disease. In any case, there are many elements of a healthy lifestyle that you can undertake at any time to help prevent the onset of a condition such as Parkinson's.

Exercise

Exercises involving weight training have been linked to increasing testosterone levels that, in turn, elevate dopamine levels. Hence, exercising is crucial in fighting Parkinson's. Exercise also reduces stress, which has been found to aggravate the symptoms of Parkinson's. Specific exercises, such as those taught by the Alexander Technique, which focuses on ridding your body of harmful tensions through improving the mechanics of moving your body in day-to-day activities, may offer particular benefit to individuals suffering from Parkinson's.

Social/Emotional

When a person first exhibits these symptoms, it is traumatic. Oftentimes, a trained professional's services are required. From a physical perspective, doctors generally treat the problems associated with motor functioning, for they are extremely alarming to someone who has never had sluggish movement of their limbs or rigidity. Though the patient is being treated for these physical symptoms, the doctor should also address the anticipated cognitive decline, for this greatly affects quality of life.

Medications

Older adults commonly develop drug-induced Parkinson's disease after having been prescribed antipsychotic drugs, such as Haldol, Thorazine, Mellaril, and Stelazine. These antipsychotics are used to sedate nursing home patients with dementia and chronic anxiety, two nonpsychotic disorders. When these drugs are discontinued, most newly diagnosed Parkinson's patients return to normal.

Environment

Studies show that toxic pesticides routinely used in agriculture and lawn care are linked to Parkinson's disease. People tend to discount low levels of exposure, but in children, the elderly, and people already ill, even small amounts can be damaging, leading to any number of problems, including nervous disorders and cancers.

As mentioned above, heavy metals damage the central nervous system. Hence, it is advisable to avoid aluminum cookware, remove amalgam dental fillings, and stay away from cigarette smoking, because cigarette papers contain cadmium.

Foods and Parkinson's Disease

A fresh, live-food diet is vital to the healing process in Parkinson's. If you suffer from this condition, your diet should incorporate mostly alkaline foods, with green drinks, such as chlorella, spirulina, barley grass, or wheatgrass, once or twice a day.

Your diet should be rich in fruits and vegetables that provide a good supply of antioxidants. Antioxidants are critical for overcoming oxidative damage to the brain and for slowing down progression of the disease. Research has shown that a combination of antioxidants can mimic chelating agents. (A chelating agent is a water-soluble molecule that can bond tightly with metal ions, keeping them from coming out of suspension and allowing them to be flushed from the system.) For maximum results, I suggest trying a combination of the C and E vitamins, polyphenols (found in green and black tea), bioflavonoids, proanthocyanidins (in grape seed extract and pine bark extract), and curcumin.

Foods such as red peppers and onions that contain glutathione (a metabolite of the essential amino acid methionine) are thought to be beneficial, as are broccoli, cauliflower, Brussels sprouts, and cabbage, which are rich in cyanohydroxybutene (a naturally occurring chemical that helps increase glutathione levels).

It is important to choose organic foods. The chemicals in nonorganic foods wreak havoc on our brains. Likewise, Parkinson's patients should consume only bottled or filtered water. Unheated extra virgin olive oil and herbs for flavoring should be used.

Sugar and fat should be avoided, as research has shown, diets high in sugar triple the risk of developing Parkinson's, while diets high in fats result in a fivefold increase in the odds of developing Parkinson's.[12]

You should also avoid wheat, dairy, and gluten products, margarine, fried foods, polyunsaturated oils, artificial sweeteners, processed food (e.g., deli meats), monosodium glutamate (MSG), alcohol (except red wine), and water containing chlorine or fluoride. (Remember, this not only applies to water you drink but also the water you bathe in; for best results, purchase a water filter, or be sure to keep your mouth closed while showering.) Do not use microwave ovens to cook your foods.

Individuals who are taking the prescription drug levodopa should limit protein intake to one meal per day, eaten late in the day, because protein hinders the absorption of levodopa.

The Latest Research

A 2012 analysis by scientists at the Harvard School of Public Health showed an association between dietary antioxidant intake and a decreased incidence of Parkinson's disease. Reviewing two decades-worth of medical records of more than 125,000 patients, the authors discovered that men who ate the highest quantities of flavonoids, a type of antioxidant abundant in berries, tea, and oranges, were 40 percent less likely to suffer from Parkinson's disease when compared to men who ate the lowest amounts of berries.[17] The study also linked the regular consumption of a particular type of flavonoid known as anthocyanins with a lower risk of developing Parkinson's disease among men and women.

Another recent study by researchers at the University of Tokyo evaluating the dietary patterns of individuals with Parkinson's disease found that patients who consumed a diet high in vegetables, fruits, and fish cut their risk of Parkinson's disease by 46 percent compared to patients who ate the lowest amounts of these foods.[18] This revelation comes on the heels of another Japanese study that linked a diet high in vitamin E (abundant in almonds, avocados, and vegetable oils) and beta carotene (abundant in apricots, carrots, and green vegetables) with a significantly lower incidence of Parkinson's disease.[19]

In the March 2012 edition of the *Harvard Health Letter*, an article titled "Another Reason to Get Out There and Get Moving!" reveals that engaging in vigorous exercise earlier in life may cut the risk of developing Parkinson's disease by 30 percent.[20] The authors arrived at their conclusion after reviewing several large cohort studies which examined the progress of tens of thousands of patients for many years. The findings suggest that middle-age people who do just twenty minutes of intense aerobic exercise several times a week can considerably decrease their odds of having Parkinson's disease twenty or thirty years in the future.

The time-honored practice of Chinese martial arts known as tai chi has been found in numerous studies to provide health benefits ranging from decreased anxiety and stress to improved flexibility. In a 2012 study published in the *New England Journal of Medicine*, researchers revealed the noteworthy effectiveness of tai chi in relieving symptoms in patients with Parkinson's disease. Lead author Fuzhong Li and his team at the Oregon Research Institute monitored the progress of three groups of patients with Parkinson's disease. One group practiced tai chi, another group did resistance training exercises, and the last group participated in stretching classes. Each group engaged in an hour-long class twice a week over the course of six months. The authors found that the ability to balance in people who practiced tai chi was two times better than it was in the group who did resistance training and four times better than it was in the stretching group.[21] Further, the individuals who spent their time doing tai chi were measured to be physically stronger than the other two groups.

Recipes

In the following list are my recommendations for easy-to-prepare meals full of nutrients that may help prevent, or slow the progression of, Parkinson's disease. The recipes are found in Appendix II of this book:

- Antioxidant Supreme
- The Big Cleanse
- Brain Juice
- Chlorophyll Boost
- Deep-Sea Juicing
- Fountain of Youth
- Free Radical Delight
- Green Power Punch
- Head Cleaner

- Pure Citrus Punch,
- Super Vegetable Cocktail
- Four-Bean Salad
- Gary's Chef's Salad with Creamy Italian Dressing
- Mixed Sprout, Bean, and Nut Salad
- Succotash Salad
- Superior Spinach Salad
- Blueberry Banana Pancakes
- Nutty Banana Breakfast
- Gary's Vegetable Pan
- Indonesian Kale
- Original Broccoli Stir-Fry
- Ratatouille
- Blackberry Nectarine Fruit Salad
- Cold Cherry Soup

Supplements

Vitamins and Minerals

Certain vitamins may be beneficial in preventing and impacting the symptoms of Parkinson's disease.

Vitamin B6. Vitamin B6 is essential in the synthesis of dopamine. When taken with zinc, B6 can help stimulate the production of dopamine. While adding foods rich in B vitamins to your diet is fine at any time, it should be noted that when you use vitamin B supplements in combination with levodopa, the vitamin B may act to stimulate production of dopamine in other areas of the body, with less reaching the brain. Therefore, if you and your health care provider decide to try supplementing with vitamin B, you should take it either at the end of the day after the last dose of levodopa, or at intervals between doses of levodopa. I recommend increasing your daily vitamin B6 supplement from 75 milligrams to 150 milligrams. Do not exceed a daily supplement of 150 milligrams.

Vitamin C. This potent antioxidant may help to slow the progression of Parkinson's symptoms. Ascorbic acid may also help to counteract severe side effects of levodopa. Vitamin C appears to be even more effective when paired with other antioxidants, such as vitamin E. I recommend increasing your daily vitamin C supplement to 500 to 1,000 milligrams to 3,000 milligrams, taken in three divided doses.

Vitamin E. Vitamin E is a potent antioxidant. When taken in combination with vitamin C, it may help slow the progression of the symptoms of Parkinson's disease. I recommend increasing your daily vitamin E supplement from 268 milligrams to 536 milligrams. Do not exceed a daily supplement of 536 milligrams.

Zinc, a cofactor of vitamin B, zinc may help with control of symptoms, such as tremors and rigidity, and may improve walking skills and bladder control. I recommend a daily supplement of 30 milligrams.

Smart Drugs and Nutrients

A number of other naturally occurring nutrients have beneficial impacts on the symptoms of Parkinson's disease.

Coenzyme Q10 (Coq10). As we age, our bodies' natural production of coenzyme Q10 (coQ10) diminishes. Our older bodies produce only 50 percent of the coQ10 they did when we were younger. This makes coQ10 one of the most important nutrients for people over thirty. Because the cells of our bodies need coQ10 to produce energy and to combat mitochondrial free radical activity, a coQ10 deficiency can result in a greater incidence of many degenerative diseases associated with aging.

Because coQ10 is a fat-soluble nutrient that goes into the mitochondria throughout the body, it should be taken with the fattiest meal of your day. When consumed in an oil-based capsule, the coQ10 can be absorbed through the lymphatic canals for better distribution throughout the entire body.

I recommend increasing your daily coQ10 supplement from 100 to 300 milligrams to 1,200 milligrams.

Glutathione. A metabolite of the essential amino acid methionine, glutathione is an important part of the body's antioxidant defense system. Studies of the substantia nigra after death in Parkinson's disease sufferers have shown the depletion of glutathione.[13] To impact the symptoms of Parkinson's, I recommend a supplement of 200 milligrams taken twice daily.

Melatonin. Melatonin is a hormone manufactured by the pineal gland in the brain. It is released into the bloodstream and is involved in synchronizing the body's hormone secretions and setting daily biorhythms. It is one of the body's most potent antioxidants. In a study conducted at Thomas Jefferson University, researchers showed that melatonin was effective in blocking the oxidative damage in dopamine-producing cells, thereby reducing or blocking Parkinsonian effects.[14] To help ease the symptoms of Parkinson's disease, I recommend supplementing with 300 micrograms to 1 milligrams, taken a half hour before bed two or three nights per week.

N-Acetylcysteine (NAC). An important amino acid that enhances the production of glutathione, N-acetylcysteine can help protect the brain from free radicals and minimize age-related deterioration of the nervous system. I recommend supplementing daily with 1,500 milligrams taken in three doses of 500 milligrams.

Nicotinamide Adenine Dinucleotide (NADH). An enzyme that helps improve neurotransmitter function, NADH is present in all living cells and plays a critical role in energy production. It helps prevent cellular degeneration, and may increase concentration and memory capacity. I recommend a supplement of 2.5 milligrams taken twice daily.

Proanthocyanidins. Proanthocyanidins (chemical relatives of bioflavonoids) serve to benefit the brain in a twofold manner: They are antioxidants, and they protect collagen.

Research has shown that proanthocyanidins are fifty times more powerful antioxidants than vitamins C and E. Intricate tests prove that proanthocyanidins are great killers of the hydroxyl radical—the free radical that is responsible for the most damage—and lipid peroxides (rancid fats).

Although proanthocyanidins can be found in the diet, the levels in food are generally insufficient to help fight the symptoms of Parkinson's disease. I recommend increasing your daily supplement from 80 milligrams to 380 milligrams, taken in three divided doses. Do not exceed a daily supplement of 380 milligrams.

Reboot Your Brain Chart of Additional Supplements for Impacting Parkinson's Disease

The following chart summarizes the supplements I recommend adding to the protocol for overall brain health from chapter 2. In some cases, I recommend increasing the dose of a particular vitamin or supplement to specifically impact Parkinson's disease. In these cases, you should increase the daily dosage from chapter 2 to the level recommended for this specific condition.

This protocol is designed for individuals who suffer from, or are specifically concerned about, Parkinson's disease. If you are concerned about additional brain conditions discussed in other chapters, consult with a health professional about how you can safely impact multiple conditions.

If you are taking medications, whether prescription or over-the-counter, or have any food restrictions, consult with your doctor before beginning any supplement program. Your health care provider should always be up-to-date on all vitamins, supplements, and herbal or homeopathic remedies you are taking. Supplement overdoses are rare, but possible, and certain combinations may affect individuals adversely.

Supplement	Dosage	Cautions
coenzyme Q10 (coQ10)	Increase daily dosage from 100–300 mg to1,200 mg. Do not exceed a daily supplement of 2,000 mg. Take with fattiest meal of the day. If going higher, do so under medical supervision.	Dosage should be gradually increased, with 300 mg daily added over a six-week period until the daily dose reaches 2,000 mg. Individuals supplementing with coQ10 at high doses should be monitored closely by their doctors.
glutathione	200 mg two times daily	Glutathione levels may also be elevated through supplementation with cysteine, N-acetylcysteine, or L-cysteine.
melatonin	300 mcg–1 mg two to three nights per week a half hour before bed	Tolerance may develop with regular use. Long-term effects of nightly use are unknown.
N-acetylcysteine	1,500 mg in three divided doses.	Regular supplementation of NAC increases urinary output of copper. If supplementing with NAC for an extended period, add 2 mg of copper and 30 mg of zinc to your daily supplement regimen.
Nicotinamide adenine Dinucleotide (NADH)	2.5 mg twice daily	High doses (10 mg per day or more) may cause nervousness, anxiety, and insomnia.

Supplement	Dosage	Cautions
proantho-cyanidins	Increase daily dosage from 80 mg to 380 mg, taken in three divided doses. Do not exceed a daily supplement of 380 mg.	
vitamin B6	Increase daily dosage from 75 mg to 150 mg. Do not exceed a daily supplement of 150 mg. Take with zinc (30 mg).	Contraindicated for use with levodopa. Discuss supplementation with your health care provider.
vitamin C	Increase daily dosage from 500–1,000 mg to 3,000 mg, taken in three divided doses.	
vitamin E	Increase daily dosage from 268 mg to 536 mg. Do not exceed a daily supplement of 536 mg.	If you have high blood pressure, limit your supplemental vitamin E to 268 mg daily. If you are taking blood thinners, consult with your doctor before taking vitamin E.
zinc	Up to 30 mg daily	Large doses (50 mg or more) can interfere with the body's absorption of essential minerals, impair blood cell function, and depress immunesystem.

Alternative Health Remedies

When suffering from a specific condition such as Parkinson's disease, we can also try some natural treatment options that are considered alternatives to traditional medicine. While a healthful lifestyle and the proper nutritional and supplement plan are vital to winning the battle against the symptoms of Parkinson's, there are some other targeted remedies that might help, too.

Herbal Remedies

Some herbal extracts and homeopathic treatments have properties similar to conventional medications, but are gentler and may lack the drugs' side effects. Always inform your medical practitioner of any herbal remedies you may be taking.

- **Atmagupta (Mucuma pruins)** is an Ayurvedic herb that contains the natural form of L-dopa. Ayurvedic herbs are commonly taken in combination to neutralize toxicity. Do not take this without consulting with your doctor.
- **Gotu kola** has been historically used in the treatment of Parkinson's disease. I recommend taking it as a tea once daily. Do not use gotu kola if you take medication for diabetes or to control cholesterol. If gotu kola is safe for you to take, I recommend 200 milligrams taken three times daily.
- **Ginkgo biloba** is an extract of the ginkgo plant used in Europe to help fight dementia and Alzheimer's disease. It is a circulatory stimulant and an antioxidant. Ginkgo can act as an anticoagulant, and individuals taking anticoagulant and antithrombotic drugs such as ASA, anti-inflammatories, and warfarin or Coumadin should consult with their doctor before taking ginkgo. If ginkgo is safe for you to use, I recommend a supplement of 120 milligrams per day, taken in three equal doses.
- **Hawthorn** acts as a circulatory stimulant and potent antioxidant. I recommend a supplement of 2 to 5 grams per day.
- **Lady's slipper** may help provide relief from tremors. I recommend 10 to 30 drops of tincture taken three or four times daily.
- **Milk thistle** can provide liver support and detoxification. I recommend a supplement of 30 to 60 drops of tincture per day.

- **Skullcap** acts to strengthen the brain. I recommend 10 to 30 drops of tincture per day.

Homeopathic Remedies

The following remedies may be used for relief from the symptoms of Parkinson's disease. When dealing with a chronic condition, homeopathic remedies must be used in conjunction with other therapies, as prescribed by a qualified health professional. Consult with your health care provider before taking any homeopathic remedy, and follow your provider's recommendation for the appropriate dosage. Always inform your medical practitioner of any homeopathic remedies you may be taking.

- **Anthimonium tartaricum** may help with trembling head and immobile hands.
- **Gelsemium** may provide relief from trembling and drooping eyelids.
- **Agarius** is for limbs that are stiff but tremble and twitch; your back and spine may be especially sensitive.
- **Rhus toxicodendron** is good for mild tremors and stiffness that feels better after movement but worse with damp weather.
- **Fish oil** is abundant in omega-3 fatty acids that have been shown to support neurological health in Parkinson's patients.[7] One study examining groups of mice injected with a Parkinson's-inducing agent found that mice fed a diet rich in omega-3s were much less likely to exhibit low levels of dopamine compared to the control group.[8] I recommend taking 2,000 to 4,000 milligrams daily of a purified fish oil concentrate. Consult with your doctor if taking anti-coagulant or anti-platelet medications or have a bleeding disorder
- **Curcumin,** derived from the turmeric spice popular in Indian cuisine, is a beneficial phytochemical that has been shown

to shield against oxidative stress and inflammation related to neurodegenerative illness.[9, 10] I recommend taking a daily supplement of 400 to 1,200 milligrams. Do not take if you have gallbladder problems or gallstones. Consult with your doctor if taking anti-coagulant or anti-platelet medications or have a bleeding disorder

Detoxification

Chelation therapy eliminates metals from the brain, as well as other toxic agents that encourage free radicals' development. A hair analysis can determine whether high levels of metals need to be chelated out of the body. Studies indicate that to properly impact Parkinson's, effective treatments must reduce oxidative stress. Chelation therapy plays an important role in eliminating iron as well as other toxins from the brain. These toxins infuse the brain with free radicals. Some think that chelation can only occur through chelation therapy. Antioxidants can also play the role of chelators, however. The C and E vitamins, bioflavonoids, polyphenols (from black and green teas), grape seed extract (specifically, the proanthocyanidins), and tocotrienols from curcumin also serve as chelators. To find out more about chelation therapy and detoxification protocols, visit my website: www.garynull.com.

Aromatherapy

Essential oils can be used in baths or inhaled to provide rebalancing effects. Do not apply essential oils directly to the skin; they must be mixed with carrier oils. Though massaging with fragrant essential oils will not cure Parkinson's, it can provide temporary relief. Experiment with various scents to see which brings you relief:

- clary sage
- marjoram
- lavender

Summary

Keep in mind that conventional medicine has defined Parkinson's as a disease that cannot be reversed. Alternative and complementary medicine has demonstrated otherwise. The Reboot Your Brain protocol for Parkinson's can help protect your brain and offer relief from the progression of the symptoms of this disease.

Chapter 8

Alzheimer's Disease

"They tell you that you'll lose your mind when you grow older.
What they don't tell you is that you won't miss it very much."

—Malcolm Cowley

When I speak to people about some of the serious conditions associated with aging, the same concern comes up over and over again: "Gary, my father [or mother, or grandparent] suffered from Alzheimer's. Is there anything I can do to keep from getting this disease as I grow older?"

Alzheimer's disease is one of the most dreaded of the numerous mental disorders associated with aging. Its slow, progressive assault on an individual's mental function robs sufferers of their memory and often their dignity. Alzheimer's advances in stages, first causing disturbances in verbal, then visual, memory before destroying the brain's executive functions, causing loss of ability to reason, plan, or organize thoughts, loss of language, and inability to recognize objects.

The severe memory impairment or dementia that occurs with Alzheimer's disease significantly interferes with daily life. Simple tasks become difficult or impossible to perform, and day-to-day functioning becomes increasingly diminished. But Alzheimer's is not a normal part of the aging process. And even if there is a history of the disease in your family, it is not inevitable that you will suffer its effects as you age.

By providing an optimal environment for brain health through a healthful lifestyle, attention to nutrition, and proper supplementation, you can preserve your mental abilities as you age. In this chapter, I talk about specific steps you can take to improve your environment and diet to protect your brain against the symptoms of cognitive decline associated with Alzheimer's. I also talk about alternative, natural treatments that may have some benefits in the fight against this serious condition.

Understanding Alzheimer's Disease

According to the Alzheimer's Association, Alzheimer's disease now affects approximately 5.4 million Americans.[1] One in eight older Americans has Alzheimer's disease, and it ranks as the sixth-leading cause of death in the United States. By the year 2050, it is projected that up to sixteen million Americans will suffer from this condition.[2]

Alzheimer's is one form of dementia, a term used to describe a group of symptoms that are caused by changes in brain function. Many different conditions can cause symptoms that mimic those of Alzheimer's disease but are not Alzheimer's. In fact, Alzheimer's has a specific, visible effect on the physical condition of the brain, as neurons, specifically those in the hippocampus, progressively degenerate, lose function, and die.

The German physician Alois Alzheimer first discovered this physical change in the brain in 1906. He presented his findings on the brain condition of a woman who had died while suffering from a rare mental disease that caused loss of memory, confusion, and hallucination before her death at age fifty-five. He described these changes in the brain as atypical clumps and twisted bundles of neurofibers accompanied by cell death as evidenced by shrinkage in the brain.

Nearly a century later, the cause of this cell death remains the subject of intense scientific scrutiny, which has provided clues, but few conclusions. Many experts believe that the cell death is related to a sticky, waxy protein called amyloid plaque, but whether the plaque causes cell death or is a by-product of it is unclear.

A second feature of Alzheimer's disease is neurofibrillary tangles consisting of tau protein (an essential protein in the infrastructure of neurons). When the tau protein disintegrates, it coils into filaments that gather in tangles. These plaques and tangles disrupt the communication in the brain, obstructing the electrical messages sent from neuron to neuron that allow us to think, remember, talk, and move.

As neurons begin to die, the amount of acetylcholine, a crucial chemical in the brain, decreases. Acetylcholine is necessary to carry the complex messages governing reactions and movement. Thus, as Alzheimer's progresses, physical impairment begins to occur along with cognitive losses.

Causes of Alzheimer's Disease

Doctors remain unable to state with certainty the cause of Alzheimer's disease. While there is no definitive cause of Alzheimer's disease, there are certain risk factors that may increase your chances of becoming a victim of this serious form of dementia. There are many health professionals who hypothesize that Alzheimer's is the result of a combination of factors. As you look at the various risk criteria outlined on the following page, it is worth noting that many of them can be proactively addressed.

Chemical Risk Factors

Imbalances in your body's delicate network of neurotransmitters, nutrient deficiencies, and metabolic deficits have all been implicated in the development and progression of the symptoms of Alzheimer's disease:

- Hyperhomocysteinemia, or high homocysteine levels, which is significantly correlated with low levels of the nutrients folic acid and vitamins B6 and B12
- Altered taurine metabolism—the body's ability to metabolize taurine, a nonessential amino acid necessary for the proper development and maintenance of the central nervous system—which may contribute to the memory loss that is characteristic of Alzheimer's when altered
- Low levels of DHEA, an adrenal hormone that declines with age
- Low levels of acetylcholine, serotonin, GABA, dopamine, and norepinephrine, which are all key neurotransmitters
- Estrogen imbalance

Environmental Risk Factors

External factors may play a role in the development and progression of symptoms of Alzheimer's disease. Such factors include exposures to neurotoxins, such as mercury, lead, pesticides, and excess iron; alcohol abuse; free radical damage; and aluminum exposure.

Social Risk Factors

Factors such as lower levels of education, lack of social contact, poor word fluency, emotional stress and/or poor stress-coping mechanisms, and the lack of willingness to learn new information and face mental challenges have all been implicated in the development and progression of the symptoms of Alzheimer's disease.

Physical Risk Factors

Possible physical risk factors include advanced age, a history of Parkinson's disease or Down's syndrome, head trauma, depression, reduced blood flow, stroke, olfactory deficits, gum disease or other markers for inflammation, or coronary disease.

Diagnosing Alzheimer's Disease

The presence of amyloid plaques and neurofibrillary tangles are the only definitive way to make a positive diagnosis of Alzheimer's disease. Progress is being made in using advanced imaging technologies and novel biomarkers to detect Alzheimer's disease and dementia before they reach the moderate stages. Unfortunately, even the powerful imaging tools used by doctors today cannot reliably scan for these markers. Only a brain biopsy or an autopsy can provide positive confirmation that Alzheimer's disease is the cause of an individual's dementia.

Because Alzheimer's is so common in the aging population, the medical profession has established some general protocols to arrive at a clinical diagnosis of Alzheimer's. By relying on a process of elimination, doctors rule out other possible causes of symptoms of cognitive failure.

Early detection of Alzheimer's disease is extremely difficult. Most clinical diagnoses are made in patients who have already developed a considerable amount of mental difficulties. Furthermore, the earliest signs of Alzheimer's disease can be extremely difficult to self-detect.

Stages of Alzheimer's Disease[2]

Experts have documented common patterns in the progression of symptoms of individuals with Alzheimer's disease and have created a system of "staging" the disease as it unfolds. The seven stages range from "no impairment" to "very severe decline." Stages 2 through 4 are considered early-stage; stages 5 and 6 are considered mid-stage, and stage 7 is considered late-stage Alzheimer's.

- Stage 1: No cognitive impairment.
- Stage 2: Very mild cognitive decline marked by memory lapses, especially forgetting familiar words or names, or the location

of everyday objects. Not generally apparent to friends, family, or coworkers.

- Stage 3: Mild cognitive decline that is noticeable to friends, family, or coworkers. Common difficulties may include problems remembering familiar names, decreased ability to remember new information, performance issues in work or social situations, inability to retain information, losing or misplacing valuable objects, and decline in ability to plan or organize.

- Stage 4: Moderate cognitive decline with clear-cut deficiencies, including decreased knowledge of recent occasions or current events; impaired ability to perform challenging mental exercises (e.g., counting backward from one hundred by sevens); decreased ability to perform complex tasks, such as bill paying, managing finances, or grocery shopping; reduced memory of personal history; and appearing subdued and withdrawn, especially in socially or mentally challenging situations.

- Stage 5: Moderately severe cognitive decline with major gaps in memory and deficits in cognitive function, including the inability to recall important details, such as address or phone number; confusion about days, dates, and the season; difficulty with less challenging mental exercises (e.g., counting backward from twenty by twos); and difficulty with performing abstract reasoning tasks, such as dressing appropriately for the season.

- Stage 6: Severe cognitive decline marked by worsening memory difficulties, significant personality changes, and need for assistance with routine daily activities.

- Stage 7: Very severe cognitive decline, with individuals unable to respond to their environment, speak recognizably, and, ultimately, control movement.

Diagnosing Alzheimer's Disease[3]

The Alzheimer's Association has developed a list of warning signs that include common symptoms of Alzheimer's. If you or someone close to you exhibits several of the symptoms listed below, you should see a doctor for a complete examination.

- memory loss, especially forgetting names, objects, places, times and dates; inability to recall recently learned information
- difficulty performing everyday tasks; forgetting to maintain personal hygiene
- problems with language; noticeable intellectual decline
- disorientation to time and place; tendency to wander from home or office
- poor or decreased judgment
- problems with abstract thinking; inability to follow simple instructions or stay focused on a task
- misplacing objects or putting things in unusual places
- changes in mood or behavior, especially rapid, unwarranted changes in emotion
- changes in personality, exhibiting extreme confusion, suspicion, fear, or dependence
- loss of initiative, depression, excessive sleeping during daylight hours

If you are concerned that you have symptoms of Alzheimer's disease, you should be thoroughly evaluated by a medical professional. Your doctor will take a current medical and psychological history, assess your neurological status, and evaluate your physical status. You should tell your doctor about any medications or supplements that you are taking. Some medications prescribed for other conditions can cause side effects that mimic some symptoms of Alzheimer's disease. Medical tests might include imaging scans, such as an MRI or CT; laboratory tests, such as blood and urine; neuropsychological tests, such as tests of memory, vision-motor coordination, and language function; and even a psychiatric evaluation to assess emotional factors.

It is important to remember that hormones are closely related to brain health. Hormone levels fluctuate with age, and the importance of consulting with an endocrinologist to assess hormone levels and balance in treating memory deterioration should not be underestimated. Hormones related to memory function include human growth hormone, vasopressin, DHEA, and pregnenolone.

To help your doctor rule out other causes of cognitive impairment, you should be prepared to discuss other possible causes of memory failure. Before settling on a diagnosis of Alzheimer's disease, carefully review the following areas with your doctor:[4]

- Medication interactions: Make a list of all substances you are taking, including prescription medications, vitamins, herbal supplements, over-the-counter products such as aspirin or cold medications, smoking cessation products, weight-loss products, and topical preparations, such as arthritis ointment.
- Physical conditions: Ask your doctor to ensure that you are not dehydrated. Dehydration can occur from episodes of vomiting or diarrhea or from heat exhaustion. Dehydration is common in older adults and can interfere with your body's ability to process medications or supplements.
- Brain traumas: Report any falls or blows to the head. Falls are common among older adults and can result in concussions and symptoms similar to those of Alzheimer's.
- Emotional status: The symptoms of depression can be remarkably similar to those of dementia. Discuss all possible

triggers, such as loss, significant life changes, or side effects of medication, all of which may be underlying causes of depression.

- Alcohol use: Consuming too much alcohol or using alcohol with certain medications may cause memory loss.

Combating Alzheimer's Disease Naturally

Scientists have not been able to point to a definitive underlying cause of Alzheimer's disease, nor have they been able to offer a cure for the symptoms. More often than not, conventional medicine recommends drug treatment with a variety of nonsteroidal anti-inflammatory drugs (NSAIDs) to stop the progression of Alzheimer's symptoms.

The progressively debilitating disease of Alzheimer's is a serious condition, and it is important to work with your health care provider to find the best treatment for your individual condition. There are safe and natural steps you can take to prevent memory loss, however. Even if you are worried you will develop Alzheimer's disease in later years, if you act now, you can help to prevent memory problems from interfering with your daily life.

Remembering and forgetting things is a perfectly normal part of daily life. But we need not fear that the extreme and progressive cognitive decline that is a symptom of Alzheimer's disease will be an inevitable part of our aging process. There are a number of things we can do to positively impact our brain health and overall mental abilities as we age.

In the Reboot Your Brain protocol for impacting Alzheimer's disease that follows, I tell you how you can make your environment more healthful, exercise your brain to retain memory and mental sharpness, and choose the best foods to help prevent the onset of Alzheimer's disease or to slow the progression of cognitive decline if you have been diagnosed with this condition.

Lifestyle

In late-stage Alzheimer's there is little that can be done to influence the mood swings, long-term memory loss, verbal outbursts, or delusions that are the hallmarks of the latest stages of the disease. There are several simple ways to prevent the onset of Alzheimer's, however, or to reduce the severity of symptoms if your doctor has diagnosed your memory loss as probable Alzheimer's disease. I have even included some coping strategies to make short-term memory loss less disruptive in your daily routine.

Environment

It is important for your environment to be free of hazardous toxins, particularly heavy metals that can accumulate in the body. High levels of aluminum and mercury are found in the brain cells of Alzheimer's patients. Limit your exposure to cookware, deodorants, antacids, and food additives that contain aluminum. Mercury is found in thermometers, thermostats, and dental amalgams. It is recommended to remove all silver fillings from your mouth. Chelation therapy—which uses certain amino acids to form strong ionic bonds with the toxic metals in your body, allowing them to be excreted from the system—may be useful in removing toxic metals and other chemicals from your body. Bentonite, a claylike substance that is used in a drink, may be taken at night to draw out toxins from the colon and assist in the detoxification process.

Installing charcoal filters on all water sources used for drinking or cooking can reduce or eliminate harmful toxins that are found in the water from our reservoirs.

Social Activity

Continued community involvement and frequent contact with friends and family may reduce your risk for Alzheimer's disease. In a paper presented at the Alzheimer's Association International Conference on the Prevention of Dementia, Jane Saczynski, PhD, of the National Institute on Aging, and colleagues presented data from a longitudinal study, conducted since 1965, that showed that subjects with decreased social activity from mid- to late life had a statistically significant risk of dementia.[5]

Exercise

Physical activity seems to play a role in slowing or preventing the progression of Alzheimer's. A National Institutes of Health news release cites research demonstrating that long-term physical activity increased the learning ability of mice and decreased the level of plaque forming beta-amyloid protein fragments in their brains.[6] Remaining physically active throughout our lifetimes offers immeasurable benefits to both body and brain. Physical activity does not have to be rigorous. Walking, dancing, or practicing yoga helps safeguard our brains against the type of cognitive decline that is a symptom of Alzheimer's disease.

Memory Skills and Brain Boosters

In addition to an active body, it is important to have an active mind. A study published in the *New England Journal of Medicine* supports the theory that mentally demanding activities can help stave off dementia.[7] The study involved 469 people ages seventy-five and older. Those participants who read, played games of strategy (e.g., checkers, backgammon, or chess), played musical instruments, or danced at least twice a week were significantly less likely to develop dementia. Those who did crossword puzzles four times a week were also found to have a significantly lowered risk. It seems clear that participating in mentally stimulating hobbies and being willing to learn new information and challenge our brains on an ongoing basis provide important benefits in preventing the symptoms of Alzheimer's disease.

Coping Strategies

If you or someone close to you has been diagnosed as being in the early stages of Alzheimer's, there are some strategies for coping with the symptoms of memory loss that may be the first hallmarks of this disease. These coping strategies will help relieve the stress and tension that arise from memory problems and can help lessen the impact of such problems on day-to-day life. Remember, in addition to practicing the strategies outlined below, you should make the lifestyle and nutritional changes I recommend in this chapter to slow or reverse the progression of these early symptoms.

- Establish a regular routine in familiar surroundings.
- Make mental associations, such as using landmarks, to help you find things.
- Repeat names when you meet people.
- Put important items, such as your keys, in the same place every time. Label or color-code doors and exits to keep from getting disoriented. Draw a map for simple routes. Write down directions.
- Make lists, use a calendar, and keep notes of important dates and financial matters.
- Set realistic daily goals.
- Keep track of when medicines are taken; use a chart or special pill box to stay current.
- Tell your doctor about all medications or supplements you are taking. Keep a list of important names and numbers near the telephone.
- Stay in frequent contact with family and friends.

Foods and Alzheimer's Disease

As research into the causes of Alzheimer's continues, researchers are concluding that there may be ways in which we can limit our risk of developing Alzheimer's disease. What these researchers are beginning to say now is something that I have said over and over again: Deficiencies of essential nutrients can lead to a variety of health problems and leave us vulnerable to serious conditions such as Alzheimer's. The good news is that it is never too early to start good nutritional habits that will help to protect the brain over a lifetime. And it is never too late to benefit from good nutritional habits.

Most Americans today eat foods that are over-processed and far from their natural state. These processed foods have been stripped of vital nutrients and filled with additives, processed sugars, and trans fats.

In addition to nutrients lost through poor diet, nutritional deficiencies may simply increase as we age. To help ensure that our bodies get the nutrients we need, we must make an effort to eat foods in their natural state. The best success that we have had helping people with Alzheimer's is to shift their diet to 75 percent raw and 25 percent lightly cooked. We begin with one 16-ounce glass of fresh, organic juice. The juice should have its primary volume filled with celery, cucumber, or apple. Then you can add into each different glass of juice any combination of grapes and berries. Begin with one 16-ounce glass per day for the first week. Add one additional juice per day for each additional week until you are at ten juices per day or as close to that many as possible. Juicing lettuce, radish, ginger, sprouts, and garlic also enhances its power. Supplement each juice with up to 1,500 milligrams of vitamin C (start with 500 milligrams until you achieve bowel tolerance).

Various studies support the efficacy of antioxidants as a method of preventing or reversing cognitive decline. Vitamins E and C are proven free radical fighters and are readily available in foods such as citrus fruits and juices; dark green, leafy vegetables; nuts; and sunflower seeds. The B vitamins, which play an important role in fighting the symptoms of Alzheimer's disease, are found in beans and animal proteins. Trace minerals, such as zinc, magnesium, and potassium, are easy to add to our diets by using whole grains, nuts, dried beans, bananas, and milk.

Essential fatty acids (EFAs) such as omega-3 and omega-6 fats, which are found in flax oil and walnuts, have significant anti-inflammatory properties and may be important in preventing Alzheimer's. It has been suggested that a dietary deficiency in fatty acids may be a risk factor for Alzheimer's. Other studies have looked at the use of EFAs in impacting Alzheimer's and found them to be beneficial.[9]

The Latest Research

Headlines were made in 2011 after a comprehensive study by researchers at the Oregon Health and Science University in Portland and the Linus Pauling Institute showed a clear link between brain deterioration, mental acuity, and our dietary choices. Lead author Dr. Gene Bowman and his colleagues discovered that seniors who consumed a diet high in the B vitamins, as well as vitamins, C, D and E, performed significantly better on mental ability tests and exhibited less brain shrinkage—an indicator of dementia—than did those who ate a poorer diet.[22] The results also suggested that higher consumption of omega-3 fatty acids improves the health of the brain, while eating trans-fats has the opposite effect.

Appearing in the *Journal of Alzheimer's Disease* in 2012 was new research into the power of two popular supplements in curbing brain degradation. Scientists at the University of California and the Scripps Institute revealed that vitamin D3 and curcumin (an antioxidant compound found in the spice turmeric) worked synergistically to help eliminate the buildup of amyloid, a toxic protein that is directly implicated in the progression of dementia and Alzheimer's disease.[23] These results are reinforced by recent articles published by researchers at the University of North Dakota and the University of Georgia College of Pharmacy, which indicated that antioxidant therapy holds great promise in mitigating cognitive decline and other symptoms associated with Alzheimer's disease.[24, 25] An additional study published in the *Journal of Alzheimer's Disease* in summer 2012 linked low blood serum levels of vitamin C and beta carotene with a higher incidence of mild dementia among seniors, once again pointing to the fundamental role of dietary nutrients in protecting against dementia and Alzheimer's disease.[26]

Numerous peer-reviewed studies published throughout the last few years offer new insight into the well-established connection between consuming unhealthy foods, overeating, and poor brain health. The dangers of a junk food diet are discussed in an article written last year by researchers at the University of Dundee in the United Kingdom. The authors highlight the association between higher fat and calorie intake and a greater incidence of cognitive degeneration in teenagers, concluding that "the increase in dementia in 'old-age' may have as much to do with 'new-age' lifestyle as it does with normal ageing."[27]

Further proof of this link was brought to light in a 2012 study by Dr. Suzanne de la Monte and fellow researchers at Brown University that examined the relationship between eating habits, brain health, and the hormone insulin. The team found that excess levels of insulin resulting from a diet rich in fatty and sugary foods decrease the brain's response to the hormone and, in turn, disrupt normal cognitive function.[28] The study, which was published in *New Scientist* magazine, implicates high insulin levels as a trigger of toxic amyloid proteins in the brain. The investigation also concluded that rats given an agent that prevented their brains from using insulin developed full-blown symptoms of Alzheimer's disease.

Research presented at the 2012 Alzheimer's Association International Conference offered strong evidence that engaging in regular physical exercise may effectively mitigate mild cognitive impairment. A group from Japan's National Center for Geriatrics and Gerontology shared new data showing that routine aerobic, strength, and balance exercise over the course of a year significantly improved language skills in adults with mild cognitive impairment over age forty-seven.[29] Another study presented by researchers at the University of British Columbia found that just six months of resistance training exercise boosted objective measurements of attention and memory in women with MCI ages seventy to eighty.[30]

Also in 2012, scientists from Rush University Medical Center in Chicago published a study in the journal *Neurology* showing a strong correlation between the physical activity levels of adults and Alzheimer's disease. Lead author Dr. Aron S. Buchman and his colleagues discovered that the individuals who were most physically active slashed their risk of Alzheimer's disease by 2.3 times compared to those people who led the least active lifestyles.[31]

A 2012 analysis undertaken by a team at the University of California, Berkeley, found that engaging in regular mental exercise can forestall cognitive degeneration on a fundamental level. Surveying a group of sixty-five adults over age sixty, the team measured how much time the subjects had devoted throughout their lives to mentally stimulating activities, such as reading books and writing letters or emails. The researchers discovered that those individuals who were mentally active over the course of their lives had significantly less buildup of the beta-amyloid protein.[32] While many studies have pointed to the short-term effectiveness of mental exercise in staving off cognitive illness, this study illustrates that keeping the mind active throughout life may help preserve brain health when we reach old age.

Recipes

In the following list are my recommendations for easy-to-prepare meals full of nutrients proven to help prevent and reduce the symptoms of Alzheimer's disease. The recipes can be found in Appendix II:

- Antioxidant Punch
- Blueberry and Pear Macadamia Nut Shake
- Brain Power
- Carrot, Pineapple, and Strawberry Juice
- Everglades Punch
- Flax Cruncher
- Free Radical Delight

- Nuts and Seeds
- Velvety Pecan Milk
- Four-Bean Salad
- Mixed Sprout, Bean, and Nut Salad
- Black Bean Soup
- Cream of Barley
- Nutty Oatmeal
- Gary's Veggieball Stew
- Indonesian Kale
- Pasta e Fagioli
- Sweet Kidney Bean Mash
- Heavenly Roasted Nuts

Supplements

Vitamins and Minerals

Certain vitamins and minerals are very important in fighting the symptoms of Alzheimer's disease.

Magnesium. Magnesium is well known for its calming properties in people with anxiety symptoms, but proper amounts of magnesium are generally lacking in the average American diet. Individuals who use oral contraceptives or diuretics, and who overuse laxatives, are at risk of magnesium deficiency. Magnesium also assists in impacting circulatory problems. For impacting the symptoms of Alzheimer's, I recommend a daily supplement of 500 to 1,000 milligrams of magnesium, taken in two equal doses on an empty stomach.

Potassium. Potassium is one of the most abundant minerals in the human body. Most of the time, supplementation with potassium is unnecessary, because it is readily available in our diet in such foods as bananas, orange juice, and potatoes. Potassium is depleted from our bodies in times of stress, thus upsetting the delicate balance of neurotransmitter communication in our brains. For this reason, potassium supplements may be useful in impacting Alzheimer's. Potassium can interact with some drugs, so if you are taking prescription medications, consult with your doctor before taking potassium supplements. If potassium is safe for you, I recommend a daily supplement of 500 milligrams.

Vitamin B-Complex. It is important that your daily vitamin B-complex contain sufficient amounts of both vitamin B9 and B12, as deficiencies in these vitamins can develop as we age, and these deficiencies can contribute to the symptoms of Alzheimer's disease. If your doctor has determined you are deficient in B vitamins, you may want to ask about receiving intravenous or injected supplements of vitamin B-complex to combat symptoms of Alzheimer's.

Vitamin C. Vitamin C may help delay the onset of Alzheimer's and slow the progression of symptoms. For best impact on the symptoms of Alzheimer's disease, I recommend increasing your daily supplement from 500 to 1,000 milligrams to 10,000 milligrams, taken in three divided doses. Do not exceed a daily supplement of 10,000 milligrams.

Vitamin E. Vitamin E has beneficial antioxidant properties, and treatment with high doses has shown initial promise in slowing the progression of symptoms in individuals with moderately severe Alzheimer's.[10] Because vitamin E has anticoagulant properties, and high doses may be associated with the risk of bleeding and interaction with anticoagulants and other medications often taken by elderly people, you should discuss high-dose vitamin E supplementation with your doctor. If you are not at risk, I recommend increasing your daily supplement of vitamin E from 268 milligrams to 536 milligrams, taken in two divided doses. Do not exceed a daily supplement of 536 milligrams.

Zinc. Many people who suffer from dementia have deficiencies in zinc. I recommend a daily supplement of 30 milligrams.

Smart Drugs and Nutrients

A number of other naturally occurring nutrients have a beneficial impact on the symptoms of Alzheimer's disease.

Acetyl-L-Carnitine (ACL). This versatile nutrient is able to permeate the blood–brain barrier to stimulate and fortify the brain's nerve cells. Acetyl-L-carnitine is a type of carnitine produced naturally in the brain. It can aid in directing fatty acids to the cell mitochondria, assisting in the creation of new cell energy. A powerful antioxidant, acetyl-L-carnitine also supplements the neurotransmitter acetylcholine. For best impact on Alzheimer's symptoms, I recommend increasing your daily supplement from 2,000 milligrams to 3,000 milligrams, taken in three equal doses. Do not exceed a daily supplement of 3,000 milligrams.

Dimethylaminoethanol (DMAE). This nutrient, found in sardines, is a powerful brain stimulant that increases acetylcholine, a neurotransmitter essential for short-term memory function and concentration. Some side effects associated with DMAE in Alzheimer's patients include drowsiness, high blood pressure, and increased confusion. If you experience these symptoms, stop taking the supplement for a few days, then return to your lower daily dose. I recommend increasing your daily supplement from 150 milligrams to 300 milligrams, taken in two equal doses with meals. Do not exceed a daily supplement of 300 milligrams.

L-Glutamine. Glutamine is one of the most abundant nonessential amino acids in the bloodstream. It is produced in the muscles and is able to pass freely through the blood–brain barrier. Once in the brain, it is converted into glutamic acid and increases GABA, a neurotransmitter essential for proper mental function. There are two types of glutamine supplements: D-glutamine and L-glutamine. L-glutamine is the form that more closely mimics the glutamine in the body. To impact the symptoms of Alzheimer's disease, I recommend supplementing with 500 milligrams, taken three times daily.

Melatonin. Melatonin is a hormone manufactured by the pineal gland in the brain. It is released into the bloodstream and is involved in synchronizing the body's hormone secretions and setting daily biorhythms. It is one of the body's most potent antioxidants.

To stabilize the sleeping cycle for Alzheimer's patients, I recommend supplementing with 300 micrograms to 1 milligram, taken nightly a half hour before bed.

N-Acetylcysteine (NAC). This amino acid protects the brain from damaging free radicals by boosting quantities of glutathione, one of the body's most powerful antioxidants. I recommend a supplement of 500 milligrams, taken three times daily.

Nicotinamide Adenine Dinucleotide (NADH). An enzyme that helps improve neurotransmitter function, NADH is present in all living cells and plays a critical role in energy production. It helps prevent cellular degeneration and may increase concentration and memory capacity. I recommend a supplement of 2.5 milligrams, taken twice a day for two or three days of the week.

Phosphatidylserine (PS). PS helps the brain use fuel more efficiently. By boosting neuronal metabolism and stimulating production of acetylcholine, PS may be able to improve the condition of patients in cognitive decline. Studies have revealed that supplementing with phosphatidylserine slows down and even reverses declining memory and concentration, or age-related cognitive impairment, in middle-aged and elderly subjects.[11]

As we grow older, aging slows the body's manufacturing of phosphatidylserine to levels that are detrimental to our functioning at our full mental capacity. For impact on memory loss, I recommend increasing your daily supplement from 300 milligrams to 400 milligrams. Do not exceed a daily supplement of 400 milligrams.

S-Adenosylmethionine (SAMe). SAMe (pronounced "sammy") has long been prescribed by European doctors as a treatment for depression. SAMe promotes cell growth and repair and maintains levels of glutathione, a major antioxidant that protects against free radicals and reduces homocysteine levels. Alzheimer patients have extremely low levels of SAMe in their brains. SAMe should not be taken if you are taking MAO inhibitor antidepressants. You should consult with your doctor before taking SAMe if you suffer from severe depression or bipolar disorder. If SAMe is safe for you to use, I recommend a daily supplement of 400 to 1,600 milligrams daily, taken in four equal doses.

Reboot Your Brain Chart of Additional Supplements for Impacting Alzheimer's Disease

The following chart summarizes the supplements I recommend adding to the protocol for overall brain health from chapter 2. In some cases, I recommend increasing the dose of a vitamin or supplement to specifically impact Alzheimer's disease. In these cases, you should increase the daily dosage from chapter 2 to the level recommended for this specific condition.

This protocol is designed for individuals who suffer from, or are specifically concerned about, Alzheimer's disease. If you are concerned about additional brain conditions discussed in other chapters, consult with a health professional about how you can safely impact multiple conditions.

If you are taking medications, whether prescription or over-the-counter, or have any food restrictions, consult with your doctor before beginning any supplement program. Your health care provider should always be up-to-date on all vitamins, supplements, and herbal or homeopathic remedies you are taking. Supplement overdoses are rare, but possible, and certain combinations may affect individuals adversely.

Supplement	Dosage	Cautions
acetyl-L-carnitine (ACL)	I recommend increasing your daily supplement from 2,000 mg to 3,000 mg, taken in three doses. Do not exceed a daily supplement of 3,000 mg.	

Supplement	Dosage	Cautions
dimethyl-aminoethanol (DMAE)	Increase daily dosage from 150 to 300 mg, taken in two equal doses with meals. Do not exceed a daily supplement of 300 mg.	Avoid if you have epilepsy or bipolar disorder, as DMAE can aggravate these conditions. If you have kidney or liver disease, consult with your doctor before taking DMAE. Some side effects associated with DMAE in Alzheimer's patients include drowsiness, high blood pressure, and increased confusion. If you experience these symptoms, stop taking the supplement for a few days, then return to your lower daily dose.
intravenous vitamin B-complex	Discuss with your health care provider whether you might benefit from injected vitamin B.	
L-glutamine	500 mg, taken three times daily	
magnesium	500–1,000 mg in two equal doses	Take on an empty stomach. If loose stools occur, decrease dosage. May take six weeks or more for effects to be felt.
melatonin	300 mcg–1 mg at night, a half hour before bed	Tolerance may develop with regular use. Long-term effects of nightly use are unknown.

Supplement	Dosage	Cautions
N-acetylcysteine (NAC)	500 mg three times daily	Regular supplementation of NAC increases urinary output of copper. If supplementing with NAC for an extended period, add 2 mg of copper and 30 mg of zinc to your daily supplement regimen.
nicotinamide adenine dinucle-otide (NADH, or coenzyme Q1)	2.5 mg twice daily, two or three times per week	High doses (10 mg per day or more) may cause nervousness, anxiety, and insomnia.
phosphatidyl-serine (PS)	Increase daily dosage from 300 mg to 400 mg. Do not exceed a daily supplement of 400 mg.	
potassium	500 mg daily	Do not take potassium supplements if you are taking medications for high blood pressure or heart disease, or if you have a kidney disorder. Consuming foods rich in potassium is okay. Do not exceed 3.5 g daily without consulting your doctor.
S-adenosyl-methionine (SAMe)	Dosage range of 400–1,600 mg	Raise the dose gradually from 200 mg twice a day to 400 mg twice a day, to 400 mg three times a day, to 400 mg four times a day, over a period of twenty days.

Supplement	Dosage	Cautions
vitamin C	Increase daily dosage from 500–1,000 mg to 10,000 mg, taken in three divided doses. Do not exceed a daily supplement of 12,000 mg.	
vitamin E	Increase daily dosage from 268 mg to 536 mg, taken in two divided doses. Do not exceed a daily supplement of 536 mg.	Vitamin E may cause increased risk of bleeding and may have adverse interactions with anticoagulants or other medications. Consult with your doctor.

Alternative Health Remedies

When suffering from a specific condition such as Alzheimer's disease, we can also try some natural treatment options that are considered alternatives to traditional medicine. While a healthful lifestyle and the proper nutritional and supplement plan are vital to winning the battle against the symptoms of Alzheimer's, there are some other targeted remedies that might help, too.

Herbal Remedies

Some herbal extracts and homeopathic treatments have properties similar to conventional medications, but are gentler and may lack the drugs' side effects. Always inform your medical practitioner of any herbal remedies you may be taking.

- **Butcher's broom** is an herb that promotes clearer focus and enhanced memory. I recommend a daily supplement of 850 milligrams, taken in two equal doses.

- **Bacopa monnieri** is a potent antioxidant that has been used in Ayurvedic medicine for centuries as a brain tonic to enhance memory, learning, development, and concentration. I recommend a daily supplement of 200 to 400 milligrams, taken in two equal doses.
- **Ginkgo biloba** is an herbal extract derived from the ginkgo biloba tree. It is commonly used in Europe to help fight Alzheimer's disease. Ginkgo biloba is a potent antioxidant that may be beneficial in impacting dementia-related symptoms. By improving circulation to the central nervous system, ginkgo biloba may help stabilize abnormal neurotransmitter communication in the brain. In a study conducted at the New York Institute for Medical Research, researchers found that almost one-third of Alzheimer's patients taking ginkgo supplements showed improvements in cognitive function during a double-blind, placebo-controlled clinical study.[12] Ginkgo can act as an anticoagulant, and individuals taking anticoagulant and antithrombotic drugs such as ASA, anti-inflammatories, and warfarin or Coumadin should consult with their doctors before taking ginkgo. If ginkgo is safe for you to take, for prevention of Alzheimer's disease I recommend a daily supplement of 120 milligrams, taken in two equal doses. For those suffering from more advanced stages of the disease, I recommend increasing your daily dose to 240 milligrams, spread out over three daily doses.
- **Kami Untan To (KUT)** is a Japanese herbal medicine that has been used for centuries in Japan to combat neuropsychiatric problems. In animal studies, KUT has been shown to increase choline acetyltransferase levels and nerve growth factor.[13] Later studies showed that KUT may be beneficial as an interventional strategy to fight Alzheimer's disease by slowing cognitive decline.[14] KUT is a blend of thirteen

different herbs and should be taken as directed by the manufacturer.

- **Huperzine A** is a compound isolated from a Chinese herb called *Hyperzia serrata*. It increases acetylcholine activity in the cortex and hippocampus sections of the brain and aids in improving memory as well as cognitive and behavioral functions. In a double-blind, placebo-controlled study conducted in China, 103 individuals with Alzheimer's disease received either huperzine A or a placebo twice daily for eight weeks. About 60 percent of the participants treated with huperzine A showed significant improvements in memory, thinking, and behavioral functions, compared to 36 percent of the placebo-treated subjects.[15] For an impact on Alzheimer's symptoms, I recommend taking a daily supplement of 100 to 200 micrograms in two equal doses.
- **St. John's wort (hypericum)** is very popular in Europe, so much so that it is actually covered by German health insurance as a prescription drug. I recommend taking a daily supplement of 300 milligrams twice per day.
- **Vinpocetine** is a derivative of an extract taken from the periwinkle shrub. It enhances circulation to the brain and may prevent or improve mild cognitive impairment. I recommend taking 10 milligrams twice daily with meals.

Homeopathic Remedies

The following remedies may be used to impact the symptoms of Alzheimer's. When dealing with a chronic condition, homeopathic remedies must be used in conjunction with other therapies, as prescribed by a qualified health professional. Consult with your health care provider before taking any homeopathic remedy, and follow their recommendation for the appropriate dosage. Always inform your medical practitioner of any homeopathic remedies you may be taking.

- **Alumina** is indicated for dealing with great weakness or loss of memory in cases where consciousness of personal identity is confused.
- **Anacardium** is used for absentmindedness; memory for names is most affected.
- **Calcarea** may help when the person is elderly, is wandering, and finds words difficult to remember.
- **Sulphur** can be used when there is difficulty remembering words or names.
- **Curcumin,** an extract from the spice turmeric, contains powerful anti-inflammatory properties that have been studied extensively in recent years. Research suggests that this compound inhibits the buildup of amyloid plaque in Alzheimer's patients.[12] I recommend taking a daily supplement of 400 to 800 milligrams. Do not take if you have gallbladder problems or gallstones. Consult with your doctor if taking anti-coagulant or anti-platelet medications or have a bleeding disorder
- **Fish Oil's** essential fatty acids are vital to healthy brain function. Studies demonstrate that these fats exert neuroprotective effects on the brain and may help slow the progression of Alzheimer's Disease.[13, 14] I recommend taking a purified fish oil supplement containing 1400 milligrams of EPA and 1000 milligrams of DHA daily. Consult with your doctor if taking anti-coagulant or anti-platelet medications or have a bleeding disorder.
- **Resveratol,** a type of antioxidant found in grapes and red wine, may help curb Alzheimer's Disease and dementia.[15] This substance has been shown to selectively target toxic amyloid plaque in brain tissue.[16] I recommend a daily dose of 250 milligrams. Consult with your doctor if taking anti-coagulant or anti-platelet medications or have a bleeding disorder.

Aromatherapy

Essential oils can be used in baths or inhaled to provide an energizing or soothing effect. Do not apply essential oils directly to the skin; they must be mixed with carrier oils. Experiment with various scents to see which help to alleviate the symptoms of Alzheimer's and increase mental clarity:

- bergamot
- clove
- frankincense
- lavender
- lemon balm

Summary

Contrary to mainstream medical belief, there are safe, natural, and nontoxic treatments for the symptoms of Alzheimer's disease. Research has demonstrated how these remedies can aid in preventing the onset of Alzheimer's or alleviating symptoms that have developed. In the past, Alzheimer's disease was considered an uncontrollable force that caused elderly patients to wither away and die. Taking action now can prevent our elder years from being characterized by cognitive degeneration and a rapid decline in health and ability.

Chapter 9

Headaches

"There are many good tunes played on an old fiddle."

—Old saying

Virtually everyone gets headaches, but not all headaches are the same. Recurring—or chronic—headaches, particularly migraine headaches, are one of the primary reasons people visit doctors. People who suffer from headaches also seek relief from hypnotherapists, chiropractors, and alternative health practitioners. Headaches, while not considered a disease, can indicate a serious underlying condition.

The good news is that as we grow older, our tendency to suffer from headaches decreases. Chronic headache onset is unusual in people older than fifty. Even migraines may lessen or disappear with age. The more concerning news is that headaches in older individuals can be a symptom of a more serious underlying illness.

Even if there is no illness causing your headaches, they can still be debilitating. Headaches can range from the pressure and pain of a tension headache to the pain of a migraine, which may be so severe that it prevents you from performing even the simplest task. According to the Migraine Awareness Group: A National Understanding for

Migraineurs (MAGNUM), approximately thirty-two million people in the United States today suffer from migraine headaches.

In this chapter, we'll look at types of headaches and their probable causes, including drug interactions or chemical changes in the brain. I discuss some important changes you can make in your lifestyle and diet to help prevent the onset of headaches. And I tell you what kinds of alternative treatments and remedies may provide you with relief from chronic headaches or migraines.

Understanding Headaches

Despite the number of trips to a doctor and missed workdays caused by severe headaches, they are not considered a disease. They can be symptoms of an illness, such as a viral or bacterial infection, allergies, or sinus infections. Fever may also cause headaches. Headaches can also be caused by factors such as hunger, stress, dehydration, drugs, sleep problems, head injuries, or certain foods.

Many doctors believe migraines are the result of a chemical or electrical problem in the brain. During a migraine, the cerebral blood vessels constrict tightly, and then quickly expand. Many believe that the nervous system, in response to a trigger such as stress, generates spasms in the nerve-rich arteries in the base of the skull. These spasms squeeze many of the arteries that supply blood to the brain, reducing the flow of oxygen-rich blood. In response to the lack of oxygen, cerebral arteries in the brain dilate, triggering the release of neurotransmitters that elicit inflammation and pain responses.

To prevent and impact occurrences of headache, it is important to understand what type of headache you may be suffering from. In the section that follows, we'll look at types of headaches that are common at any age.

Types of Headaches

In the discussion of types, diagnosis, and ways to impact headaches that follows, I briefly discuss several types of headache, but focus primarily on tension headaches—the most common type of headache—and migraine headaches—the most severe type of headache. Both have commonly identified triggers and generally exhibit positive responses to changes in nutrition and lifestyle.

Hypnic Headaches

This newly described type of headache, which occurs in elderly patients, is easy to recognize. Hypnic headaches—so called because they arise out of sleep—present as bilateral pain that lasts for thirty to sixty minutes, awakening patients from sleep one or two times each night. Hypnic headaches occur primarily in individuals over age sixty-five and respond well to treatment with medication (most often lithium, taken at bedtime).

Cluster Headaches

Cluster headaches come in groups. They can last for extended periods of time for days, weeks, or even months. Sufferers usually experience one or more headaches per day. Each headache may be relatively brief, lasting for thirty to ninety minutes, and may escalate in intensity during that time. In general, cluster headaches affect one side of the head, and the pain is centralized in the eye area on the affected side.

Exertion Headaches

Exertion headaches are connected to physical activities such as exercise, sex, laughing, and coughing. They generally occur during or just after the activity. In and of themselves they are not dangerous, but frequent exertion headaches may indicate an underlying physical state conducive to stroke or another serious condition.

Organic Headaches

Headaches that are the symptoms of a serious underlying physical condition, such as high blood pressure or brain tumors, are considered organic headaches. In addition to the headache pain, the sufferer may have fever, confusion, and/or trouble speaking or moving.

The pain tends to grow worse, increasing with each headache or striking more frequently.

Migraine Headaches

Migraines are less common in individuals over the age of fifty, but may first occur in our later years. Migraine headaches are characterized by severe, throbbing pain—often on one side of the head, though the entire head may be involved—and may be accompanied by lightheadedness and nausea and/or vomiting. Sufferers of migraines may be sensitive to sound, light, and smells. The pain from a migraine can last from a few hours to a few days.

Classic migraines strike on one side of the head and are preceded by warning signs called auras, which are commonly experienced as spots of light or changes in vision, although visual, auditory, and olfactory hallucinations also rarely occur. These auras precede the migraine attack by ten to thirty minutes.

A migraine attack can leave the sufferer listless, exhausted, and vulnerable to other mental or physical conditions.

Tension Headaches

Tension headaches are characterized by a dull, aching pain that radiates throughout the entire head. Some sufferers describe the feeling as having a tight band wrapped around their head. Tension headaches can start in the shoulders and neck and move upward to the back of the head. Stress, arguments, repressed anger, poor posture, depression, social problems, or major life changes can induce tension headaches. Tension headaches may also be a symptom of depression, especially in the elderly who have experienced a potentially traumatic or stressful event, such as retirement, forced relocation, reduced mobility or independence, or a serious illness.

Diagnosing Headaches

Chronic headaches, or headaches that change in character or suddenly develop in an older person, should be carefully evaluated. They may be the result of a drug interaction or carbon monoxide poisoning. Headaches may also be the symptom of a more serious condition, such as giant cell arteritis (a condition of the arteries of the optic nerves that can result in blindness), brain tumors, spinal degeneration, lung disease, or even a warning sign of stroke. Determining if you are suffering from tension headaches and migraine headaches can let you take steps to prevent future occurrences. Both of these types of headache also respond well to both conventional and alternative treatments.

Keeping a daily journal of headache occurrences may help you and your doctor to understand what is causing your headaches. I counsel migraine sufferers in my support groups to keep a detailed record of all medications and supplements they are taking, as well as all food and drink they consume. In addition to these daily accounts, I encourage them to record the frequency, location, duration, and timing of the headaches, as well as the type of pain and any tangential symptoms (e.g., nausea or vision disturbances) that accompany or precede the headache. Because a combination of triggers may be responsible for the occurrence of chronic headache, a journal such as the one I've described can reveal areas in lifestyle and nutrition where you need to make changes.

Women tend to suffer more from migraines, and hormones may play a role. Some women suffer from migraines during their menstrual periods. Other migraine sufferers may find that the headaches stop when they are pregnant. Women who take oral contraceptives may also be susceptible to migraines.

A number of medications, many of which are commonly prescribed as we grow older, may cause headaches. Your doctor may ask if you are taking any over-the-counter medications. He or she may also want to know if you take or have changed your dosage of any of the following commonly prescribed medications: cardiovascular drugs, such as vasodilator or nitroglycerin; anti-arrhythmia drugs; blood pressure medications; Parkinson's drugs, such as L-dopa; sedatives; stimulants, including caffeine; nonsteroidal anti-inflammatory drugs (NSAIDs); some analgesics; histamine blockers, such as Tagamet or

Zantac; bronchodilators; or antibiotics, especially trimethoprimsul-famethoxazole (Bactrim, Septa).

If you are worried about your headaches, or if they are disruptive to your daily functioning, you should consult with your health care provider. If your headaches follow a recent head injury, are associated with seizures, are so severe they prevent you from doing activities you want to do, wake you from sleep, cause blurred vision, eyespots, or other visual changes, or are associated with fever, vomiting, stiff neck, or tooth, jaw, or sinus pain, you should consult with your doctor immediately.

Tension and migraine are the most commonly diagnosed chronic headache conditions, and I discuss the symptoms of each in more detail below.

Symptoms of Tension Headaches

Tension headaches may happen daily or episodically. Episodic occurrences are usually the result of stressful events. This type of headache is generally of moderate intensity and responds well to nonprescription drugs or alternative treatment. Chronic tension headache usually occurs daily, and is associated with contracted muscles of the neck and scalp. Other symptoms of tension headaches are:

- feeling of pressure or tightness
- pain in the front of the head or eye area
- mild to moderate intensity
- duration of thirty minutes up to seven days
- no nausea or vomiting
- sensitivity to sound or light
- minimum of ten previous episodes; fewer than 180 days per year with headache
- occurs acutely when you are under emotional distress or intense worry
- may cause insomnia
- often occurs upon waking, or shortly thereafter
- not aggravated by physical activity

Symptoms of Migraine Headaches

Migraine headaches can be caused by heredity or by specific triggers—or by a combination of triggers. The pain may be felt in the whole head or just on one side. Some people experience an aura before a migraine attack, but most people do not have warning of when a migraine will strike unless they are aware of their own specific triggers for this type of headache. Symptoms of a migraine include:

- predictive aura, such as blind spots, flashing lights, and wavy or tunnel vision
- visual, auditory, or olfactory hallucination (rare)
- physical weakness or exhaustion
- throbbing pain
- duration of four to seventy-two hours
- nausea
- vomiting
- sensitivity to light or sound
- lightheadedness
- neurological abnormalities, such as confusion, seizures, or impairment of consciousness
- ocular muscle paralysis (rare)
- aphasia (rare)

Combating Headaches Naturally

Although the onset of debilitating headaches becomes less common as we grow older, those individuals who are prone to tension headaches or migraines may continue to experience them as they age. Taking steps to prevent these headaches at any age will lessen the chances of headaches becoming a factor in your brain health as you grow older. As I pointed out above, however, a medical professional should evaluate any sudden onset of headache in an elderly person to rule out drug interactions, an underlying medical condition, or the unusual syndrome of hypnic headaches.

In the Reboot Your Brain protocol for impacting headaches that follows, I suggest ways to use alternative therapies and nutritional strategies to prevent severe and debilitating headaches at any age.

Lifestyle

Attention to specific areas of your lifestyle can be crucial in preventing headache. Any behavior that promotes a healthful lifestyle, such as regular sleeping schedules, managing stress, practicing relaxation techniques, and staying physically fit, can reduce the frequency and intensity of both tension and migraine headaches. When the pain is in your brain, the importance of the mind–body connection becomes paramount.

Exercise

Studies have shown that moderate exercise can release endorphins and natural cortisol, which act to elevate mood and reduce stress. Aerobic exercise, such as dancing, walking, biking, or swimming, can help reduce the frequency of tension headaches. Gentle exercises, such as stretching, yoga, or even walking, can reduce discomfort while releasing stress. Exercise is also beneficial in normalizing sleep patterns and enhancing self-confidence. To ensure that you stay on a regular exercise regimen, I suggest that you choose a pleasurable activity and stick with it.

Meditation

Meditation acts to calm the mind and relieve stress. Twenty minutes, twice a day, of mindful meditation is recommended to prevent and reduce tension and stress. Engaging in breathing exercises and being generally aware of your breathing patterns throughout the day can be beneficial in eliminating headaches. Focusing on the positive aspects of life and nurturing an optimistic outlook will reduce the effects of stress on the body and aid in coping with headaches.

Posture

It may sound simple, and it is. Standing and sitting correctly can keep your muscles from tensing and triggering a tension headache. Good posture supports and protects all of your body, allowing you to move efficiently and with less fatigue. When standing, make sure your weight is evenly distributed on both feet, hold your shoulders back, and tuck in your chin. Pull in your abdomen and buttocks. When sitting, make sure your thighs are parallel to the ground and your head is not slumped forward. Try to avoid standing or sitting in one position for long periods of time. Take frequent breaks to move around and stretch. Make sure your shoes fit correctly, and do not make a habit of wearing high heels regularly.

Nutrition

An identical diet to that recommended for Alzheimer's, Parkinson's, ALS, and depression can be used here also—75 percent raw, 25 percent lightly cooked, and lots of juices daily.

Foods and Headaches

Studies indicate that a poor diet may be a significant factor in triggering headaches, particularly migraines. To prevent and impact migraine headaches, I recommend some very specific dietary guidelines.

One of the most important steps is the elimination of caffeine from your diet. Caffeine and caffeine-like substances found in coffee, tea, and many soft drinks can cause symptoms of anxiety, such as nervousness, fear, heart palpitations, nausea, restlessness, and tremors. Caffeine overstimulates the adrenal system and can deplete your body of important B-complex and C vitamins. It can cause stress and anxiety reactions in users. One study shows that patients with anxiety experienced a degree of anxiety that directly correlated with their consumption of caffeine. Even more astonishing, this report suggested that the persons most at risk for suffering from anxiety effects have a heightened sensitivity to the effects of just one cup of coffee.

Ironically, the process of eliminating caffeine from your diet may cause withdrawal headaches, as your body compensates for the lack of caffeine by producing more adenosine, a neurotransmitter that helps to regulate the diameter of the arteries in your head. As adenosine levels increase, your arteries dilate, and the excessive blood flow can then cause a throbbing headache. Once your body begins to regulate adenosine levels, however, the withdrawal headache will cease and you should remain headache-free.

Hypoglycemia (lowered blood glucose levels) is also directly correlated to headache and its related symptoms. To compensate for lowered glucose levels, your body releases insulin, a hormone that encourages glucose to move from the bloodstream into the cells. A sudden drop in blood sugar may cause the arteries in your brain to constrict, contributing to high blood pressure and headache. Maintaining proper blood sugar levels by avoiding refined carbohydrates is essential to controlling headaches.

Another common trigger for headaches is sensitivity to certain chemicals in foods. These chemicals include monosodium glutamate (MSG), a common flavor enhancer found in many processed foods; artificial sweeteners found in diet foods and diet soft drinks; nitrites, preservatives found in processed meats and some cheeses; and amines, a common compound found in a wide range of foods, including spinach, tomato, potato, tuna, liver, dark chocolate, and alcohol.

Phenols, a serotonin-depleting compound found in red wine, may also trigger migraines. Of course, drinking too much alcohol may not only trigger migraine headaches, but may also cause the headache of a hangover, which is due largely to dehydration.

Headache sufferers should be conscious of the foods they eat. Choose organic, chemical-free foods and eat regular meals to avoid hypoglycemic reactions. Keep a food journal that lets you see if there are food-related patterns to your headaches. When a headache occurs, review the foods you ate in the seventy-two hours prior to its onset to see whether you can identify any trends. If you suspect a particular food may cause headaches, try eating that specific food for a week and see whether it triggers a headache. If it does, avoid it in the future.

The Latest Research

The power of an herbal homeopathic treatment to alleviate migraines was the subject of a recent study published in the journal *Headache*. In the study, researchers administered a homeopathic blend of ginger and feverfew to patients suffering from migraine headaches. The results showed that 63 percent of those who took the herbal preparation experienced a reduction in pain, while only 39 percent in the placebo group noticed improvement. Compared to the placebo group, those who took the herbal treatment were twice as likely to be pain-free after two hours.[33]

A new study out of Sweden sheds light on the benefits of exercise in staving off migraine headaches. To carry out the study, scientists at the Sahlgrenska Academy at the University of Gothenburg divided ninety-one people into three groups. One group engaged a physical exercise regimen for forty minutes, three times a week; one practiced relaxation techniques; and one took the prescription medication topiramate (Topamax). All three groups witnessed a decrease in migraine frequency after three months, but in their conclusion, the authors focused on the promising outcomes of the exercise group.[34] Researcher Emma Varkey stated that "our conclusion is that exercise can act as an alternative to relaxations and topiramate when it comes to preventing migraines, and is particularly appropriate for patients who are unwilling or unable to take preventative medicines."[35]

Recipes

In the following list are my recommendations for easy-to-prepare meals full of nutrients proven to help prevent headaches. The recipes can be found in Appendix II:

- Antioxidant Supreme
- Apple Pear Ginger Ale

- The Big Cleanse
- Brain Juice
- Chlorophyll Boost
- Cucumber Coolade
- Delicious Detox
- Fatigue Buster
- Fountain of Youth
- Gingermint Tea
- Pure Citrus Punch
- Relax Your Mind
- Sleep Insurer
- Gary's Chef's Salad
- Nature's Total Salad
- Pasta Salad
- Chilled Cantaloupe Soup
- Creamy Tomato Soup
- Blueberry Breakfast Treat
- Gary's Vegetable Pan
- Original Broccoli Stir-Fry
- Blackberry Nectarine Fruit Salad

Supplements

Vitamins and Minerals

Certain vitamins and minerals are very important in the prevention of headache.

Magnesium. About half of the people who suffer migraines are deficient in the free and active form of magnesium called ionized magnesium.[2] Magnesium's role in fighting migraines is undeniable. It has the ability to relax muscles, including those that encircle the arteries. Magnesium also affects serotonin receptors.

A double-blind study conducted to examine the effectiveness of magnesium on migraines showed that when given to patients on a daily basis, it reduced migraine attacks by 42 percent after nine weeks.[3] If you suffer from migraines, I recommend a daily supplement of 1,000 milligrams of free-form magnesium from citrate. Be sure you are taking a daily B-complex vitamin along with the magnesium, as vitamin B3 plays an important role in aiding the absorption of magnesium.

Vitamin B2 (Riboflavin). Vitamin B2 is important in mitochondrial energy production. In individuals suffering from migraine, mitochondrial energy production may be low. To optimize this cellular energy production, I recommend increasing your daily supplement from 50 milligrams to 150 milligrams. Do not exceed a daily supplement of 150 milligrams.

Vitamin B3 (Niacin). Vitamin B3 may aid in preventing migraine headaches by opening constricted arteries and increasing blood flow. At the onset of a migraine aura, I recommend taking a supplement of 100 to 150 milligrams of vitamin B3.

Smart Drugs and Nutrients

Other naturally occurring nutrients may have beneficial impacts on headaches.

5-Hydroxytryptophan (5-HTP). 5-HTP is a form of the amino acid tryptophan that the body converts into serotonin and can be effective in preventing migraines. I recommend 50 to 100 milligrams daily.

Melatonin. Research has shown that migraine sufferers are low in melatonin,[4] a hormone produced by the pineal gland to aid in sleep and setting our circadian rhythms. Melatonin also has an anti-inflammatory effect and is a powerful antioxidant. To prevent migraines, I recommend a supplement of 300 micrograms to 1 milligram, taken a half hour before bed, two to three nights per week.

Reboot Your Brain Chart of Additional Supplements for Impacting Headache

The following chart summarizes the supplements I recommend adding to the protocol for overall brain health from chapter 2. In some cases, I recommend increasing the dose of a particular vitamin or supplement to specifically impact headache. In these cases, you should increase the daily dosage from chapter 2 to the level recommended for this specific condition.

This protocol is designed for individuals who suffer from, or are specifically concerned about, headache. If you are concerned about additional brain conditions discussed in other chapters, consult with a health professional about how you can safely impact multiple conditions.

If you are taking medications, whether prescription or over-the-counter, or have any food restrictions, consult with your doctor before beginning any supplement program. Your health care provider should always be up-to-date on all vitamins, supplements, and herbal or homeopathic remedies you are taking. Supplement overdoses are rare, but possible, and certain combinations may affect individuals adversely.

Supplement	Dosage	Cautions
5-hydroxytry pto-phan (5-HTP)	50–100 mg	Several months of treatment may be needed for maximum benefit. Nausea is the main side effect, but if it occurs, it usually dissipates within several days. Do not combine with prescription antidepressants. If you are taking prescription medication for depression, you should consult with your doctor before taking 5-HTP. Excess levels of serotonin in the blood can be dangerous in case of coronary artery disease.
magnesium	Up to 1,000 mg	May take six weeks or more for effects to be felt.

Supplement	Dosage	Cautions
melatonin	1–5 mg two to three nights per week	Tolerance may develop with regular use. Long-term effects of nightly use are unknown.
vitamin b2	Increase daily dosage from 50 mg to 150 mg. Do not exceed a daily supplement of 150 mg.	Must build up to a therapeutic level. May not show results for several months.
vitamin b3	At the onset of migraine aura, take 100–150 mg.	High doses of niacin may cause a "hot flash" sensation. Some varieties are advertised as "flush free" and prevent this effect.

Alternative Health Remedies

When suffering from a specific condition like headache, we can also try some natural treatment options that are considered alternatives to traditional medicine. While a healthful lifestyle and the proper nutritional and supplement plan are vital to winning the battle against headaches, there are some other targeted remedies that might help, too.

Herbal Remedies

Some herbal extracts and homeopathic treatments have properties similar to conventional medications, but are gentler and may lack the drugs' side effects. Always inform your medical practitioner of any herbal remedies you may be taking.

- **Butterbur** is an herb native to Europe, Asia, and Africa. It is used in Germany to alleviate migraines. Butterbur's principal components are petasin and isopetasin, which are believed to slow the body's production of leukotrines substances that can cause an inflammatory response and constricted blood cells. I recommend a daily supplement of 75 milligrams.

- **Feverfew** is an herb with anti-inflammatory and pain-relieving properties commonly used in Europe to impact migraine headache, especially the type with vomiting and sensitivity to noise and light. I recommend a daily dose of 250 milligrams.
- **Ginkgo biloba** enhances cerebral circulation and oxygen flow to the brain tissue. I recommend a daily dose of 120 milligrams, taken in two equal doses with meals. Ginkgo can act as an anticoagulant, and individuals taking anticoagulant and antithrombotic drugs such as ASA, anti-inflammatories, and warfarin or Coumadin should consult with their doctor before taking ginkgo.
- **Valerian** acts as a mild sedative and may play a role in helping lower blood pressure. For migraine relief, I recommend taking 300 to 500 milligrams.
- **White willow bark** is commonly used in Germany as an alternative to aspirin for headache pain. I recommend taking 60 to 120 milligrams per day for relief of headache pain.

Homeopathic Remedies

The following remedies may be used for both temporary and acute cases of headache. When dealing with a chronic condition, homeopathic remedies must be used in conjunction with other therapies, as prescribed by a qualified health professional. Consult with your health care provider before taking any homeopathic remedy, and follow your provider's recommendation for the appropriate dosage. Always inform your medical practitioner of any homeopathic remedies you may be taking.

- **Bryonia** is indicated when the headache is left-sided, over the left eye or forehead, and worse when coughing.

- **Ferrum** is suggested for a continuous headache lasting two to three days. Headache can be in one spot on the left temple or a general frontal headache.
- **Gelsemium** is used for a headache that begins at the neck and gradually moves to the forehead.

Acupuncture

Acupuncture may provide relief from chronic headache pain. By listening to your symptoms and examining your appearance and pulse, acupuncturists can diagnose and impact headaches.

Acupuncture releases tension in the muscles. It causes a relaxation response in the body, resulting in lowered blood pressure and heart rate. Acupuncture increases the flow of blood, lymph, and nerve impulses to affected areas and decreases stress while promoting feelings of well-being and energy.

Therapeutic Touch

A variety of treatments involve the transfer of energy from the practitioner to the patient, which can help relieve pain and anxiety. In one study, massage reduced anxiety and lowered saliva cortisol levels (a key measurement of stress). Massage can be very effective at removing tension from the muscles and may provide relief from headache pain.

Reiki. Pronounced "ray-kee," this method employs a powerful, hands-on healing technique in which the universal life force energy is channeled through the practitioner and transferred to the patient. Chronic stress and anxiety can deplete the energy in our bodies. Reiki is used to support the body's natural ability to heal itself. It releases spiritual and emotional blocks and brings a feeling of harmony and vitality.

Massage. This popular technique can enhance general relaxation and provide an outlet for stress and tension. Massage therapy can reduce feelings of anxiety, promote better sleep patterns, and increase feelings of well-being.

Shiatsu. This form of physical therapy combines traditional Chinese medical theory and various Japanese massage techniques. The therapist uses direct pressure with hands and fingers to redirect the flow of energy throughout the body. Shiatsu treatment is deeply relaxing and can be beneficial in both chronic and acute conditions.

Dental Devices. Many people who experience tension or migraine headaches also grind their teeth during sleep—a practice called bruxism. A device called an NTItension suppression system (NTItss) is created and fit by a dentist and is worn while sleeping as a guard against tooth grinding and jaw clenching.

Craniosacral Therapy. This gentle form of manipulation is a hands-on healing technique that manipulates the craniosacral system the soft tissues and bones of the head (cranium), the spine down to its tail (sacrum), and the pelvis, as well as the membranes and cerebrospinal fluid that surround these areas to reestablish the normal flow of the cerebrospinal fluid. The practitioner uses an extremely light touch to palpate, or feel, areas to detect a fluctuation in the cerebrospinal fluid, and then manipulates the area to clear blockages and correct the flow. This therapy is beneficial in reducing stress, improving the quality of sleep, and enhancing the general functioning of the body's organs.

Neurofeedback

Also known as brainwave training or EEG biofeedback, this technique is being used as a safe, drug-free alternative to impact stress, migraines, chronic pain, seizures, and more. Painless electronic sensors are placed on the scalp and earlobes. These sensors record the brain's activity, registering relaxed and focused brain waves with a video game–like pattern on a computer screen. When the mind drifts, the screen goes blank. Neurofeedback is being used to reset particular brain patterns associated with certain illnesses or conditions, so that the brain is able to perform at optimal levels. The effects that are experienced with the computerized biofeedback device are practiced and learned until the exercise and its effect on the brain can be reproduced at home without the device.

Aromatherapy

Essential oils can be used in baths or inhaled to provide rebalancing effects. Do not apply essential oils directly to the skin; they must be mixed with carrier oils. Some of the scents below may be effective in easing headache pain:

- eucalyptus
- ginger
- lavender
- peppermint
- rosemary
- sandalwood
- wintergreen

Summary

The Reboot Your Brain program in this chapter stresses the importance of nutrition and lifestyle modification, both in preventing and impacting chronic headaches. Remember, anything that impacts this disorder can be used to prevent it from occurring. Headaches have many causes, and the appropriate treatment will vary from person to person. Addressing all aspects of physical, mental, and emotional health will help prevent chronic and debilitating headache pain.

Chapter 10

Brain Trauma

"40 is the old age of youth; 50 is youth of old age."

—Victor Hugo

Trauma to the brain can result from even the mildest of head injuries. In fact, approximately 80 percent of patients with traumatic brain injury (TBI) have the condition as a result of a seemingly innocuous accident or event.[1] Blows to the head, falls, automobile accidents, and even whiplash can cause our brains to suffer harm sufficient enough to cause physical, mental, or emotional symptoms that range from moderate to severe.

Unlike some of the other conditions discussed in this book, there is not always something you can do to prevent an accident from happening. If you do have an accident that causes head injury and possibly brain trauma, you must treat the situation with appropriate concern. Rehabilitation can be a long process, and your symptoms and needs may change as your recovery progresses. If you have suffered a trauma to your head, and are being treated for or recovering from a brain injury, you need to take it seriously. Consult with your doctor and be sure to inform him or her of any methods you are utilizing to speed recovery and support your brain's health.

In this chapter I focus on ways you can help your brain heal from a trauma, including which nutrients and supplements fortify and protect the brain, and alternative measures that may provide relief from some of the symptoms of brain trauma.

Understanding Brain Trauma

Severe brain injuries can be permanently disabling, leaving the individual with a host of symptoms that must be addressed. More mild injuries, if left untreated, can also have serious consequences. Secondary cell death may cause wide and diffuse damage for months or years after the initial injury. The cortex, thalamus, and hippocampus—areas of the brain critical to memory and cognitive processing—are particularly vulnerable to such cellular decay.

In addition to ongoing damage to brain cells, one of the most serious aspects of TBI is that the trauma not only kills or injures the brain cells either at the time of the injury or during some interval thereafter, but also hampers brain plasticity, which is the ability of damaged brain cells to repair themselves.[2]

Studies have also established a link between TBI and Parkinson's disease.[3] Individuals with TBI may also have a higher incidence of psychiatric conditions.[4] The study reported that the rate of psychiatric disorders one year after a TBI is considerably higher when measured against members of the general population who have not suffered a brain injury. Depression was found to be nearly seven times more likely in the brain injury group than in the general population.

Let's look at the areas of your brain that may be affected by trauma and the types of symptoms that may result.

Types of Brain Trauma

Trauma to the brain results in a variety of physical, mental, and emotional symptoms, depending on which part of the brain is injured.

Following are some of the most common symptoms of brain trauma related to specific areas of injury in the brain.

Frontal Lobe (Forehead)

Trauma to the frontal lobe of the brain can result in difficulty with movement or paralysis. It can interfere with your ability to orchestrate complex or multiple movements. A person with injury to the frontal lobe may become fixed on a single thought or be unable to concentrate while working on a particular task. He or she may have trouble finding the correct words or otherwise communicating with language. Emotional instability and personality changes are also characteristic of trauma to the frontal lobe.

Parietal Lobe (Top Back of Head)

An injury to the parietal lobe affects memory, causing sufferers to be unable to recall the correct names of objects or find the correct word when writing. They may experience difficulty in reading and simple mathematics. Difficulty in hand–eye coordination may occur and drawing can be difficult. An individual with parietal lobe injury may be unable to discern left from right and often experiences extreme difficulty in multitasking.

Occipital Lobe (Back of Head)

Trauma to the occipital lobe commonly results in vision problems, including the inability to recognize colors, words, or the movement of an object. A person with an occipital lobe injury may hallucinate and may have trouble reading or writing.

Temporal Lobe (Above the Ears)

Injury to the temporal lobe of the brain causes short-term memory loss and may cause problems with long-term memory. Individuals may have difficulty recognizing faces and understanding spoken words. Fluctuations in an individual's sex drive may occur. Damage to the right temporal lobe may result in persistent talking.

Brain Stem (Deep Inside the Brain)

Injuries that cause trauma to the brain stem are very serious and often life-threatening. A decreased capacity for breathing may limit an individual's ability to speak. The person may experience dizziness and nausea, problems with balance and movement, and difficulty perceiving and organizing the environment. Sleeping difficulties, such as insomnia and sleep apnea, may occur. More serious problems include the inability to swallow food or liquids.

Cerebellum (Base of the Skull)

Traumatic injury to the cerebellum causes the loss of fine motor abilities, tremors, dizziness, and even the ability to walk. It can cause an individual to have difficulty in reaching out and grabbing objects or making rapid movements. Slurred speech is a common symptom of trauma to the cerebellum.

Diagnosing Brain Trauma

TBI happens when a sudden event harms the brain. Such trauma can be the result of an external blow to the head, such as might be suffered in a car accident or when an object goes through the skull, damaging the brain tissue. When a TBI occurs and the skull has not been fractured, it is referred to as a closed-head injury.

An accident does not have to fracture your skull or cause lacerations or broken bones, or even cause you to lose consciousness, for brain trauma to result. Whiplash or a seemingly innocuous blow to the head can cause serious injury, without your ever losing consciousness.

Traumatic brain injuries are usually rated as mild, moderate, or severe, depending on how long the symptoms last and whether you lose consciousness. But my contention is that any damage to the brain is serious damage and needs to be treated with appropriate concern. Hippocrates, the father of medicine, said it best: "No head injury is too severe to despair of nor too trivial to ignore."

If you experience an injury to your head, a medical professional should carefully assess the level of trauma sustained by your brain. Experienced medical staff can stabilize your condition. In any head injury, it is crucial that the brain continues to receive the proper amount of oxygen and blood flow. This is important, both in treating the immediate condition of brain trauma and for your future brain health.

Being informed about the type of trauma to your brain will let you take preventive steps that will protect your brain as it heals and keep it healthy for a lifetime.

Symptoms of Brain Trauma

The symptoms of traumatic brain injury depend on the extent of the injury suffered. Such symptoms may include:

- persistent headache
- disorientation
- confusion
- lightheadedness
- vertigo
- blurred vision
- ringing in the ears
- change in sleeping patterns
- mood or personality changes
- difficulty concentrating or maintaining attention
- memory lapses
- nausea
- seizures
- dilated pupils
- slurred speech

Combating Brain Trauma Naturally

Combating brain trauma naturally depends foremost on getting an accurate medical assessment of the type of injury the brain has sustained and the prognosis for the individual's recovery from a wide range of symptoms. A medical professional should immediately evaluate any head injury. A doctor can order X-rays, MRI, or PET scans and the tests necessary to determine the extent and seriousness of the injury and can assure that the brain receives vital oxygen and nutrients immediately following a traumatic incident.

While you must follow your doctor's orders for treating a head or brain injury, there are certain things you can do to help protect your brain during this vulnerable time and speed healing and recovery. In the Reboot Your Brain protocol that follows, I recommend natural techniques for relief from symptoms of brain injury, as well as methods for revitalizing and rebuilding the vital brain connections that may have been interrupted by brain trauma.

Lifestyle

While no one can prevent every accident that may result in a traumatic brain injury, there are a few simple safety rules that can offer important protection against head injury:

- Wear helmets when participating in such sports as baseball, hockey, or horseback riding.
- Wear helmets when riding bicycles or motorcycles.
- Wear a seat belt when riding in a car.
- Make sure area rugs are nonslip to prevent falls.
- Use caution in the bathtub and shower; be sure to use a bathmat to help prevent falls.
- If you are experiencing dizziness or vertigo, consult with a medical professional to treat conditions that may cause a fall.
- Use caution when walking in slippery conditions such as ice or snow or on wet floors. Older people can have difficulty with their balance and should be especially careful when the footing is treacherous.

Nutrition

Foods and Brain Trauma

The proper nutrition can keep your brain strong and can help it to recover from damage from trauma. After a TBI, your brain is particularly vulnerable as it struggles to halt or repair cell damage. Diets rich in antioxidants can aid in the recovery of memory, halt brain cell loss, and improve the brain's function in all areas. Scientists believe the free radical cleansing effect of antioxidants is vital in preventing damage to the brain on a cellular level. In the nutritional plan provided in chapter 2, I give you guidelines for a brain-healthy eating plan. To help your brain recover from an injury and help support its return to optimal functioning, I recommend that you review this chapter and the following plan for healthy eating, with a focus on antioxidant-rich foods.

Recipes

In the following list are my recommendations for easy to prepare meals full of nutrients proven to help the brain recover from trauma. The recipes can be found in Appendix II:

- Antioxidant Punch
- Antioxidant Supreme
- Brain Juice
- Brain Power
- Chlorophyll Boost
- Enzyme Enhancer
- Fountain of Youth
- Green Power Punch
- Super Vegetable Cocktail
- Wisdom Drink
- Herbed Tomato Salad
- Superior Spinach Salad

- Cream of Sweet Potato Soup
- Papaya Nectar Soup
- Blueberry Breakfast Treat
- Gary's Veggieball Stew
- Macaroni Marconi
- Potato Chowder
- Tantalizing Tempeh Dinner
- Carob Power Brownies
- Cold Cherry Soup

Supplements

Vitamins and Minerals

Certain vitamins and minerals are very important in protecting the brain from the symptoms of brain trauma.

Lecithin/Choline. Choline, a key component of lecithin, is a building block of acetylcholine, a key neurotransmitter that may aid in brain injury rehabilitation.[5] By encouraging brain wiring growth, acetylcholine can help the brain regain plasticity and repair damaged circuitry. Levels of acetylcholine are known to decline with age, and studies have shown that supplementation with choline can improve memory and learning. I recommend increasing your daily lecithin supplement from 1 gram to 2.5 grams for men and 2 grams for women. Take in two divided doses and do not exceed a daily supplement of 2.5 grams for men and 2 grams for women.

Vitamin C. In one study that examined the effects of free radical damage in patients with TBI, plasma levels of vitamin C were determined to be appreciably lower in patients with TBIs than in the control patients in the study. Furthermore, the vitamin C levels in TBI patients were inversely related to the diameter of the injury. In cases of brain trauma, I recommend increasing your daily supplement from 1 gram to 3 grams. Do not exceed a daily supplement of 3 grams.

Smart Drugs And Nutrients

Other naturally occurring nutrients may have beneficial impacts on the symptoms of brain trauma.

Curcumin. According to a recent study, this antioxidant, found in foods such as mustard and turmeric, has the potential to combat the effects of a TBI.[6] The study found that curcumin decreased the accumulation of damaging beta-amyloid proteins that can interfere with neural functioning in the brain.

Another study conducted at the UCLA labs looked at curcumin's protective benefits following a traumatic brain injury.[7] In this study, rats were placed on a curcumin-based diet for three weeks prior to experiencing a concussion similar to that which an individual might experience in an auto accident. With this type of injury, most rats experienced a decrease in capacity for learning and memory. The brains of the rats maintained on the curcumin diet, however, were protected. To impact traumatic brain injury, I recommend a supplement of 500 milligrams, taken three times daily.

Nimodipine. Nimodipine dramatically improves blood flow in the brain by acting as a barrier to calcium in blood cells, allowing the cells to relax and raising the amount of blood and oxygen available to the brain. I recommend taking 100 milligrams four times daily.

Dimethylaminoethanol (DMAE). This nutrient, found in sardines, is a powerful stimulant that increases acetylcholine levels. Acetylcholine is an important neurotransmitter in the brain. It plays a role in memory, concentration, and focus. I recommend increasing your daily supplement from 150 milligrams to 650 to 1,650 milligrams.

N-Acetylcysteine (NAC). This amino acid protects the brain from damaging free radicals by boosting quantities of glutathione, one of the body's most powerful antioxidants. I recommend a supplement of 500 milligrams taken three times a day.

Picamilon. Picamilon is used in Russia to treat brain inflammation, enhance cognitive abilities, and promote brain energy. Picamilon is a compound substance consisting of niacin and the neurotransmitter

GABA. The niacin facilitates the passage of GABA through the blood–brain barrier, enhancing cerebral circulation and improving overall brain function. I recommend taking 100 milligrams, three times daily.

Phosphatidylserine (PS). PS helps the brain use fuel more efficiently. It boosts neuronal metabolism and stimulates production of acetylcholine. As we grow older, aging slows the body's manufacturing of phosphatidylserine to levels that are detrimental to functioning at our full mental capacity. In the case of a brain trauma, it is even more critical for our brains to be able to access this vital neurotransmitter. To help your brain recover from a TBI, I recommend increasing your daily supplement from 300 milligrams to 400 milligrams. Do not exceed a daily supplement of 400 milligrams.

Reboot Your Brain Chart of Additional Supplements for Impacting Brain Trauma

The following chart summarizes the supplements I recommend adding to the protocol for overall brain health from chapter 2. In some cases, I recommend increasing the dose of a vitamin or supplement from chapter 2 to impact a specific condition.

This protocol is designed for individuals who suffer from, or are specifically concerned about, brain trauma. If you are concerned about additional brain conditions discussed in other chapters, consult with a health professional about how you can safely impact multiple conditions.

If you are taking medications, whether prescription or over-the-counter, or have any food restrictions, consult with your doctor before beginning any supplement program. Your health care provider should always be up-to-date on all vitamins, supplements, and herbal or homeopathic remedies you are taking. Supplement overdoses are rare, but possible, and certain combinations may affect individuals adversely.

Supplement Dosage Cautions: Consult your physician before beginning any major treatment protocol.

Supplement	Dosage	Cautions
Lecithin/choline	Increase daily dosage from 1 g to 2.5 g for men and 2 g for women. Take in two divided doses, and do not exceed a daily supplement of 2.5 g for men and 2 g for women.	Side effects may include nausea, bloating, vomiting, sweating, and diarrhea; extremely large doses can cause a heart-rhythm abnormality. Do not use if you have bipolar disorder.
curcumin	500 mg up to three times daily	
dimethylaminoethanol (DMAE)	Increase daily dosage from 150 mg to 650–1650 mg.	May be overstimulating for some people. Headaches, muscle tension, and irritability may occur. Do not take if you have epilepsy, or a history of convulsions, or bipolar disorder. If you have kidney or liver disease, consult your doctor before taking this supplement.
N-acetylcysteine (NAC)	500 mg three times daily	Regular supplementation of NAC increases urinary output of copper. If supplementing with NAC for an extended period, add 2 mg of copper and 30 mg of zinc to your supplement routine.

Supplement	Dosage	Cautions
nimodipine	100 mg four times daily	
picamilon	100 mg three times daily	If taking prescription drugs or MAO inhibitors, consult with your doctor before using.
phosphatidylserine (PS)	Increase daily dosage from 300 mg to 400 mg. Do not exceed a daily supplement of 400 mg.	
vitamin C	Increase daily dosage from 1 to 3 g. Do not exceed a daily supplement of 3 g.	

Alternative Health Remedies

When suffering from a specific condition such as brain trauma, we can also try some natural treatment options that are considered alternatives to traditional medicine. While a healthful lifestyle and the proper nutritional and supplement plan are vital to winning the battle against brain trauma, there are some other targeted remedies that might help, too.

Herbal Remedies

Some herbal extracts and homeopathic treatments have properties similar to conventional medications, but are gentler and may lack the drugs' side effects. Always inform your medical practitioner of any herbal remedies you may be taking.

Ginkgo biloba enhances cerebral circulation and oxygen flow to the brain tissue. I recommend a daily dose of 120 milligrams, taken in two equal doses with meals. Ginkgo can act as an anticoagulant, and individuals taking anticoagulant and antithrombotic drugs such as ASA, anti-inflammatories, and warfarin or Coumadin should consult with their doctor before taking ginkgo.

Homeopathic Remedies

The following remedy may be used for both temporary and acute cases of brain trauma. Depending on the nature of the symptoms caused by a TBI, other homeopathic remedies may be appropriate to impact specific conditions, such as memory loss or depression. A qualified homeopathic practitioner will be able to advise you regarding specific remedies for impacting the after-effects of a brain injury. When dealing with a chronic condition, homeopathic remedies must be used in conjunction with other therapies, as prescribed by a qualified health professional. Consult with your health care provider before taking any homeopathic remedy, and follow your provider's recommendation for the appropriate dosage. Always inform your medical practitioner of any homeopathic remedies you may be taking.

Arnica can help in controlling bleeding and swelling in the brain. It should be given as soon as possible after the brain injury occurs.

Therapeutic Touch

A variety of treatments involve the transfer of energy from the practitioner to the patient, which can help to relieve pain and anxiety and may be helpful in promoting healing of a brain suffering from a traumatic injury.

Reiki. Pronounced "ray-kee," this method employs a powerful, hands-on healing technique in which the universal life-force energy is channeled through the practitioner and transferred to the patient. Chronic stress and anxiety can deplete the energy in our bodies. Reiki is used to support the body's natural ability to heal itself. It releases spiritual and emotional blocks and brings a feeling of harmony and vitality.

Shiatsu. This form of physical therapy combines traditional Chinese medical theory and various Japanese massage techniques.

The therapist uses direct pressure with hands and fingers to redirect the flow of energy throughout the body. Shiatsu treatment is deeply relaxing and can be beneficial in both chronic and acute conditions.

Craniosacral Therapy. This gentle form of manipulation is a hands-on healing technique that manipulates the craniosacral system—the soft tissues and bones of the head (cranium), the spine down to its tail (sacrum), and the pelvis, as well as the membranes and cerebrospinal fluid that surround these areas—to reestablish the normal flow of the cerebrospinal fluid. The practitioner uses an extremely light touch to palpate, or feel, areas to detect a fluctuation in the cerebrospinal fluid, and then manipulates the area to clear blockages and correct the flow. This therapy is beneficial in reducing stress, improving the quality of sleep, and enhancing the general functioning of the body's organs.

Neurofeedback

Also known as brainwave training or EEG biofeedback, this technique is being used as a safe, drug-free alternative to prevent stress, migraines, chronic pain, seizures, and more. Painless electronic sensors are placed on the scalp and earlobes. These sensors record the brain's activity, registering relaxed and focused brain waves with a video game–like pattern on a computer screen. When the mind drifts, the screen goes blank. Neurofeedback is being used to reset particular brain patterns associated with certain illnesses or conditions, so that the brain is able to perform at optimal levels. The effects that are experienced with the computerized biofeedback device are practiced and learned until the exercise and its effect on the brain can be reproduced at home without the device.

Prayer

For centuries people have been debating the efficacy of the role of prayer in healing. A scientific study, however, showed that those who prayed demonstrated healthier behaviors than those who did not.[8] Another study has shown that those in a test group who had a stronger belief in prayer had better physical functioning and higher mental health scores.[9] Traditional medicine practitioners may not point you in the direction of prayer; they prefer neatly boxed, quantifiable solutions to healing injuries. My feeling is that when an effective treatment for a condition is reported, whether it fits into the scientific box or not, it must be given some credit. When combating TBIs with alternative modalities, I urge you not to be afraid to think outside the box.

Hyperbaric Oxygen Therapy (HBOT)

Hyperbaric oxygen therapy improves the body's natural healing mechanism process by increasing oxygen levels in the blood. HBOT is a process of inhalation therapy that utilizes 100 percent oxygen in a total body chamber where atmospheric pressure can be increased and controlled. This direct delivery of oxygen allows the body's white blood cells to attack bacteria; it lessens swelling and enables new blood vessels to grow at a faster rate in injured parts of the body. HBOT can be used for both preventive and curative purposes.

Aromatherapy

Essential oils can be used in baths or inhaled to provide rebalancing effects. Do not apply essential oils directly to the skin; they must be mixed with carrier oils. Some of the scents below may be effective in easing the symptoms of brain trauma:

- chamomile
- geranium
- juniper
- lavender
- marjoram
- myrrh
- rose
- tea tree

Summary

No two individuals will experience the effects of brain trauma in the same way. Treatment and rehabilitation will need to be tailored to specific symptoms and resulting conditions. If you have suffered a traumatic brain injury, you need to support your brain's healing process with good nutrition and complement your doctor's prescribed programs and treatments with alternative healing modalities.

Chapter 11

Brain Allergies

"No wise man ever wished to be younger."

—Jonathan Swift

When I talk about brain allergies, I am talking about allergic reactions most commonly triggered by ingestion of foods, food additives, or other chemicals that affect the brain. Most people readily accept the assertion that what they eat can affect their bodies. What may be more difficult for them to believe is that food can have a strong impact on their brains. The fact is that our brains use approximately 30 percent of all the energy our bodies obtain from food.

Almost everyone has seen, or experienced firsthand, the effects of allergens. Dust, pollen, pet dander, and smoke are just some of the triggers that cause people to sniffle, sneeze, wipe at watery eyes, or break out in hives. As the scope of these symptoms show, allergic reactions can be manifested in any part of the body. Generally, allergies occur as a result of a hyperaggressive immune response that perceives a generally benign substance as harmful. The body tags the substance as harmful, and white blood cells are mobilized to fight the perceived infection. In common allergic reactions, such as hay fever, a chemical reaction causes the release of histamines, which cause tissues in the eyes and nose to swell, causing the characteristic stuffy nose and watery eyes that accompany a hay fever attack.

What I specifically discuss in this chapter are allergic reactions that target the brain. These reactions are caused most often by particular foods or certain chemicals found in prepared foods. This type of allergic response is often difficult to diagnose, because the symptoms do not usually appear right after eating the offending food, but can take hours or days to manifest. The symptoms are not as easily diagnosed as the hives that might break out in a fixed allergic reaction to a single, particular food, such as nuts. The symptoms of a masked, or cyclic, food-related brain allergy can present as other brain conditions, such as depression, insomnia, mental fog, or even schizophrenia.

In the sections that follow, I suggest ways in which you can identify and eliminate triggers for brain allergies, and tell you which nutrients and supplements will strengthen your body's immune system and your brain's capacity to resist an allergic attack.

Understanding Brain Allergies

When the response to a specific allergen has a detrimental effect on an individual's behavior, attitude, or emotions, it is likely that the sufferer is experiencing an allergic reaction in the brain.

There are certain biochemical reactions that are attributed to brain allergies, including excessive histamine release in the brain, alterations of levels of vitamins in the brain, changes in blood sugar levels, and neurochemical effects specific to certain food additives, such as NutraSweet, which contains phenylalanine.

Diagnosing Brain Allergies

The reactions to brain allergies can be extremely specific to each individual, with the same allergen producing very different symptoms in different people. But there are several methods for testing whether brain allergies are the underlying cause of certain medical or physical symptoms.

Brain allergies can be diagnosed using hair mineral testing, skin testing, blood tests that measure immunoglobulin food antibody levels and white blood cell reactions to antigens, and applied kinesiology. A method of removing specific foods or chemicals from your diet for a specific period of time before reintroducing them and noting the effect is a frequent diagnostic tool in testing for brain allergies. This "elimination diet" approach should be done under the supervision of a professional health care provider, especially if your symptoms are severe.

If you are undergoing a thorough medical workup to determine if you are suffering from brain allergies, I recommend you be tested for parasitic invasions, candida, and insufficient digestive enzymes. If any of these conditions exist, treatment can help improve your ability to absorb food nutrients and lessen systemic reactivity to certain foods.

Good dental care can play a role in reducing allergic reactions, too. Infections hidden in root canal–treated teeth, undetected abscesses, periodontal disease, or infection of dental implants can all trigger allergy-like symptoms.

Symptoms of Brain Allergies

In children, brain allergies are thought to play a role in hyperactivity, learning disorders, and attention deficit disorders. In adults, manic-depressive disorders, hyperactivity, and various phobias may be symptoms of brain allergies. Severe psychotic reactions may occasionally occur. Food or chemical intolerances are thought to play a role in schizophrenia.

The effects of brain allergies are defined by both positive and negative reactions. An individual suffering from brain allergies might exhibit symptoms that vacillate between behaviors on both ends of the scale. This type of "roller coaster" of symptoms is a hallmark of brain allergies. In the scale that follows, the levels designated as positive (+) are levels of stimulation. The negative (–) levels are degenerative reactions.

+4: mania, excitement, agitation, possibly convulsions

+3: hypomania, anxiousness, aggressiveness, loquaciousness, apprehension, clumsiness

+2: tension, thirst, talkativeness, argumentativeness, oversensitivity, hyperactivity, irritability, hunger

+1: alert, active, lively, apparently symptom-free

 0: homeostasis (even-keeled, in balance)

 0: homeostasis (even-keeled, in balance)

–1: physical manifestation of runny nose, hives, gas, diarrhea, eye and ear symptoms

–2: systemic reactions such as tiredness, mild depression, swelling, pain, cardiovascular effects

–3: deepening depression, disturbed mental processes, confusion, moodiness, withdrawal

–4: severe depression, possibly paranoia or suicidal tendencies

Combating Brain Allergies Naturally

In individuals suffering from brain allergies, the delicate chemical balance of the brain has become hypersensitive to foods or environmental chemicals. Poor nutrition, stress, toxic metal poisoning, and environmental pollution may all serve to heighten the brain's sensitivity to allergenic substances. When treating brain allergies, all these factors must be considered, in addition to removing the substance that is the primary trigger for the brain's allergic reaction.

Lifestyle

The best way to avoid allergic reactions is to stay away from the substances that provoke them. While I am specifically focusing on symptoms triggered by brain allergies in this chapter, if you are prone to allergic reactions in general, your immune system may benefit from specific allergen-removing techniques.

Removing Allergens from Your Home

Wash your bedding frequently in very hot water (at least 135°F) to remove allergens such as dust mites. Sheets, blankets, pillows, and comforters should be laundered weekly. Special covers that are dustmite–proof and can easily be removed and washed can be purchased to go over mattresses and pillows.

Reduce allergens in your home and improve the air quality by using an air filtration system. Units with three to four filtering systems work best. These systems remove bacteria, mold, pollens, and animal dander from the air. Placing a filter directly in a window and sealing the sides will limit the amount of pollutants coming into a room.

Plants are also invaluable and inexpensive air filters. Spider plants will filter out toxins, including formaldehyde, and produce oxygen in return. Other helpful plants include Brazilian palms, wide-leaf wandering Jews, and marigolds.

New technologies such as ozone disinfection, can purify water, including drinking water, saunas, whirlpools, swimming pools, and private bathing facilities.

Other steps you can take to remove allergens from your home include using natural, rather than chemical, products for daily grooming and cleaning:

- Use soaps without artificial scents or colors.
- Make homemade shampoos and conditioners using castile soap and olive or avocado oils; sesame oil makes an effective hair conditioner. Use peppermint and baking soda instead of commercial toothpaste. Use cornstarch instead of deodorant.

- Use cornstarch instead of talcum powder. Use sesame oil as a skin moisturizer.
- Use lemon oil and vinegar as room deodorizers. Use baking soda as a room or refrigerator freshener.
- Avoid the use of pesticides. Boric acid can be spread in a thin line (out of reach of children and pets) to discourage roaches and ants. In the garden, use insecticidal soap to kill pests without harming beneficial bugs.
- Create nontoxic surface cleaners using three tablespoons of vinegar to one quart of water for glass and smooth surfaces. Use baking powder instead of abrasive scrubs.
- In the laundry, pure baking soda will remove residues of detergent from clothing, and one cup of vinegar added to the rinse cycle will serve as a fabric softener and rinse out without leaving an odor. Look for natural detergents that do not have chlorine bleach or other chemical additives.
- Avoid drycleaning clothing whenever possible. If clothes must be drycleaned, remove them from the plastic cleaning bags and allow them to air out in the sun before wearing.

Nutrition

Foods and Brain Allergies

If you suffer from brain allergies, you should avoid refined sugars and carbohydrates, caffeine, and alcohol. Eat a diet with sufficient protein, and make sure you get sufficient amounts of essential fatty acids from the right sources. EFAs have inflammation-fighting properties that are beneficial to allergy sufferers. Depending on what foods trigger your reaction, your diet must be carefully tailored to limit your exposure to certain foods. A clinical nutritionist can help you determine allergic triggers and create an eating plan that will reduce your allergic potential.

The most common brain allergy inducers are sugar, wheat, dairy, beef, potatoes, shellfish, eggs, tomatoes, coffee, peanuts, soy nuts, corn, yeast, and citrus. A rotation diet, in which different foods are eaten each day, without repeating any single item for four to seven days, can help you determine which foods may be triggers. If you have a slight sensitivity to a wide range of foods, this type of dietary approach can keep your body from overreacting to some foods. Others may have to be excluded from your diet on a permanent basis.

I recommend keeping a food diary to determine the specific chemicals and foods that produce allergic reactions. You should notice if you feel bloated or tired, or if you have headaches after consuming particular foods. Even if these symptoms are not immediate, you should note them in your diary. If you are allergic to a food or additive, a pattern will emerge.

Recipes

In the following list are my recommendations for easy-to-prepare meals full of nutrients proven to help you prevent and impact brain allergies. The recipes can be found in Appendix II:

- The Big Cleanse
- Brain Juice
- Brain Power
- Delicious Detox
- Detox Tonic
- Fatigue Buster
- Head Cleaner
- Relax Your Mind
- Sleep Insurer
- Fabulous Wild Rice Salad
- Black Bean Soup
- Chinese Mushroom Soup
- Cinnamon Fruit Soup
- Papaya Nectar Soup

- Blueberry Breakfast Treat
- Rice and Strawberries
- Brazilian Rice
- Good Shepherd's Pie
- Blackberry Nectarine Fruit Salad

Supplements
Vitamins and Minerals

Calcium. To balance the effects of the magnesium supplement below, I recommend taking a daily supplement of 400 to 600 milligrams of elemental calcium from citrate.

Magnesium. Magnesium is well known for its calming properties in people with anxiety symptoms, but proper amounts of magnesium are generally lacking in the average American diet. Individuals who overuse laxatives or use oral contraceptives or diuretics are at risk of magnesium deficiency. Magnesium also assists in impacting circulatory problems. For impacting the symptoms of brain allergies, I recommend a daily supplement of 500 milligrams from citrate.

Manganese. This essential trace mineral supports the immune system. Low levels of manganese may accentuate the symptoms of brain allergies. I recommend a daily supplement of 20 milligrams, taken in two equal doses.

Vitamin A. Vitamin A is a great supporter of the immune system, and taking a daily supplement of vitamin A may reduce the possibility of developing allergies. I recommend supplementing with 6,700 milligrams daily.

Vitamin C. Vitamin C works to reduce histamine levels in the blood, detoxifies, and strengthens the immune system. I recommend increasing your daily supplement from 500 to 1,000 milligrams to 3,000 milligrams, taken in three equal doses. Do not exceed a daily supplement of 3,000 milligrams.

Zinc. Zinc may fight food allergies by increasing production of hydrochloric acid in the stomach. Zinc also boosts the immune system. I recommend a daily supplement of 30 milligrams.

Smart Drugs and Nutrients

Other naturally occurring nutrients may have beneficial impacts on the symptoms of brain allergies.

Bromelain. Derived from pineapple, this enzyme is a potent anti-inflammatory that helps strengthen the immune system. To combat the symptoms of brain allergies, I recommend a daily supplement of 1,000 milligrams while the symptoms are present.

Glutathione. A metabolite of the essential amino acid methionine, glutathione is an important part of the body's antioxidant defense system and enhances the immune system. To impact the symptoms of brain allergies, I recommend a daily supplement of 400 milligrams, taken in two equal doses.

L-Glutamine. Glutamine is one of the most abundant nonessential amino acids in the bloodstream. It is produced in the muscles and is able to pass freely through the blood–brain barrier. Once in the brain, it is converted into glutamic acid and increases GABA, a neurotransmitter essential for proper mental function. There are two types of glutamine supplements: D-glutamine and L-glutamine. L-glutamine is the form that more closely mimics the glutamine in the body. For relief from symptoms of brain allergies, I recommend supplementing with 1,500 milligrams, taken daily in three divided doses while symptoms last.

Methionine. Methionine is an essential amino acid and a powerful antioxidant and helps protect the body from toxic substances as well as destructive free radicals. Methionine also acts to decrease the blood level of histamine, which, in brain allergies, can interfere with neurotransmitter messages. I recommend a daily supplement of 1,000 milligrams taken up to three times daily.

Methylsulfonylmethane (MSM). MSM contains bionutritional sulphur, which plays an important role in the body's functioning. It assists in restoring the immune system and also supports the respiratory system. I recommend a daily supplement of 1,000 milligrams.

Reboot Your Brain Chart of Additional Supplements for Impacting Brain Allergies

The following chart summarizes the supplements I recommend adding to the protocol for overall brain health from chapter 2. In some cases, I recommend increasing the dose of a particular vitamin or supplement to specifically impact brain allergies. In these cases, you should increase the daily dosage from chapter 2 to the level recommended for this specific condition.

This protocol is designed for individuals who suffer from, or are specifically concerned about, brain allergies. If you are concerned about additional brain conditions discussed in other chapters, consult with a health professional about how you can safely impact multiple conditions.

If you are taking medications, whether prescription or over-the-counter, or have any food restrictions, consult with your doctor before beginning any supplement program. Your health care provider should always be up-to-date on all vitamins, supplements, and herbal or homeopathic remedies you are taking. Supplement overdoses are rare, but possible, and certain combinations may affect individuals adversely.

Supplement	Dosage	Cautions
bromelain	1,000 mg daily while symptoms are present	
calcium	400–600 mg elemental calcium daily	

Supplement	Dosage	Cautions
L-glutamine	1,500 mg daily in three divided doses while symptoms are present	Take while symptoms persist, but not for more than one month.
glutathione	400 mg daily in two equal doses	
magnesium	500 mg daily	May take six weeks or more for effects to be felt.
manganese	20 mg daily in two equal doses	
methionine	1,000 mg up to 3 times daily	
methyl-sulfonylmethane (MSM)	1,000 mg	
vitamin A	6,700 mg daily	
vitamin C	Increase daily dosage from 500–1,000 mg to 3,000 mg, taken in three equal doses. Do not exceed a daily supplement of 3,000 mg.	
zinc	30 mg daily	Large doses (50 mg or more) can interfere with the body's absorption of essential minerals, impair blood cell function, and depress the immune system.

Alternative Health Remedies

When suffering from a specific condition such as brain allergies, we can also try some natural treatment options that are considered alternatives to traditional medicine. While a healthful lifestyle and the proper nutritional and supplement plan are vital to protecting the brain against allergens, there are some other targeted remedies that might help, too.

Herbal Remedies

Some herbal extracts and homeopathic treatments have properties similar to conventional medications, but are gentler and may lack the drugs' side effects. Always inform your medical practitioner of any herbal remedies you may be taking.

- **Astragalus** is one of the best immune system stimulants now available. I recommend taking 250 milligrams, four times per day.
- **Chamomile** reduces inflammation by decreasing the body's production of histamines, prostaglandins, and other inflammatory agents. I recommend taking 325 milligrams, three times per day, preferably with food.
- **Garlic** builds immunity and serves as a natural antiseptic agent. Add to your diet or take prepared capsules as directed by the manufacturer.
- **Goldenseal** was used by Native Americans for allergy- or infection-induced conditions. Rich in alkaloids, it is stimulating to the immune system. I recommend taking 125 milligrams, twice a day for three weeks at the first sign of symptoms. (Note: Goldenseal is not to be used if you are pregnant or lactating.)
- **Ginkgo biloba** is an extract of the ginkgo plant and is a potent antioxidant. I recommend a supplement of 120 milligrams per day, taken in three equal doses.

- **Licorice root extract** has been used by the Chinese for more than five thousand years to support the adrenal system. I recommend 100 milligrams, taken one to three times daily. (Note: Licorice root extract is not to be taken if you have high blood pressure.)
- **Marshmallow root** soothes inflamed tissues and contains key immune system boosters, including vitamins A and C. Marshmallow root is commonly taken as a tea and should be prepared and ingested according to the manufacturer's directions.
- **Schisandra** is an adaptogenic herb that helps rebalance the body, build strength, and reduce fatigue. I recommend 100 milligrams, taken twice daily.

Homeopathic Remedies

The following remedies may be used for both temporary and acute cases of brain allergies. When dealing with a chronic condition, homeopathic remedies must be used in conjunction with other therapies, as prescribed by a qualified health professional. Consult with your health care provider before taking any homeopathic remedy, and follow their recommendation for the appropriate dosage. Always inform your medical practitioner of any homeopathic remedies you may be taking.

- **Conium maculatum** is useful in cases with impaired thinking, dull and sluggish mind, weakness of memory, and headaches.
- **Ignatiahomaccord** is a preparation containing ignatia and several active substances in a specific balance of potency.

Therapeutic Touch

A variety of treatments involve the transfer of energy from the practitioner to the patient, which can help relieve pain and anxiety, and may be helpful in promoting healing of a brain suffering from an allergic reaction.

Craniosacral therapy is a hands-on healing technique that manipulates the craniosacral system—the soft tissues and bones of the head (cranium), the spine down to its tail (sacrum), and the pelvis, as well as the membranes and cerebrospinal fluid that surround these areas—to reestablish the normal flow of the cerebrospinal fluid. The practitioner uses an extremely light touch to palpate, or feel, areas to detect a fluctuation in the cerebrospinal fluid, and then manipulates the area to clear blockages and correct the flow. This therapy is beneficial in reducing stress, improving the quality of sleep, and enhancing the general functioning of the body's organs.

Detoxification

Many brain allergies can be traced to an impaired digestive system, which results from a toxic buildup in the intestines. An internal cleansing therapy can become the first step in overcoming the problems. The following detoxification programs should be undertaken only under the supervision of a medical health professional: bentonite clay detoxification; hydrotherapy, including colonic enema therapy; and juice fasts (watermelon in particular is a great detoxifier).

Aromatherapy

Essential oils can be used in baths or inhaled to provide rebalancing effects. Do not apply essential oils directly to the skin; they must be mixed with carrier oils. Experiment with some of the scents below to see if they bring you relief from symptoms of brain allergies:

- chamomile
- lavender
- lemon balm

Summary

Throughout the years, I have repeatedly emphasized the importance of the milieu—the environment of a person's body and immune system—in maintaining physical health on a cellular level. To protect your body against brain allergies and to combat the symptoms that may occur, it is important to protect your immune system by paying careful attention to triggers in your environment and foods. A strong immune system is your best defense against brain allergies.

Chapter 12

Insomnia

"Care keeps his watch in every old man's eye,
And where care lodges, sleep will never lie."

—William Shakespeare

Sleep is an important part of our lives. While we sleep, our bodies are able to recharge and repair themselves at a cellular level. The effects of lack of sleep are swift and apparent, especially as they relate to functions of our minds. Forgetfulness, irritability, lack of focus, and inability to concentrate are some of the most common manifestations of an exhausted brain.

It is not unusual to have trouble sleeping at times. But if you begin to consistently feel that you do not get enough sleep, or do not feel refreshed when you awaken, you may suffer from insomnia. Insomnia is the most common sleep complaint. Insomnia is not defined by the number of hours of sleep you are able to log per night. The amount of sleep needed to recharge each night varies from person to person; some people need less sleep, some need more, with the average "good night's sleep" being seven to nine hours per night. If you suffer from insomnia, you are not alone. Approximately sixty million Americans have trouble falling, or staying, asleep.

Insomnia is more common in women, especially those who have reached menopause, and in the elderly. You may have heard it said that as we age we require less sleep. Unfortunately this is not true. Our ability to sleep may decrease, but our bodies' need for rest does not. When you are dealing with insomnia, it is important to consider lifestyle, diet, and nutritional changes that will allow us to achieve the complete and restful sleep necessary for good health. In this chapter, I offer some strategies for preventing and limiting insomnia and show you how you can change your environment and diet to promote the type of sleep necessary for mental and physical health.

Understanding Insomnia

Insomnia can encompass many sleep complaints, including difficulty falling asleep, difficulty falling back to sleep if awakened, sleeping too lightly, sleep disrupted by multiple spontaneous awakenings each night, or early morning waking with an inability to fall back to sleep. Often insomnia is a symptom of an underlying physical or psychological condition. Let's look at the different types of insomnia and what causes them.

Types of Insomnia

Insomnia is categorized based on both cause and duration. It can occur as a result of one factor or a combination of factors that may be biological, physical, psychological, or environmental.

Primary and Secondary Insomnia

If a person is having sleep problems that are not directly linked to another health condition or problem, the insomnia is categorized as "primary." If the person is experiencing sleep problems because of a physical condition (e.g., heartburn, asthma, arthritis, or restless leg syndrome), a mental condition (e.g., depression), or medication or other substances they are using (e.g., alcohol, caffeine), the person is said to have "secondary" insomnia.

Transient Insomnia

Insomnia that lasts up to one week but then abates is called transient, or intermittent, insomnia. It is often caused by situational stress, such as that associated with a move, an upcoming deadline, or beginning a new job. People who suffer from transient insomnia often find that it recurs with new or similar stressful situations. Good sleep habits and proven stress reducers are often effective in preventing transient insomnia, even when you are under stress.

Acute Insomnia

This type of short-term insomnia lasts for a week to several months and is usually associated with persistent stressful situations, such as a death or serious illness of a loved one, or with environmental factors, such as noise, light, or extreme temperature. Acute insomnia may also be caused by changes in a normal sleeping schedule, such as those experienced when switching from a day shift to a night shift at work or suffering from jet lag.

Chronic Insomnia

Chronic insomnia occurs when a person has insomnia at least three nights a week for at least one month. It can be caused by many things, but most commonly occurs as a result of another health problem, such as depression, chronic stress, pain, and discomfort, such as that from arthritis. Heart disease, Parkinson's disease, sleep apnea, and hyperthyroidism are other serious health problems that may cause insomnia. Chronic insomnia can last for six months or longer.

Diagnosing Insomnia

If you think you have insomnia, you should talk to your health care provider. A medical history, physical examination, and sleep history will help to determine if there is a specific underlying cause. In the case of chronic insomnia, a psychiatric evaluation may be helpful in determining if your insomnia is a symptom of depression.

Keeping a sleep diary that keeps track of your sleep patterns and notes your perception of the quality and quantity of your sleep may be helpful in making a diagnosis. Be sure to provide your doctor with a list of all medications (both over-the-counter and prescription) that you may be taking. Some medications may contribute to insomnia.

Insomnia becomes more prevalent as we age, and most health care professionals look at four main areas when determining the cause of insomnia in older individuals:

- Physical: may include cardiovascular disease, asthma or other lung problems, chronic pain, bladder or prostate problems, epilepsy, sleep apnea, Alzheimer's disease or other dementia, and gastroesophageal reflux.
- Environmental: noise, late-night eating, late-night exercise, or inactivity during the day.
- Medical: drugs such as caffeine, alcohol, nicotine, antidepressant medications, stimulants, or medication schedules.
- Mental: depression (life changes and events that become more common as we age, such as retirement or death of a spouse or friends, may trigger depression), stress (health-related, financial), and anxiety.

Common tests to determine causes of insomnia may include:

- EEG sleep studies
- overnight oximetry (testing oxygen levels while you are asleep)
- minimental state exam
- cardiopulmonary exam
- neurological exam
- blood and urine tests

Symptoms of Insomnia

Insomnia is characterized by one or a combination of the following symptoms:

- difficulty falling asleep
- awaking often (more than three or four times) with a memory of being awake
- moving suddenly from sleep to wakefulness
- light, restless sleep that does not leave you refreshed, even if you sleep the same number of total hours as usual
- shifting sleep patterns (often a cycle of waking very early without being able to return to sleep, then having to go to bed earlier, causing even earlier morning wakings)
- confusion between day and night in terms of your body's levels of tiredness and energy

Combating Insomnia Naturally

Rather than becoming dependent on medications that induce sleep, it is important to prevent insomnia by making changes in your waking and sleeping habits and environment. For older people especially, the types of medications (called hypnotics) typically prescribed for insomnia can be metabolized at a slower rate, resulting in a rebound effect that may lead to carryover effects, such as daytime sleepiness, that could result in falls and injuries.

If your insomnia is caused by one of the underlying conditions addressed in the other chapters of this book, consult the relevant chapter for natural treatment options.

Quality sleep is essential in repairing and rejuvenating our brains and our bodies. In the Reboot Your Brain protocol for impacting insomnia that follows, I tell you how you can make your environment conducive to a restful night's sleep and suggest natural techniques for promoting relaxation and reducing stress. My nutritional and supplement plan in this section is specifically designed to prevent insomnia and allow you to get the optimal rest you need each night.

Lifestyle

Three main areas can impact our ability to get a good night's sleep. Our environment, our "sleep hygiene" habits, and our daytime activities are all factors in promoting or preventing insomnia. The suggestions below are proven insomnia fighters.

Environment

It is important that your nighttime environment is conducive to quality sleep. The following suggestions may help to prevent or overcome insomnia:

- Make sure your bedroom is dark, quiet, peaceful, and comfortable.
- Do not turn your bedroom into an office or den.
- Make sure your mattress is comfortable.
- Your bedroom should be well ventilated and slightly cool.
- Use a white noise machine or earplugs to cover any external sounds.

Sleep Hygiene

How you prepare for sleep will influence the quality of your rest.

- Avoid nicotine, caffeine, and alcohol late in the day.
- Avoid heavy meals late in the day. A light snack before bedtime may help regulate glucose during the night and help you sleep.
- Go to bed at the same time each night and wake up at the same time each morning. Avoid naps if possible.
- Do not go to bed until you feel tired.
- Follow a bedtime routine to help you relax before bed. A warm bath before bed can relax both your body and your mind.

- Avoid using your bed for any activities other than sleep or sex. Sex before bedtime may have the effect of either promoting or impeding sleep.
- Read or watch television (not in your bedroom, however!) until you feel drowsy. If you do not fall asleep after going to bed, get up again and engage in a nonstimulating activity (e.g., listening to relaxing music) for another half hour, then return to bed.

Daytime Activities

Your activities during the day can have an impact on the quality of your rest at night. To prevent insomnia:

- Exercise daily. Moderate exercise releases endorphins and natural cortisol, which reduce stress. Do not exercise in the three hours before your bedtime.
- Reduce stress by making a to-do list before you go to bed.
- Writing your worries in a journal can free you from worrying about them after you turn out the light.
- Practice relaxation techniques, such as meditation or breathing exercises, throughout the day so that you are able to call on them at night when you want to "turn off" your stressful thoughts.

Nutrition

Foods and Insomnia

If you suffer from insomnia, you should avoid any foods or beverages that may be stimulating, especially those that contain caffeine, sugar, or alcohol. To prevent any unnecessary stimulation to your system, you should avoid coffee, tea, cola, chocolate, spicy foods, refined carbohydrates, and prepared food with preservatives, especially those containing MSG. Sugar and foods high in sugar raise glucose levels and may create a burst of energy that disturbs sleep. Foods that are high in protein can inhibit sleep by blocking the synthesis of serotonin.

Do not combine too many ingredients in your last meal of the day, and avoid consuming too much food at night. Try not to eat within three hours of going to bed.

The Latest Research

The link between oxidative stress and insomnia was seen in a 2012 study by researchers at Ataturk University in Turkey, which showed that individuals suffering from insomnia were significantly more likely to have low levels of the key antioxidant glutathione and higher levels of malondialdehyde, a biomarker of oxidative stress. The results reinforce the notion that taking antioxidant supplements and consuming a diet rich in antioxidants is particularly important for insomnia patients.[36]

Recipes

In the following list are my recommendations for easy-to-prepare meals full of nutrients proven to help you prevent and impact insomnia. The recipes can be found in Appendix II:

- Brain Juice
- Chilling Relaxer
- Chlorophyll Boost
- Deep-Sea Juicing
- Free Radical Delight
- Green Power Punch
- How Green Is Your Juice
- Relax Your Mind
- Sleep Insurer
- Fabulous Wild Rice Salad
- Nature's Total Salad
- Pasta Salad
- Chinese Mushroom Soup
- Blueberry Breakfast Treat
- Cream of Barley
- Rice and Strawberries

- Brazilian Rice
- Good Shepherd's Pie
- Macaroni Marconi
- Blackberry Nectarine Fruit Salad
- Cherry Grape Kanten

Supplements
Vitamins and Minerals

Calcium. Calcium can have a sedative effect on the body, and a calcium deficiency can cause restlessness and wakefulness. To impact insomnia, I recommend taking a daily supplement of 2,000 milligrams, divided into four equal doses after meals and at bedtime.

Iron. An iron deficiency may impact the quality of your sleep. If your doctor determines that you are deficient in this important mineral, I recommend adding a daily iron supplement of 15 milligrams for menstruating women and 10 milligrams for men and nonmenstruating women.

Magnesium. Magnesium is well known for its calming properties in persons with anxiety symptoms, but proper amounts of magnesium are generally lacking in the average American diet. Individuals who use oral contraceptives or diuretics, and who overuse laxatives, are at risk of magnesium deficiency. Magnesium also assists in impacting circulatory problems. If you are suffering from insomnia, I recommend a daily supplement of 1,000 milligrams, taken in four equal doses, along with the calcium supplement.

Zinc. A growing body of scientific evidence suggests that zinc helps promote restful sleep. One recent study discovered that women who had higher levels of zinc slept for longer periods of time compared to women who were deficient in this mineral.[17] I recommend taking up to 30 milligrams daily. If taken chronically, large doses (50 milligrams or more) can interfere with the body's absorption of essential minerals, impair blood cell function, and depress the immune system.[18]

Smart Drugs and Nutrients

Other naturally occurring nutrients may have beneficial impacts on insomnia.

L-Tryptophan. A building block for the sleep-enhancing neurotransmitter serotonin, L-tryptophan may help to enhance relaxation and promote sleep. Tryptophan also enhances the brain's ability to produce melatonin, the hormone that regulates your body clock. I recommend taking 1,000 milligrams a half hour before you go to bed.

Melatonin. This hormone is produced by the pineal gland to aid in sleep and setting our circadian rhythms. Low levels can cause interrupted or restless sleep. To prevent insomnia, I recommend supplementing with 300 micrograms to 1 milligram, taken a half hour before bed two or three nights per week.

Reboot Your Brain Chart of Additional Supplements for Impacting Insomnia

The following chart summarizes the supplements I recommend adding to the protocol for overall brain health from chapter 2. In some cases, I recommend increasing the dose of a particular vitamin or supplement to specifically impact insomnia. In these cases, you should increase the daily dosage from chapter 2 to the level recommended for this specific condition.

This protocol is designed for individuals who suffer from, or are specifically concerned about, insomnia. If you are concerned about additional brain conditions discussed in other chapters, consult with a health professional about how you can safely impact multiple conditions.

If you are taking medications, whether prescription or over-the-counter, or have any food restrictions, consult with your doctor before beginning any supplement program. Your health care provider should always be up-to-date on all vitamins, supplements, and herbal or homeopathic remedies you are taking. Supplement overdoses are rare, but possible, and certain combinations may affect individuals adversely.

Supplement	Dosage	Cautions
calcium (from citrate)	1,000 mg from citrate, taken in four equal doses	
iron	15 mg daily for menstruating women, 10 mg daily for men and nonmenstruating women	
L-tryptophan	1,000 mg, taken a half hour before bed	
magnesium	1,000 mg, taken in four equal doses along with calcium	May take up to six weeks for effects to be felt.
melatonin	300 mcg–1mg taken a half hour before bed	Tolerance may develop with regular use. Long-term effects of nightly use are unknown.
zinc	Dosage is up to 30 mg daily	Large doses (50 mg or more) can interfere with the body's absorption of essential minerals, impair blood cell function, and depress the immune system.

Alternative Health Remedies

When suffering from a specific condition such as insomnia, we can also try some natural treatment options that are considered alternatives to traditional medicine. While a healthful lifestyle and the proper nutritional and supplement plan are vital in preventing insomnia, there are some other targeted remedies that might help, too.

Herbal Remedies

Some herbal extracts and homeopathic treatments have properties similar to conventional medications, but are gentler and may lack the drugs' side effects. Always inform your medical practitioner of any herbal remedies you may be taking.

- **Chamomile** reduces restlessness and irritability at bedtime. I recommend taking up to 650 milligrams an hour before bed, preferably with a little food. Chamomile may also be used as a tea, taken in the hours before bed.

- **Skullcap** has a calming effect on the nerves and muscles and can act as a mild sedative. It may be particularly useful in easing the symptoms of "restless leg syndrome." Consult with your doctor if you are taking any other medications, including over-the-counter medications, such as antihistamines. If skullcap is safe for you to use, I recommend taking 1 to 2 grams up to three times daily. Skullcap is often combined with other mildly sedative herbs, including valerian, passionflower, hops, and lemon balm. If you are taking such a preparation, follow the manufacturer's instructions.

- **St. John's wort** is very popular in Europe, where double-blind, placebo-controlled studies support its efficacy in helping fight depression. It has a calming and mildly sedative effect on the nervous system. To help impact insomnia, I recommend taking 450 milligrams twice a day.

- **Valerian** may help to improve sleep. It has a reputation for easing anxiety and relaxing tense muscles. I recommend taking 400 to 450 milligrams half an hour before bedtime. Do not take valerian for more than two consecutive weeks. Although the herb has no addictive properties, it is unwise to rely on any sleep aid exclusively. Valerian is often combined with other mildly sedative herbs, including skullcap, passionflower, hops, and lemon balm. If you are taking such a preparation, follow the manufacturer's instructions.

Homeopathic Remedies

The following remedies may be used for both temporary and acute cases of insomnia. When dealing with a chronic condition, homeopathic remedies must be used in conjunction with other therapies, as prescribed by a qualified health professional. Consult with your health care provider before taking any homeopathic remedy, and follow their recommendation for the appropriate dosage. Always inform your medical practitioner of any homeopathic remedies you may be taking.

- **Arnica** is good for insomnia brought about by physical overwork.
- **Aconite** is recommended in cases of insomnia caused by shock, grief, fright, or bad news.
- **Arsenicum album** is for feelings of sleepiness during the day and restlessness at night.
- **Cocculus** is recommended when insomnia is brought about by overtiredness or exhaustion.
- **Ignatia** is used to prevent insomnia brought about by emotional stress.
- **Kali phosphoricum** is beneficial when insomnia is caused by excitement or mental strain.
- **Nux vomica** may be helpful when insomnia is caused by too much alcohol or food.
- **Pulsatilla** is recommended for early waking with an overactive mind and/or recurrent thoughts.
- **Sulphur** is suggested to treat night wakings followed by difficulty returning to sleep.

Acupuncture

Acupuncture may provide relief from insomnia. By listening to your symptoms and examining your appearance and pulse, acupuncturists can diagnose and impact insomnia.

Acupuncture releases tension in the muscles. It causes a relaxation response in the body, resulting in lowered blood pressure and heart rate. Acupuncture increases the flow of blood, lymph, and nerve impulses to affected areas, and decreases stress while promoting feelings of well-being and energy.

Therapeutic Touch

A variety of treatments involve the transfer of energy from the practitioner to the patient, which can help to relieve pain and anxiety. In one study, massage reduced anxiety and lowered saliva cortisol levels (a key measurement of stress). Massage can be very effective at removing tension from the muscles and may provide relief from insomnia.

Reiki. Pronounced "ray-kee," this method employs a powerful, hands-on healing technique in which the universal life force energy is channeled through the practitioner and transferred to the patient. Chronic stress and anxiety can deplete the energy in our bodies. Reiki is used to support the body's natural ability to heal itself. It releases spiritual and emotional blocks, and brings a feeling of harmony and vitality.

Massage. This popular technique can enhance general relaxation and provide an outlet for stress and tension. Massage therapy can reduce feelings of anxiety, promote better sleep patterns, and increase feelings of well-being.

Shiatsu. This form of physical therapy combines traditional Chinese medical theory and various Japanese massage techniques. The therapist uses direct pressure with hands and fingers to redirect the flow of energy throughout the body. Shiatsu treatment is deeply relaxing and can be beneficial in both chronic and acute conditions.

Craniosacral Therapy. This gentle form of manipulation is a hands-on healing technique that manipulates the craniosacral system—the soft tissues and bones of the head (cranium), the spine down to its tail (sacrum), and the pelvis, as well as the membranes and cerebrospinal fluid that surround these areas—to reestablish the normal flow of the cerebrospinal fluid. The practitioner uses an extremely light touch to palpate, or feel, areas to detect a fluctuation in the cerebrospinal fluid, and then manipulates the area to clear blockages and correct the flow. This therapy is beneficial in reducing stress, improving the quality of sleep, and enhancing the general functioning of the body's organs.

Yoga and Meditation

Many have discovered the joy of yoga and meditation in helping clear the mind of thoughts and stress that can cause insomnia. Brief periods of meditation throughout the day can help refocus the mind and reinvigorate mental energy. The practice of walking meditation is particularly useful for achieving a restful state, as it combines both meditation and simple exercise.

To practice walking meditation, focus your attention on each foot as it contacts the ground. When the mind wanders away from your feet or legs, or the feeling of your body walking, refocus your attention. To deepen your concentration, don't look around, but keep your gaze forward and soft.

Aromatherapy

Essential oils can be used in baths or inhaled to provide rebalancing effects. Do not apply essential oils directly to the skin; they must be mixed with carrier oils. Experiment with some of the scents below to see if they bring you relief from insomnia:

- chamomile
- jasmine
- lavender
- lemon balm
- marjoram
- neroli

- rose
- sandalwood
- ylangylang

Summary

In the previous sections, I focused on ways to impact insomnia when it occurs, but it is important to remember that insomnia itself is a symptom, not a disease. Insomnia is associated with a wide variety of mental and physical disorders, and these underlying conditions must be diagnosed and treated accordingly. Good sleep is crucial in supporting the functions and protecting the health of our minds and bodies.

Chapter 13

Senile Dementia

"His memory is like wares at the auction—going, going, and anon
it will be gone."

—Herman Melville

When people talk to me about growing older, they tell me that one
of their greatest fears is that they will become forgetful. They fear
that memory loss is the first sign of Alzheimer's disease and that it
signals an inevitable mental and physical decline. For as long as I
can remember, and for long before that, traditional medicine practitioners have told us that memory loss and confusion are simply
normal parts of growing older. They implied that we should simply
accept such changes in our mental capacities as an inevitable part of
the aging process.

But I have known, and now modern medicine is beginning to
admit, that remaining alert and able as we age can be the norm,
rather than the exception. Many people experience memory lapses.
Some are serious and others are not. People who have serious
changes in their memory, personality, and behavior may suffer from
dementia.

Dementia (from the Latin for "irrationality") describes a group of symptoms that are caused by changes in the way the brain functions. Senile (meaning old) dementia refers to the onset of these symptoms in older people. Dementia can strike anyone at any age—as Dr. Eric Braverman puts it, "We have a neurodegenerative disease epidemic in this country where thirty-year-olds and forty-year-olds begin the process of dementia and 50 percent of our older Americans are demented by eighty and dementing by fifty."[19] We have to be vigilant at all ages in adulthood. However, the most common conditions with dementia as a symptom include Alzheimer's disease and vascular disease, both of which are specific to older individuals.

By providing an optimal environment for brain health, and through a healthful lifestyle, attention to nutrition, and proper supplementation, you can preserve your mental abilities as you age. In this chapter, I talk about specific steps you can take to improve your environment and diet to protect your brain against the symptoms of cognitive decline associated with senile dementia. I will also talk about alternative, natural treatments that may have some benefits in the fight against this age-related condition.

Understanding Senile Dementia

Individuals suffering from senile dementia have impaired memory as well as changes in other areas of cognition, such as language, vision, and abstract thinking, that prevent them from functioning properly on a daily basis.[1] The signs and symptoms of dementia occur primarily in the absence of delirium and may be associated with an organic cause.

The classic indicators of dementia are short-term memory loss, inability to think through problems or to finish complex tasks, difficulty concentrating, confusion, and abnormal behavior.

While some types of dementia, such as that caused by Alzheimer's disease, often cause a steady and progressive decline in patients, other types of dementia can be prevented, treated, or reversed by addressing the underlying conditions.

Causes of Senile Dementia

Many disorders can cause dementia. Some, such as Alzheimer's disease—which accounts for approximately 60 percent of all dementia cases in the elderly—are characterized by steadily progressive loss of first cognitive, and then physical, functions. Other causes of dementia are treatable and easily reversible, once the underlying condition is addressed. Reactions to medications, emotional stress, metabolic imbalances, problems in optical or auditory processing, nutritional deficiencies, hormone imbalances, diabetes, AIDS, Huntington's disease, head trauma, brain tumors, or inflammation or infection can all trigger symptoms of dementia. In the sections that follow, I discuss several of the most common conditions that can result in symptoms of dementia.

Alzheimer's Disease

This form of dementia encompasses a group of symptoms caused by changes in brain function. Alzheimer's disease is characterized by a specific, visible effect on the physical condition of the brain caused by the degeneration and death of neurons in the hippocampus. A sticky, waxy plaque called amyloid and neurofibrillary tangles are also present in the brains of Alzheimer's patients. For a detailed discussion of Alzheimer's disease, see chapter 8.

Lewy Body Dementia

Lewy body dementia (LBD) is named after Frederick Lewy, who first discovered this form of dementia in 1914. LBD resembles Alzheimer's disease, but the abnormal brain cells, called cortical Lewy bodies, that are characteristic of this disease are found in the cortex and substantia nigra regions of the brain. Lewy body disease produces symptoms similar to Alzheimer's but may progress more rapidly.

Pick's Disease

Pick's disease affects the frontal and temporal lobes of the brain and is sometimes referred to as frontotemporal dementia (FTD). This illness is also similar in symptoms to Alzheimer's and generally affects individuals between ages forty and sixty. It is characterized by a gradual loss of social skills and personality alteration, as well as damage to the memory and language functions. Pick's disease is characterized in the brain by swollen neurons.

Vascular Disease

Vascular dementia is the second most common type of dementia after that caused by Alzheimer's disease. Vascular problems in the brain or body (most commonly strokes) are the main causes of this type of dementia. In general, this type of dementia occurs suddenly, frequently after a stroke. It generally does not progress steadily, however, like Alzheimer's-related dementia. The patient may have long periods of stability or even improvement, but quickly develop new symptoms if more strokes occur.

Pseudodementia

Some elderly people may suffer anxiety and fear that their mental abilities and memory are declining. These feelings may trigger a severe depression called pseudodementia. Cognitive changes, memory loss, and slowed motor movements are typical of this condition. This type of depression may also trigger other symptoms, like those of senile dementia, including apathy, inability to answer simple questions correctly, poor eye contact, or little spontaneous movement. Treatment of the underlying depression will cause the dementia-like symptoms to disappear.

Diagnosing Senile Dementia

Because there are so many conditions that have symptoms similar to those caused by senile dementia, and because there is no definitive test that can accurately diagnose dementia, diagnosis is often made by excluding other conditions that may present similar symptoms.

Symptoms of Senile Dementia

- forgetfulness at work
- difficulty with familiar activities; unwillingness to learn new things
- language problems
- problems with getting lost
- inability to keep track of days of the week
- impaired judgment
- problems with abstract thinking
- misplacing objects, or putting them in unusual places
- extreme or inappropriate mood swings
- personality changes
- paranoia
- loss of initiative, loss of interest in previously pleasurable activities
- motor skills impairment

Individuals suffering from the onset of senile dementia are usually unable to identify the problem themselves. If you or an elderly person close to you is exhibiting some of the symptoms above, a health care provider should be consulted and provide a thorough physical, neurological, and psychological workup as described in the following section.

A doctor will take a current medical and psychological history, assess neurological status, and evaluate physical status. You should tell your doctor about any medications or supplements you are taking. Some medications prescribed for other conditions can cause side effects that mimic dementia. Medical tests might include imaging scans, such as an MRI or CT; laboratory tests, such as blood and urine tests; neuropsychological tests, such as tests of memory, vision, motor coordination, and language function; and even a psychiatric evaluation to assess emotional factors.

It is important to remember that hormones are closely related to brain health. Hormone levels fluctuate with age, and the importance of consulting with an endocrinologist to assess hormone levels and balance in treating memory deterioration should not be underestimated. Hormones related to memory function include human growth hormone, vasopressin, DHEA, and pregnenolone.

To help your doctor rule out other causes of cognitive impairment, you should be prepared to discuss other possible causes of memory failure. Before settling on a diagnosis of senile dementia, carefully review the following areas with your doctor:[2]

- Medication interactions: Make a list of all substances you are taking, including prescription medications, vitamins, herbal supplements, over-the-counter products, such as aspirin or cold medications, smoking cessation products, weight loss products, and topical preparations, such as arthritis ointment.
- Physical conditions: Ask your doctor to ensure that you are not dehydrated. Dehydration can occur from episodes of vomiting or diarrhea or from heat exhaustion. Dehydration is common in older adults and can interfere with your body's ability to process medications or supplements.
- Brain traumas: Report any falls or blows to the head. Falls are common among older adults and can result in concussions and symptoms of dementia.
- Emotional status: The symptoms of depression can be remarkably similar to those of dementia. Discuss all possible triggers, such as loss, significant life changes, or side effects of medication, which may be underlying causes of depression.
- Alcohol use: Consuming too much alcohol or using alcohol with certain medications may cause memory loss.

- Tobacco use: Cigarette smoking is linked to changes in the flow of blood supply to the lungs and brain. Vascular disease is one of the primary causes of dementia.

Combating Senile Dementia Naturally

Remembering and forgetting things is a perfectly normal part of daily life. But we need not fear that the extreme and progressive cognitive decline that is a symptom of senile dementia will be an inevitable part of our aging process. There are a number of things we can do to positively impact our brain health and overall mental abilities as we age.

In the Reboot Your Brain protocol for impacting senile dementia that follows, I tell you how you can make your environment more healthful, exercise your brain to retain memory and mental sharpness, and choose the best foods to help prevent the onset of senile dementia or to slow the progression of cognitive decline if you have been diagnosed with this condition.

Lifestyle

Making healthful changes to your lifestyle can be crucial in preventing the onset of dementia and keeping your memory sharp as you grow older. There are several simple things you can do to prevent the onset of senile dementia or to slow or prevent the progression of symptoms. In the following sections, I offer suggestions for improving your living environment, your physical health, and your social support system changes that can help you fight age-related memory loss and dementia. I have even included some coping strategies to make short-term memory loss less disruptive in your daily routine.

Environment

It is important for your environment to be free of hazardous toxins, particularly heavy metals, that can accumulate in the body. Limit your exposure to cookware, deodorants, antacids, and food additives that contain aluminum. Mercury is found in thermometers, thermostats, and dental amalgams. Chelation therapy, which uses certain amino acids to form strong ionic bonds with the toxic metals in your body, allowing them to be excreted from the system, may be useful in removing toxic metals and other chemicals from your body. Bentonite, a claylike substance that is used in a drink, may be taken at night to draw out toxins from the colon and assist in the detoxification process.

Installing charcoal filters on all water sources used for drinking or cooking can reduce or eliminate harmful toxins that are found in the water from our reservoirs.

Social Activity

Continued community involvement and frequent contact with friends and family may reduce your risk for senile dementia. In a paper presented at the Alzheimer's Association International Conference on the Prevention of Dementia,[3] Jane Saczynski, PhD, of the National Institute on Aging, and colleagues presented data from a longitudinal study conducted since 1965 that showed that subjects with decreased social activity from mid- to late life had a statistically significant risk of dementia. Continue to set goals for yourself. Having a reason to get up and get going each day can enhance your overall quality of life and contribute to mental fitness.

Exercise

Physical activity seems to play a role in slowing or preventing the progression of senile dementia. A National Institutes of Health news release cites research demonstrating that long-term physical activity increased the learning ability of mice and decreased the level of plaque-forming beta-amyloid protein fragments in their brains.[4] Remaining physically active throughout our lifetimes offers immeasurable benefits to both body and brain. Physical activity does not have to be rigorous. Walking, dancing, or practicing yoga all help safeguard our brains against age-related cognitive decline.

Memory Skills and Brain Boosters

In addition to an active body, it is important to have an active mind. A study published in the *New England Journal of Medicine* supports the theory that mentally demanding activities can help stave off dementia.[5] The study involved 469 people ages 75 and older. Those participants who read, played games of strategy (e.g., checkers, backgammon, or chess), played musical instruments, or danced at least twice a week were significantly less likely to develop dementia. Those who did crossword puzzles four times a week were also found to have a significantly lowered risk. It seems clear that participating in mentally stimulating hobbies and being willing to learn new information and challenge our brains on an ongoing basis provide important benefits in preventing the onset of senile dementia.

Weight Management

A recent study published in the *British Medical Journal* examined more than ten thousand members of a medical insurance program in California. The study followed subjects from their early forties until their late sixties and seventies. According to the results, those individuals who were obese at the start of the study were 74 percent more likely to develop dementia than their slimmer counterparts.[6]

Coping Strategies

If you or someone close to you has been diagnosed as having senile dementia, there are some strategies for coping with the symptoms of memory loss that may be the first hallmarks of this disease. These coping strategies will help relieve the stress and tension that arise from memory problems and can help lessen the impact of such problems on day-to-day life. Remember, in addition to practicing the strategies outlined on the next page, you should make the lifestyle and nutritional changes I recommend in this chapter to slow or reverse the progression of these early symptoms.

- Establish a regular routine in familiar surroundings.
- Make mental associations, such as using landmarks, to help you find things.
- Repeat names when you meet people.
- Put important items, such as your keys, in the same place every time.
- Label or color-code doors and exits to keep from getting disoriented.
- Draw a map for simple routes; write down directions.
- Make lists, use a calendar, and keep notes of important dates and financial matters.
- Set realistic daily goals.
- Keep track of when medicines are taken; use a chart or special pill box to stay current.
- Tell your doctor about all medications or supplements you are taking.
- Keep a list of important names and numbers near the telephone.
- Stay in frequent contact with family and friends.

Nutrition

Foods and Senile Dementia

As research into the causes of dementia continues, researchers are concluding that there may be ways in which we can limit our risk of developing senile dementia as we age. What is now being proposed is something that I have said over and over again: Deficiencies of essential nutrients can lead to a variety of health problems and leave us vulnerable to serious conditions such as senile dementia. The good news is that it is never too early to start good nutritional habits that will help to protect the brain over a lifetime. And it is never too late to benefit from good nutritional habits.

Most Americans today eat foods that are over-processed and far from their natural state. These processed foods have been stripped of vital nutrients and filled with additives, processed sugars, and trans fats.

In addition to nutrients lost through poor diet, nutritional deficiencies may simply increase as we age. To help ensure that our bodies get the nutrients we need, we must make an effort to eat foods in their natural state. For people suffering from senile dementia it is vitally important to purchase organic foods whenever possible, because these foods are more likely to have trace minerals like chromium, magnesium, selenium, and zinc, which are vital to the brain's health.

Various studies support the efficacy of taking antioxidants as a method of preventing or reversing cognitive decline. Vitamins E and C are proven free radical fighters and readily available in foods like citrus fruits and juices; dark green, leafy vegetables; nuts; and sunflower seeds. The B vitamins, which play an important role in fighting the symptoms of Alzheimer's disease, are found in fish, eggs, beans, and animal proteins. Trace minerals such as zinc, magnesium, and potassium are easy to add to our diets by using whole grains, nuts, dried beans, bananas, and milk.

Essential fatty acids (EFAs) such as omega-3 and omega-6 fats, which are found in flax oil and walnuts, have significant anti-inflammatory properties and may be important in preventing senile dementia.

Recipes

In the following list are my recommendations for easy-to-prepare meals full of nutrients proven to help prevent the onset of senile dementia. The recipes can be found in Appendix II:

- Antioxidant Punch
- Blueberry and Pear Macadamia Nut Shake

- Brain Power
- Carrot, Pineapple, and Strawberry Juice
- Everglades Punch
- Flax Cruncher
- Free Radical Delight
- Nuts and Seeds
- Velvety Pecan Milk
- Four-Bean Salad
- Mixed Sprout, Bean, and Nut Salad
- Black Bean Soup
- Cream of Barley
- Nutty Oatmeal
- Gary's Veggieball Stew
- Indonesian Kale
- Pasta e Fagioli
- Sweet Kidney Bean Mash
- Heavenly Roasted Nuts

Supplements

Vitamins and Minerals

Certain vitamins and minerals are very important in fighting the onset of senile dementia.

Calcium. Calcium from citrate can have a calming effect on the body, and a calcium deficiency can cause restlessness and wakefulness. To impact restlessness associated with senile dementia, I recommend taking a daily supplement of 1,000 milligrams, divided into four equal doses after meals and at bedtime.

Magnesium. Magnesium is well known for its calming properties in persons with anxiety symptoms, but proper amounts of magnesium are generally lacking in the average American diet. Individuals who use oral contraceptives or diuretics, and who overuse laxatives, are at risk of magnesium deficiency. Magnesium from citrate also assists in impacting circulatory problems. I recommend a daily supplement of 500 to 1,000 milligrams of magnesium, taken in two equal doses on an empty stomach.

Potassium. Potassium is one of the most abundant minerals in the human body. Most of the time, supplementation with potassium is unnecessary, because it is readily available in our diet in such foods as bananas, orange juice, and potatoes. Potassium is depleted from our bodies in times of stress, thus upsetting the delicate balance of neurotransmitter communication in our brains. For this reason, potassium supplements may be useful in impacting senile dementia. Potassium can interact with some drugs, so if you are taking prescription medications, consult with your doctor before taking potassium supplements. If potassium is safe for you, I recommend a daily supplement of 300 milligrams.

Vitamin B-Complex. It is important that your daily vitamin B-complex contain sufficient amounts of both vitamin B5 and B2, because deficiencies in these vitamins can develop as we age, and these deficiencies can contribute to the symptoms of senile dementia. If your doctor has determined that you are deficient in B vitamins, you may want to ask about receiving intravenous or injected supplements of vitamin B-complex to prevent or combat symptoms of senile dementia.

Vitamin C. Vitamin C may help delay the onset of senile dementia and slow the progression of symptoms. I recommend increasing your daily supplement from 500 to 1,000 milligrams to 3,000 milligrams, taken in three equal doses. Do not exceed a daily supplement of 3,000 milligrams.

Vitamin E. Vitamin E has beneficial antioxidant properties, and treatment with high doses has shown initial promise in slowing the progression of symptoms in individuals with dementia associated with moderately severe Alzheimer's.[7] Because vitamin E has anticoagulant properties, and high doses may be associated with the risk of bleeding and interaction with anticoagulants and other medications often taken by elderly people, you should discuss high-dose vitamin E supplementation with your doctor. If you are not at risk,

I recommend increasing your daily supplement from 268 milligrams to 536 milligrams, taken in two equal doses. Do not exceed a daily supplement of 536 milligrams.

Zinc. Many people who suffer from dementia have deficiencies in zinc. I recommend a daily supplement of 30 milligrams.

Smart Drugs and Nutrients

A number of other naturally occurring nutrients may have beneficial impacts on the symptoms of senile dementia.

Acetyl-L-Carnitine (ACL). This versatile nutrient is able to permeate the blood–brain barrier to stimulate and fortify the brain's nerve cells. Acetyl-L-carnitine is a type of carnitine produced naturally in the brain. It can aid in directing fatty acids to the cell mitochondria, assisting in the creation of new cell energy. A powerful antioxidant, acetyl-L-carnitine also supplements the neurotransmitter acetylcholine. I recommend increasing your daily supplement from 2,000 milligrams to 3,000 milligrams, taken in three equal doses. Do not exceed a daily supplement of 3,000 milligrams.

L-Glutamine. Glutamine is one of the most abundant nonessential amino acids in the bloodstream. It is produced in the muscles and is able to pass freely through the blood–brain barrier. Once in the brain, it is converted into glutamic acid and increases GABA, a neurotransmitter essential for proper mental function. There are two types of glutamine supplements: D-glutamine and L-glutamine. L-glutamine is the form that more closely mimics the glutamine in the body. To impact the symptoms of senile dementia, I recommend supplementing with 500 milligrams, taken three times daily.

N-acetylcysteine (NAC). This amino acid protects the brain from damaging free radicals by boosting quantities of glutathione, one of the body's most powerful antioxidants. I recommend a supplement of 500 milligrams, taken three times daily.

Phosphatidylserine (PS). PS helps the brain use fuel more efficiently. By boosting neuronal metabolism and stimulating production of acetylcholine, PS may be able to improve the condition of patients in cognitive decline. Studies have revealed that supplementing with phosphatidylserine slows down and even reverses declining memory and concentration, or age-related cognitive impairment, in middle-age and elderly subjects.

As we grow older, aging slows the body's manufacturing of phosphatidylserine to levels that are detrimental to our functioning at our full mental capacity. For treatment of memory loss that accompanies senile dementia, I recommend increasing your daily supplement from 300 milligrams to 400 milligrams. Do not exceed a daily supplement of 400 milligrams.

S-Adenosylmethionine (SAMe). SAMe (pronounced "sammy") has long been prescribed by European doctors as a treatment for depression. SAMe promotes cell growth and repair, and maintains levels of glutathione, a major antioxidant that protects against free radicals and reduces homocysteine levels. Alzheimer patients have extremely low levels of SAMe in their brains. SAMe should not be taken if you are taking MAO inhibitor antidepressants. You should consult with your doctor before taking SAMe if you suffer from severe depression or bipolar disorder. If SAMe is safe for you to use, I recommend a daily supplement of 400 to 1,600 milligrams, taken in four equal doses.

Reboot Your Brain Chart of Additional Supplements for Impacting Senile Dementia

The following chart summarizes the supplements I recommend adding to the protocol for overall brain health from chapter 2. In some cases, I recommend increasing the dose of a particular vitamin or supplement to specifically impact senile dementia. In these cases, you should increase the daily dosage from chapter 2 to the level recommended for this specific condition.

This protocol is designed for individuals who suffer from, or are specifically concerned about, senile dementia. If you are concerned about additional brain conditions discussed in other chapters, consult with a health professional about how you can safely impact multiple conditions.

If you are taking medications, whether prescription or over-the-counter, or have any food restrictions, consult with your doctor before beginning any supplement program. Your health care provider should always be up-to-date on all vitamins, supplements, and herbal or homeopathic remedies you are taking. Supplement overdoses are rare, but possible, and certain combinations may affect individuals adversely.

Supplement	Dosage	Cautions
acetyl-L-carnitine (ACL)	Increase daily dosage from 2,000 mg to 3,000 mg, taken in three equal doses. Do not exceed a daily supplement of 3,000 mg.	
calcium	1,000 mg daily, in four equal doses after meals and at bedtime	
intravenous vitamin B-complex	Discuss with your health care provider whether you might benefit from injected vitamin B.	
L-glutamine	500 mg, taken three times daily	
magnesium	500–1,000 mg, in two equal doses	May take up to six weeks for effects to be felt.

Supplement	Dosage	Cautions
Potassium	300 mg daily	Do not take potassium supplements if you are taking medication for high blood pressure or heart disease or if you have a kidney disorder. Consuming foods rich in potassium is okay. Do not exceed a supplementary dose of 500 mg daily without consulting your doctor.
N-acetylcysteine (NAC)	500 mg, three times daily	Daily supplementation of NAC increases urinary output of copper. If supplementing with NAC for an extended period, add 2 mg of copper and 30 mg of zinc to your daily supplement regimen.
phosphatidylserine (PS)	Increase daily dosage from 300 mg to 400 mg. Do not exceed a daily supplement of 400 mg.	

Supplement	Dosage	Cautions
S-adenosylmethionine (SAMe)	Dosage range of 400–1,600 mg	Raise the dose gradually from 200 mg twice a day to 400 mg twice a day, to 400 mg three times a day, to 400 mg four times a day, over a period of twenty days.
vitamin C	Increase daily dosage from 500–1,000 mg to 3,000 mg	
vitamin E	Increase daily dosage from 268 mg to 536 mg, taken in two equal doses. Do not exceed a daily supplement of 536 mg.	Vitamin E may cause increased risk of bleeding and may have adverse interactions with anticoagulants or other medications. Consult with your doctor before beginning high-dose supplementation with vitamin E.
zinc	Up to 30 mg daily	Large doses (50 mg or more) can interfere with the body's absorption of essential minerals, impair blood cell function, and depress the immune system.

Alternative Health Remedies

When suffering from a condition such as senile dementia, we can also try some natural treatment options that are considered alternatives to traditional medicine. While a healthful lifestyle and the proper nutritional and supplement plan are vital to winning the battle against dementia, there are some other targeted remedies that might help, too.

Herbal Remedies

Some herbal extracts and homeopathic treatments have properties similar to conventional medications, but are gentler and may lack the drugs' side effects. Always inform your medical practitioner of any herbal remedies you may be taking.

- **Butcher's broom** is an herb that promotes clearer focus and enhanced memory. I recommend a daily supplement of 850 milligrams, taken in two equal doses.
- **Bacopa monnieri** is a potent antioxidant that has been used in Ayurvedic medicine for centuries as a brain tonic to enhance memory, learning, development, and concentration. I recommend a daily supplement of 200 to 400 milligrams, taken in two equal doses.
- **Ginkgo biloba** is an herbal extract derived from the ginkgo biloba tree. It is commonly used in Europe to combat Alzheimer's disease. Ginkgo biloba is a potent antioxidant that may be beneficial in impacting dementia-related symptoms. By improving circulation to the central nervous system, ginkgo biloba may help to stabilize abnormal neurotransmitter communication in the brain. In a study conducted at the New York Institute for Medical Research, researchers found that almost one-third of Alzheimer's patients taking ginkgo supplements showed improvements in cognitive

function during a double-blind, placebo-controlled clinical study.[9] For prevention of senile dementia, I recommend a daily supplement of 120 milligrams, taken in two equal doses. For those suffering from this condition, I recommend increasing your daily dose to 240 milligrams, spread out over three equal doses.

- **Huperzine A** is a compound isolated from a Chinese herb called Hyperzia serrata. It increases acetylcholine activity in the cortex and hippocampus sections of the brain, and aids in improving memory as well as cognitive and behavioral functions. In a double-blind, placebo-controlled study conducted in China, 103 individuals with Alzheimer's disease received either huperzine A or a placebo twice daily for eight weeks. About 60 percent of the participants treated with huperzine A showed significant improvements in memory, thinking, and behavioral functions, compared to 36 percent of the placebo-treated subjects.[12] For impacting senile dementia, I recommend taking a daily supplement of 100 to 200 micrograms in two equal doses.

- **St. John's wort (hypericum)** is very popular in Europe, so much so that it is actually covered by German health insurance as a prescription drug. I recommend taking a daily supplement of 300 milligrams, twice per day.

- **Vinpocetine** is a derivative of an extract taken from the periwinkle shrub. It enhances circulation to the brain and may prevent or improve mild cognitive impairment. I recommend taking 10 milligrams, twice daily with meals.

Homeopathic Remedies

The following remedies may be used for both temporary and acute cases of senile dementia. When dealing with a chronic condition, homeopathic remedies must be used in conjunction with other therapies, as prescribed by a qualified health professional. Consult with your health care provider before taking any homeopathic remedy, and follow your provider's recommendation for the appropriate dosage. Always inform your medical practitioner of any homeopathic remedies you may be taking.

- **Alumina** is indicated for impacting great weakness or loss of memory in cases where consciousness of personal identity is confused.
- **Anacardium** is used for absentmindedness; memory for names is most affected.
- **Argentum nitricum** is for dementia with irritability and lack of control over impulses.
- **Helleborus** impacts stupefaction, when a person answers questions slowly and stares vacantly.
- **Silica** is best for mental deterioration with anxiety over small details.
- **Sulphur** can be used when there is difficulty remembering words or names.

Aromatherapy

Essential oils can be used in baths or inhaled to provide an energizing or soothing effect. Do not apply essential oils directly to the skin; they must be mixed with carrier oils. Experiment with various scents to see which help to alleviate the symptoms of senile dementia and increase mental clarity.

- bergamot
- clove
- frankincense
- lavender
- lemon balm

Summary

Contrary to mainstream medical belief, safe, natural, and nontoxic treatments can alleviate the symptoms of senile dementia. Research has demonstrated how these remedies can aid in preventing the onset of senile dementia. In the past, dementia was considered an uncontrollable outcome of aging. Taking action now can prevent our elder years from being characterized by cognitive degeneration and a rapid decline in health and ability.

Chapter 14

Menopause Study

A Comprehensive Lifestyle Intervention to Manage Menopause-Andropause and Improve Functions Affected by Aging

"I am a friend of life; at 80 life tells me to behave like a woman and not like an old woman."

—Chavela Vargas

The Study

The objective of all my Menopause-Andropause Health Study groups over the years has been to measure the effects of a comprehensive lifestyle program on common symptoms of menopause and andropause. The three-month study was the latest phase of a larger, ongoing intervention that we have conducted for more than fifteen years to determine how lifestyle choices affect daily functioning and well-being.

In keeping with this larger purpose, the menopause-andropause study also evaluated the impact of our lifestyle protocols on various aspects of mental, physical, and energy functioning and hair and skin status that may be negatively affected as we age. The lifestyle changes we studied encompassed diet and juicing, supplementation, exercise, stress management, and modification of behaviors and attitudes.

An important aspect of our lifestyle studies is that participants make these changes concurrently. We believe that a multicomponent approach to lifestyle change best reflects the way people improve their health in everyday lives. However, our multifactorial intervention also means that we do not (and cannot) determine which specific lifestyle factor is responsible for a given improvement. The multiple inputs—diet, physical activity, stress reduction, and so forth—work together to achieve the positive effect.

We chose to focus on menopause and andropause in our continuing study of lifestyle change because we wanted to evaluate the potential benefits of natural, nontoxic therapies during this transitional phase of life. Conventional medicine has traditionally approached menopause as a disease and has favored the use of pharmaceutical, synthetic hormone replacement therapy as a "cure." Two popular hormone replacement products are Premarin, a synthetic estrogen derived from the urine of pregnant horses, and Provera, a synthetic progestin. Unfortunately, clinical studies have confirmed that the use of synthetic hormones can increase the risk of breast cancer by up to 33 percent. The treatment of andropause, when the symptoms are recognized and evaluated, usually centers on the administration of testosterone.

Our goal was to determine how much improvement in menopause or andropause symptoms could be achieved with lifestyle changes alone. If women can minimize their symptoms with these natural interventions, they may have less need for hormone replacement therapy. Even bioidentical hormone products, such as estriol and estradiol—which are natural versions of the synthetic hormones used by mainstream medicine—may be needed in lesser amounts if lifestyle changes prove useful. The same philosophy applies to andropause. To the extent that lifestyle choices can help men manage the symptoms, they may be able to reduce the amount of testosterone replacement they require.

Background on Menopause

Menopause is a biological event common to women around the world. It can be defined as the conclusion of the female reproductive phase of life. The onset typically occurs between the ages of forty-five and fifty, although it may occur anywhere between forty and sixty or be initiated at an earlier age because of ovarian surgery and certain types of illnesses. The periods of pre-menopause and post-menopause can be thought of as processes lasting several years or more.

The Symptoms

Hot flashes are a common symptom of menopause. In addition, women may have dry skin, irritability, vaginal dryness, night sweats, urinary tract infections, mood swings, fatigue, and sleep disturbances. It should be noted that some women do not have any troublesome symptoms during menopause.

Nonetheless, this period in a woman's life cycle is characterized by a diminishing production of estrogen by the ovaries. When this occurs, the manufacture of estrogen is transferred to the adrenal glands and, to a lesser extent, the body's fat cells. Consequently, women with healthy adrenal glands often are less susceptible to acute symptoms.

A common misconception is that women will lose their sexual drive once they experience menopause. In fact, only a small percentage lose their ability to become aroused, and these cases can be effectively treated. Many women report heightened sexuality because the risk of pregnancy is absent. Another outdated belief is that, after this hormonal change occurs, life will no longer be enjoyable. Many women mistakenly fear that their later years will be marked by intense psychological problems.

Many studies have shown that women in Asian countries tend to adapt more easily to the hormonal changes involved in menopause because they accept the aging process as a natural transition. Age is associated with wisdom and respect in Asian countries, and therefore women do not dread this stage of life. In the United States and other post-industrial Western countries, women have a profound fear of advanced age due to cultural conditioning. This negative outlook is often correlated with the acquisition of acute menopausal symptoms. Asian women also may avoid such symptoms in part because their diets contain high quantities of soy products.

Background on Andropause

While menopause has traditionally been defined as a female condition, men experience a similar condition called andropause, which is caused by low testosterone levels. This is commonly referred to as male menopause. It typically begins as men enter their forties.

At this stage in life, many men begin to experience physical and emotional changes. The exercise routine that formerly held their body together alone is no longer sufficient. Fat slowly appears in places where muscle used to be. Sexual activity and interest wane, and a man's enthusiasm for living may decrease along with his sexual desire. When men have low levels of testosterone, it has a domino effect on mood, mental skills, memory, and sexual desire. Reports indicate that approximately twenty-five million men in the United States between forty and fifty-five years of age suffer from andropause.

Methods of the Menopause-Andropause Study

The Menopause-Andropause Health Study lasted for three months. We held regular support group meetings as participants followed the program's multiple lifestyle protocols. Of fifty-one people who participated in the group, thirty had sufficient data to be included in our analysis of results.

At the conclusion of the three-month period, participants rated the degree of change (or lack thereof) they had experienced in thirty-seven outcome measures that we listed in a preformatted questionnaire. The thirty-seven measures were divided into five major areas of assessment: (1) menopause or andropause symptoms, (2) mental function, (3) energy function, (4) body fat percentage, infections, allergies and digestion, and (5) hair and skin condition. Our rating scale included five degrees of change for participants to select for each outcome measure: worse, unchanged, improved, slightly improved, or much improved.

In addition to the data we collected by questionnaire, we followed up with participants by telephone for up to six months after the formal intervention period had ended. We also obtained testimonials and compliance information from twenty-two participants through videotaped or in-person statements or telephone interviews.

The Intervention Protocols

The menopause-andropause intervention recommended the following protocols:

1. DIET AND JUICING

Our nutritional protocols featured a largely vegetarian diet. The focus was on the consumption of complex carbohydrates—such as grains, legumes, fruits, vegetables, and nuts and seeds—and on daily juicing. The goals of the diet, juicing, and supplementation protocols were to turn off inflammatory reactions, to stop the process of glycation, which creates a cross-linking of proteins and sugars that has a negative effect on cells, and to rebalance hormones.

We permitted fish as an optional food choice because the omega-3 fatty acids found in various types of fish protect against heart disease and stroke and provide other health benefits. However, any fish containing high levels of mercury or polychlorinated biphenyls were to be avoided. We also recommended that participants consume healthy fats, which tend to be low in the American diet.

Specifically, the study asked participants to make the following dietary changes:

- Eliminate meat, including beef and poultry, and shellfish, swordfish, catfish, and shark. Replace with fresh, non-farmed, coldwater fish (including Pacific or Alaskan salmon, orange roughy, trout, sole, mackerel, sardines, calamari, octopus, cod, sea bass, halibut, mahi-mahi and snapper) and with vegetarian sources of protein, including organic nuts, nut butters, seeds, soybeans and soy products, quinoa (a high-protein grain), veggie burgers, soy chicken patties, sunshine burgers (made with sunflower seeds), seaweeds (e.g., wakame, arame, hijiki, dulse, and kelp) and protein shakes. Mix beans with grains such as brown rice, kamut, buckwheat, millet, and amaranth.

• Eliminate dairy, including milk, yogurt, cheese, butter, ice cream, cream sauces, and anything containing casein. Replace with nondairy milks (rice, soy, nut, and silken tofu). Replace butter with coconut oil, almond oil, Earth Balance spread, or Spectrum spread. Replace ice cream with rice or soy ice cream without added sugar.

• Eliminate nonorganic produce. Replace with organically grown fruits, vegetables, grains, and beans. We recommended nine servings of fruits and vegetables a day and four servings of beans/legumes and grains.

• Eliminate wheat. Replace with spelt bread, sprouted whole-grain bread, rice bread, millet bread, and Essene bread, as well as pastas, pancakes, and waffles made from spelt, buckwheat, quinoa, and rice.

• Eliminate sugar and artificial sweeteners (including maple syrup). Replace with stevia, Agave nectar, organic kiwi sugar, raw honey, molasses, barley malt, and brown rice syrup. (Chromium picolinate, 200 micrograms, was recommended to relieve sugar cravings.)

• Eliminate caffeine and alcohol, including chocolate, coffee, tea, colas, wines, hard liquor, and so forth. Replace with herbal teas, Mu tea, twig tea, Japanese teas, grain beverages (e.g., Cafix), green tea, and white tea (not black or oolong tea).

- Eliminate carbonated drinks, including soda and seltzer. Replace with spring, distilled, or filtered water, lemon water, fresh-squeezed organic fruit juice, iced herbal tea or Teeccino or soy coffee, and coconut juice or water.
- Eliminate fried and processed foods. Replace with steamed, sautéed, stir-fried, grilled, or broiled foods.
- Eliminate chemicals, including food additives, preservatives, coloring agents, and artificial flavorings. Avoid MSG and miso. Use nonirradiated spices and flavorings such as Herbamare, sea salt, granulated dulse and other sea vegetables, sesame seeds, organic, wheat-free soy sauces, and salad dressings consisting of olive oil, lemons, spices, and balsamic vinegar.
- *Include* the following beneficial foods in the diet, as well: sprouts, sea vegetables, onions, garlic, and healthy oils. For cooking, use coconut, macadamia, and mustard seed oils (but not olive oil). For baking, use hazelnut and macadamia oils. For salads and to add to cooked foods, use flax seed oil, extra virgin, cold-pressed olive oil, safflower oil, seed oils (grape, sesame, sunflower), avocado, and nut oils (almond, walnut, hazelnut, peanut).
- *Include* fresh juices. Participants started with one glass of green juice per day and built up to eight glasses per day in week twelve. The juice consisted of four ounces of dark and light green vegetables and six ounces of fluid, or one tablespoon of chlorophyll-rich green powder and ten ounces of fluid (e.g., milk substitute, cooled herb tea, diluted vitamin water, organic fruit juice, or filtered water). To this, one ounce of aloe concentrate and one teaspoon of red fruit powder were added.
- The program suggested that participants make a gallon of fresh green juice to be used over a week. Ingredients included one to two bunches of organic celery, one to two bunches of

organic parsley, four to five organic cucumbers, four organic lemons or limes, four to five organic apples, and optional foods such as cruciferous vegetables (purple cabbage, cauliflower, broccoli), green leafy vegetables (kale, chard, collards, mustard greens, arugula, spinach, bok choy), ginger, dill weed, fennel, scallions, onions, garlic, mint, cilantro, and other natural spices/flavorings. Carrots, tomatoes, or beets could be added for sweetness, but only in limited amounts for people with imbalances related to sugar consumption.

Discussion of Nutrition

Complex carbohydrates are beneficial in several ways. First, they are high in fiber and therefore can prevent common afflictions associated with aging, such as constipation, hemorrhoids, intestinal diseases, high blood pressure, and colorectal cancer. They also are rich in phytochemicals, antioxidant substances found in plants that help us prevent everything from cancer to arthritis and heart disease. Phytonutrients may be among the principal agents of repair to DNA damage.

Polyphenols, a type of phytonutrient, have a great neuroprotective effect. They also have anti-inflammatory properties and are powerful iron chelators. Polyphenols can be obtained from blueberries, bilberries, any deep-colored berries, plums, grapes, and black currants. Color can be used as a guide; in general, the stronger and more vibrant the color, the more nutritional value a fruit or vegetable has.

Sea vegetables and algae may not be household words, but the sea vegetables dulse, kelp, and nori are exceptionally high in minerals, particularly calcium, iodine, potassium, and magnesium, and in trace elements, as well. Garlic and onions are health superstars because they contain sulfur compounds that have an anti-aging and anticancer effect.

In terms of menopause, dietary choices can help manage symptoms and avert the need for synthetic hormone replacement therapy.

Women who incorporate natural estrogen-containing foods into their diets can experience dramatic relief from hot flashes. Studies have shown that plant estrogens, such as those found in soy products (e.g., tofu, tempeh, soybeans), are quite helpful in combating symptoms. Other foods that enhance estrogen, although in more modest amounts, are cashews, almonds, alfalfa, flax seeds, apples, grapefruit, lemons, pears, peaches, kuzu (a thickener used in place of flour), and boron-containing items such as green leafy vegetables, fruits, nuts, and legumes.

In addition, an increased dietary intake of fiber and reduced quantities of animal products can limit irritability. Sunflower seeds, walnuts, hazelnuts, cabbage, asparagus, broccoli, and barley are also additional combatants of menopausal symptoms.

Nutrition is an important component of mental functioning during menopause and andropause. Just as positive dietary choices help maintain good health, poor dietary habits can negatively impact emotions and exacerbate or bring on an episode of depression. Someone suffering from depression may have little or no appetite for food. The first step in eating a brain-healthy diet is to eliminate fast foods, simple carbohydrates, alcohol, artificial sweeteners, white flour products, and caffeine.

Detoxification

An important benefit of drinking juices daily and eating a well-balanced diet, with an emphasis on organically grown fruits and vegetables, is to help detoxify the body. The green juices included in the menopause-andropause study help with this process by supplying the body with chlorophyll, the ultimate blood purifier.

No matter how well we take care of ourselves, the air, water, food, and household products we come in contact with every day tend to be increasingly full of highly toxic chemicals. These manmade chemicals—which may number in the hundreds of thousands—have profound adverse effects on human health. Once they are absorbed, they are never fully eliminated, except by means of a comprehensive detoxification regimen.

During menopause and andropause, it is especially important to counter the group of toxic chemicals known as endocrine disruptors, which directly target the hormonal system. The endocrine system comprises all of the body's glands, including the thyroid and parathyroids, reproductive glands (testes and ovaries), adrenal glands, pancreas, hypothalamus, pituitary gland, and pineal glands. These glands and others secrete hormones that are responsible for a great deal of the body's regulatory activities. Many of the glands work in unison, and the hormones create a network of communication. Consequently, a disruption of one gland or hormone creates the potential for great disturbance throughout the body that will affect other internal systems.

There are numerous endocrine disruptors in our modern, industrial environment: emissions from factories and automobiles; incineration plants; household products; cosmetics, sunscreens, soaps, and perfumes; solvents; dental sealants; plastics; polystyrene (better known as Styrofoam); and, most important, pesticides.

Detrimental health effects associated with endocrine-disrupting chemicals include immunological disorders; cancer of the breast, colon, cervix, vagina, and testicles; abnormalities of the uterus, cervix, and vagina; non-Hodgkin's lymphoma; reduced sperm count and male infertility; prostate gland dysfunction; and behavioral and mental disorders. In women, endocrine disruptors accumulate faster and are stored in more concentrated amounts because they are attracted to fatty cells. Synthetic chemicals also can be passed easily to the bloodstream of a developing baby. Some endocrine disruptors convert into metabolites, a more toxic form of the original chemical, as they pass to the child.

2. SUPPLEMENTATION

This component of the study recommended a core group of vitamins, minerals, and herbs for both men and women. To that, we added a smaller group of supplements targeted specifically to women or specifically to men. The protocols were as follows:

SUPPLEMENTS FOR BOTH **MEN AND WOMEN**:

Vitamin A	6,700 mg
Vitamin B1 (Thiamine Mononitrate)	25 mg
Vitamin B2	50 mg
Vitamin B6	50 mg
Vitamin B12 (Cyanocobalamin)	1,000 mcg
Vitamin C (in Divided Doses)	5,000 mg
Vitamin E	402 mg
Vitamin D3	670 mg
Pantothenic Acid (D-Calcium Pantothenate)	300 mg
Choline Bitartrate	150 mg
Inositol	150 mg
Calcium Citrate	500 mg
Magnesium Citrate	500 mg
Zinc	15 mg
Selenium	100 mcg
Copper	2 mg
L-Carnitine	500 mg
Acetyl-L-Carnitine Arginate HCL	500 mg
L-Carnosine (in Divided Doses)	1,500 mg
L-Cysteine	200 mg
L-Glutamine	500 mg
L-Taurine	100 mg

L-Tyrosine 1	100 mg
N-Acetyl Cysteine	800 mg
Alpha Lipoic Acid	500 mg
Co-enzyme Q10	300 mg
Glucerophosphorylcholine	250 mg
Quercetin	1,000 mg
Phosphatidyl-Serine	200 mg
Pycnogenol	100 mg
DHEA (if Blood Chemistry or Saliva Level Shows Deficiency)	15 mg
Astaxanthin	25 mg
Benfotiamine	50 mg
Bromelain	100 mg
Lutein	25 mg
Lycopene	25 mg
Rutin	100 mg
Tocotrienols	200 mg
Bilberry Fruit Extract	25 mg
Blue Cohosh	100 mg
Broccoli Stem	25 mg
Cabbage Leaf	25 mg
Carrot Root	25 mg
Cayenne	50 mg
China Green Tea Leaf Powder	200 mg
Citrus Bioflavonoid	300 mg
Ginkgo Biloba Leaf	100 mg

Grape Seed Extract (Resveratrol, 300 mg)	150 mg
Licorice Root	25 mg
Milk Thistle Leaf	25 mg
Raspberry Leaf Powder	5 mg
Red Wine Concentrate	100 mg
Rosemary Leaf Powder	25 mg
Siberian Ginseng Root	100 mg

ADDITIONAL SUPPLEMENTS FOR **WOMEN** ONLY:

Black Cohosh Root	100 mg
Chasteberry Fruit Powder	100 mg
Dong Quai Root	100 mg
EPA/DHA	1,400/1,000 mg
Flax Seed Oil	1–3 tbsp
GLA	285–1,425 mg
L-Theanine	100–200 mg
L-Tryptophan	500–1,000 mg
Pomegranate Extract	200 mg
Red Clover Blossom Extract	100 mg
Soy Bean Extract	500 mg
St. John's Wort	300 mg
Vitex Berry Extract	625 mcg

ADDITIONAL SUPPLEMENTS FOR **MEN** ONLY:

Acetyl-L-Carnitine	1,000–2,000 mg
Cernitin	100 mg
Chrysin (do not take if you have prostate cancer)	1,500 mg

Citrus Pectin	220 mg
Milk Thistle Seed	200 mg
Muira Puama	600 mg
Phytosterol Complex	100 mg
Piperine	10 mg
Pygeum Bark Extract	160 mg
Saw Palmetto Berry Extract	250 mg
Soy Germ Powder	120 mg
Stinging Nettles	200 mg

Discussion of Supplementation

Vitamin D is an important nutrient for menopausal women. It can be supplemented in quantities of 670 milligrams or more per day and also is absorbed directly from sunlight. Vitamin E is beneficial in reducing vaginal dryness and thinning, as well. Natural sources of vitamin E, including the various mixed tocopherols, are more efficient than artificial versions.

Adequate quantities of essential fatty acids should be consumed because they act as natural hormone supplements, prevent cancer, and can alleviate the symptoms of aging. People on low-fat diets often suffer essential fatty acid deficiency and, consequently, need to incorporate certain foods into their diet to raise fatty acid levels. Omega-3 fatty acids are found in fish, fish oil, and flax seed oil. Many Americans have an excess of omega-6 fatty acids in relation to omega-3s. However, one type of beneficial omega-6 that *is* deficient in many women is gamma linoleic acid (GLA). GLA is available as evening primrose oil, borage oil, and black currant seed oil.

Calcium supplements may help prevent or reduce bone loss (osteoporosis). Calcium supplementation is particularly beneficial when started before menopause. While many women have difficulty assimilating dairy products, calcium citrate and amino acid chelate offer alternative calcium sources that can be easily digested. Regardless of the source, a woman's body requires 1,300 milligrams of calcium on a daily basis. Boron also may help with maintenance of bones.

Finally, certain soy products have high amounts of isoflavones, which are phytoestrogens that perform like a weaker version of estrogen. Several studies have found that soy significantly reduces the occurrence of hot flushes. A double-blind, placebo-controlled study showed that women who received 60 grams of soy protein isolate per day lessened their hot flash episodes by 45 percent. The results of one study showed a significant decrease in the occurrence of hot flashes after a six-week period among women who had taken 400 milligrams of soy extract and 50 milligrams of isoflavone daily.

Herbal Treatments

In addition to natural supplements, there are many herbs that can enhance a woman's ability to cope with menopause. They include chasteberry or vitex, black cohosh—which has been shown to help relieve menopausal symptoms—and dong quai. Traditional Asian physicians have used dong quai forcenturies to balance female hormones and avoid problems associated with menopause.

Menopausal Hormone Issues

Menopause is not just a deficiency of estrogen. The levels of four hormones—estrogen, testosterone, DHEA, and progesterone—must be balanced during menopause to ensure proper mental and physical functioning. The hormones affect the entire body and are linked to energy levels, brain electrical activity and cognitive function, healthy sexual function, vaginal lubrication, proper sleep, mood, skin and hair, muscle tone, and a general feeling of well-being.

3. EXERCISE

The exercise protocol included both aerobic and resistance training. For the aerobic portion, we recommended forty-five minutes of cardiac conditioning per day in which participants sustained 70 percent of their optimal heart rate. Although exercise produces harmful free radicals, our protocols emphasized the consumption of antioxidant-rich foods that help neutralize free radicals. Resistance training (free weights, circuit training, and calisthenics) was to be done for a half hour per day, working on every muscle group in the body.

Discussion of Exercise

Research demonstrates that exercise can diminish the occurrence of hot flashes in menopausal women. Exercise can also be a good counter to menopausal depression and mood swings because it enhances the production of endorphins and serotonin in the brain. Women who want to completely reap time benefits of physical fitness should initiate regular exercise significantly before the onset of menopause, although any time is a good time to begin—with medical guidance.

Similarly, a regular exercise routine can help men counteract the physical impact of andropause on the body. Numerous studies have documented that high-intensity exercise helps men keep their testosterone levels elevated.

Regular aerobic exercise assists with detoxifying the body, as well. Waste products are removed from the system with each exhalation. Exercise facilitates lung functioning and enables us to detoxify, as we sweat, through the outlet of our skin. Along with an adequate intake of water, it also helps detoxify the lymphatic system, which is part of the body's immunological function.

In addition, exercise allows more blood to flow to the tissues throughout the body. By oxygenating brain cells, exercise enhances brain function. It also improves metabolism, so that the body can easily maintain a normal weight. Finally, weight-bearing exercises, such as walking, jogging, and weightlifting, enhance bone density and thus help prevent osteoporosis.

Beneficial forms of exercise include biking, running, swimming, walking, and dancing. An effective option is power walking, which provides the aerobic benefits of running without putting stress on the joints. Cross-training also can be advantageous, but it is important to perform different exercises on different days of the week to avoid overexerting any one part of the body.

4. STRESS REDUCTION

The relaxation/meditation aspect of the intervention recommended a minimum of two half hour sessions per day of techniques such as Tai Chi, qi gong, meditation, prayer, yoga, journal writing, listening to calming music, or walking.

Discussion of Stress Management

Stress overtaxes the adrenal system and is a major contributor to premature aging, degenerative disease, and early death. In these hurried times, we need to make a conscious effort to slow down and find satisfaction in life. Meditation and relaxation techniques help with that effort. In addition, biofeedback uses the body's own signals to help combat stress. Massage also is an excellent way to relax.

5. BEHAVIOR MODIFICATION

Participants learned to identify their problem areas—such as overworking, overeating, unclear life goals, or dysfunctional relationships—and seek to modify that behavior. They kept journals in which they wrote about life issues and challenges. This regular practice helped them recognize life-affirming goals and determine how to achieve them in the face of obstacles.

In addition, it was important for participants to change their attitude toward lifestyle practices required by the study, such as vegetarian eating and daily exercise, and toward any toxic relationships they had. In some cases, they had to develop new social networks to gain support for the lifestyle changes they were making. The intervention program supported participants in adopting new lifestyle behaviors through group meetings in which questions and concerns were addressed; education on diet, exercise, stress management, and other topics was presented; exercise was demonstrated; and a "buddy system" that encouraged support within small groups was promoted.

Study Results

More than half of participants—and usually a substantial majority—reported improvement in thirty-five of the thirty-seven outcome measures listed in our questionnaire. These included all ten of our measures of menopause and andropause symptoms. In a noteworthy finding, 100 percent of participants saw improvement in three measures of functioning: overall energy function, overall mental function, and concentration. In fact, participants fared well across the board in our measures of mental functioning and energy functioning.

In the charts to follow, we provide a detailed presentation of the study results. As noted earlier, participants rated the degree of change they had experienced in each of the thirty-seven measures at the end of their participation. The rating scale provided to them included five choices: worse, no change, slightly improved, improved, or much improved. In two of the charts presented on the following pages, we have combined the three levels of improved condition—slightly improved, improved, and greatly improved—into one "improved" category.

In addition to the chart data, testimonials from participants confirm the many positive changes associated with lifestyle interventions. Almost all participants were enthusiastic in reporting their personal experiences, frequently citing additional benefits such as weight loss, joint disorder relief, new hair growth, renewed menstrual cycles, first-time marathon training, and increased self-esteem. Participants typically reported remarkable, and often outstanding, results.

The following six charts present the findings of our study:

CHART 1: Change in Menopause Symptoms

Female participants rated the degree of change they experienced in five symptoms of menopause. A majority reported improvement in all five measures. Two common symptoms of menopause—night sweats and hot flashes—were improved in 87 percent and 71 percent of women, respectively. About two-thirds scored positive change in incontinence (69 percent) and vaginal secretion/dryness (67 percent). Least often improved was painful intercourse (55 percent).

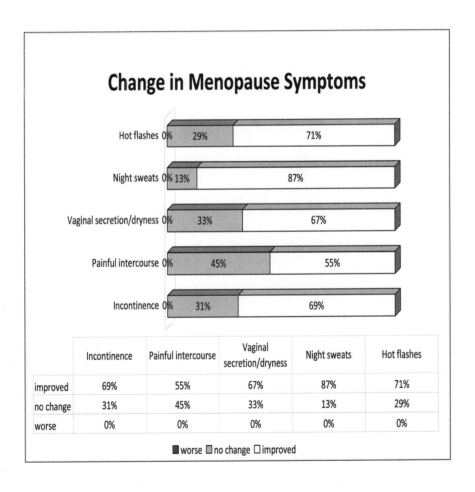

Change in Menopause Symptoms

	Incontinence	Painful intercourse	Vaginal secretion/dryness	Night sweats	Hot flashes
improved	69%	55%	67%	87%	71%
no change	31%	45%	33%	13%	29%
worse	0%	0%	0%	0%	0%

■ worse ■ no change ☐ improved

CHART 2: Change in Andropause Symptoms

Male participants rated their degree of change in five symptoms of andropause. More than half reported improvement in all five measures. The reversal of a loss of interest in sex was the most frequent improvement (84 percent of participants), including all three levels of improvement. This was followed by a reversal of weight gain (78 percent), sleep difficulty (76 percent), and general loss of interest (65 percent). The lowest rate of change was in irritability (51 percent).

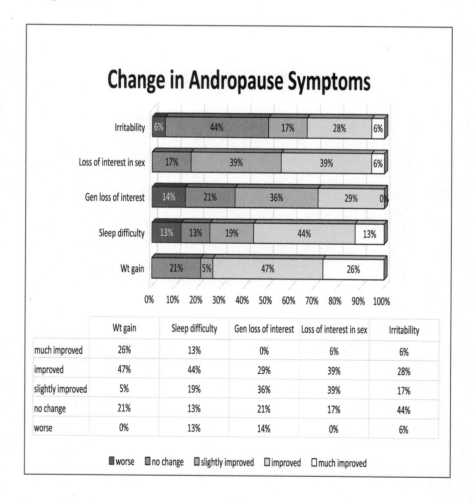

Change in Andropause Symptoms

	Wt gain	Sleep difficulty	Gen loss of interest	Loss of interest in sex	Irritability
much improved	26%	13%	0%	6%	6%
improved	47%	44%	29%	39%	28%
slightly improved	5%	19%	36%	39%	17%
no change	21%	13%	21%	17%	44%
worse	0%	13%	14%	0%	6%

■ worse　■ no change　□ slightly improved　□ improved　□ much improved

CHART 3: Change in Mental Function

This category saw high levels of improvement in six measures of functioning that may be affected during menopause/andropause and the aging process in general. Two of the measures—overall mental function and concentration—improved in 100 percent of participants. The other measures show frequent improvement across the board: short-term memory (93 percent of participants), clarity of thought (90 percent), brain fog (80 percent), and mood swings (78 percent).

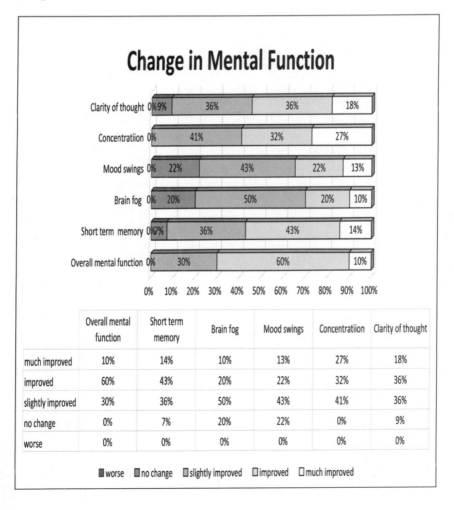

Change in Mental Function

	Overall mental function	Short term memory	Brain fog	Mood swings	Concentratiion	Clarity of thought
much improved	10%	14%	10%	13%	27%	18%
improved	60%	43%	20%	22%	32%	36%
slightly improved	30%	36%	50%	43%	41%	36%
no change	0%	7%	20%	22%	0%	9%
worse	0%	0%	0%	0%	0%	0%

■ worse ■ no change ■ slightly improved □ improved □ much improved

CHART 4: Change in Energy Function

This category also generated high rates of positive change. Eighty percent or more of participants scored improvements in seven of our eight energy measures, with 100 percent reporting improvement in their overall energy function. Also improved: evening energy (91 percent), energy decrease (88 percent), strength (84 percent), p.m. energy (82 percent), a.m. energy (80 percent), consistency (80 percent), and, least often, stamina (55 percent).

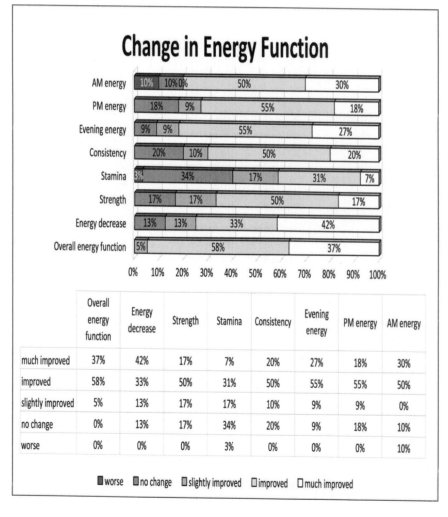

	Overall energy function	Energy decrease	Strength	Stamina	Consistency	Evening energy	PM energy	AM energy
much improved	37%	42%	17%	7%	20%	27%	18%	30%
improved	58%	33%	50%	31%	50%	55%	55%	50%
slightly improved	5%	13%	17%	17%	10%	9%	9%	0%
no change	0%	13%	17%	34%	20%	9%	18%	10%
worse	0%	0%	0%	3%	0%	0%	0%	10%

CHART 5: Change in Body Function

More than three-fourths of participants reported improvement in four of five measures of body functioning. Most often improved was percentage of body fat (95 percent of participants), followed by digestion (86 percent), infection (77 percent), and, least often, allergy (33 percent).

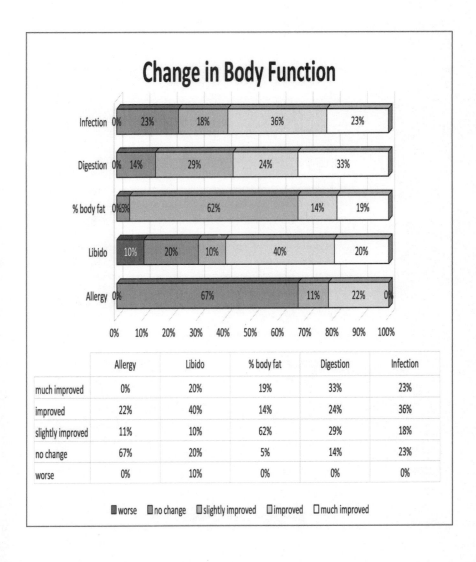

	Allergy	Libido	% body fat	Digestion	Infection
much improved	0%	20%	19%	33%	23%
improved	22%	40%	14%	24%	36%
slightly improved	11%	10%	62%	29%	18%
no change	67%	20%	5%	14%	23%
worse	0%	10%	0%	0%	0%

■ worse ■ no change ▨ slightly improved ▢ improved ▢ much improved

CHART 6: Change in Hair and Skin Condition

A majority of participants saw improvement in seven of eight measures of hair, skin, and nail condition. Quality of nails was improved in 100 percent of participants and quality of skin in 77 percent. The remaining six measures concerned hair status, and more than 70 percent said four of them had improved: hair texture/luster (77 percent), thinning of hair (75 percent), hair color (75 percent), and loss of hair (71 percent). Three in ten saw improvement in balding (29 percent).

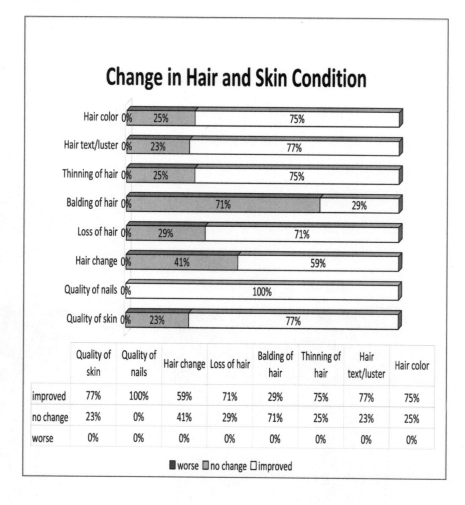

Change in Hair and Skin Condition

	Quality of skin	Quality of nails	Hair change	Loss of hair	Balding of hair	Thinning of hair	Hair text/luster	Hair color
improved	77%	100%	59%	71%	29%	75%	77%	75%
no change	23%	0%	41%	29%	71%	25%	23%	25%
worse	0%	0%	0%	0%	0%	0%	0%	0%

■ worse ▨ no change ☐ improved

Conclusion

The Menopause-Andropause Health Study demonstrates that natural, nontoxic lifestyle interventions—including diet, exercise, supplementation, stress management, and behavior modification—can help manage symptoms associated with this transitional stage of life. In addition to these positive results, the program generated high levels of improvement in various aspects of mental and energy functioning that may be negatively affected by menopause-andropause and the aging process in general. It is worth noting that participants were able to make the necessary lifestyle changes despite the comprehensive nature of the intervention. Support provided by the program was an important part of this process.

These findings suggest that the medical field should consider a more wellness-oriented approach to helping patients minimize the symptoms of menopause-andropause and counter the effects of aging on everyday functioning. A more natural approach may be especially important for women because of the health questions surrounding the use of synthetic hormone replacement therapy. By using lifestyle changes as a tool to manage menopausal symptoms, women may have less need for synthetic hormones or even bioidentical hormone products. Similarly, men may have a reduced need for testosterone therapy. In this way, a lifestyle approach may help shift the perspective of the medical establishment—and the patients it serves—toward a wellness paradigm.

Chapter 15

Psychoneuro-
immunology

"The greatest discovery of my generation is that man can alter his
life simply by altering his attitude of mind."

—William James

"Man is what he believes."

—Anton Chekhov

In the preceding chapters of this book, I stressed the importance of
the mind–body connection. I talked about how ensuring the health
of your body can protect the health of your brain, I explained how
underlying physical conditions can have negative effects on your
mental health, and I provided you with nutritional and lifestyle
strategies that enhance and protect the interrelationship between
good physical health and good brain health. I hope you see clearly
that the ways in which you treat your body can positively influence
the health of your brain. Now I want to talk to you about the other

side of the coin: how your brain can have a dramatic impact on your body's health.

In the beginning of this book, I challenged you to be part of a paradigm shift in defining the concept of successful aging and in quality of life as we grow older. What I want to leave you with is my thoughts on another equally potent paradigm that is emerging.

Psychoneuroimmunology (PNI) is the scientific study of the interconnections between the body's most complex systems, the emotions, the brain, and the immune system. My interest in psychoneuroimmunology and its applications for optimal health was sparked by a 1973 study conducted at Johns Hopkins University.[1] This study reported the discovery of receptors on our immune cells for neuropeptides. Neuropeptides are chemicals produced by the brain that fluctuate according to our emotions. The results of this study indicate that a person's immune system is affected by a person's thoughts. In essence, how you think you feel is how you feel.

This scientific discovery reaffirms my personal philosophy that there is no more important force in human history than belief. Jesus, Mohammad, Moses, Buddha, Copernicus, Mother Teresa, Martin Luther King, Jr., Thomas Edison, and Winston Churchill—all of these great historical figures had unshakable belief systems as their anchors.

We all have heard about individuals experiencing dramatic improvements in their health as a result of taking a placebo. Many attribute the positive effects of placebos to psychological forces—a strong belief that the treatment will work or a feeling that it is working. Irving Kirsch, a psychologist at the University of Connecticut, attributes the effectiveness of Prozac and other drugs almost entirely to the placebo effect. Kirsch conducted an experiment in which he analyzed nineteen clinical trials of antidepressants, concluding that the belief in improvement of the condition, as opposed to the alterations in brain chemistry, was responsible for 75 percent of the drugs' effectiveness.[2]

Studies indicate the existence of a circuit that connects the immune system and the brain, connecting illness or stress and thought. Traditional medicine has dismissed the notion that going outside in the cold can result in one catching a cold; nonetheless, there is much anecdotal evidence that contradicts this belief. New research is on the horizon that may make those "old wives' tales" (as described by those who discount this anecdotal evidence) accepted by traditional medicine.

Steven Maier, PhD, a University of Colorado distinguished professor and the director of the Center for Neuroscience, has explored two broad areas of research in the connection between stress and immunity functions. Dr. Maier studies the manner in which the brain regulates the immune system and how immune system cells send signals to the brain. The primary focus of his studies concerns comprehending the mechanisms of immune-to-brain signaling at various levels.[3]

The other major area of Dr. Maier's study concerns the variables that regulate the impact stressors have on brain chemistry and the neurochemical mechanisms that allow these stressors to change behavior, mood, and the organism's reactions to drugs.[4] This aspect of the study is primarily concerned with the degree to which behavioral control organisms are able to exercise control over stressors. The research indicates that stress—perhaps even the stress of being cold—appears to connect to the same immune system nervous system mechanism that ignites common cold symptoms.

For more than a decade, researchers have known that behavioral and psychological events can influence the immune system. What the study of psychoneuroimmunology tells us is that our beliefs cannot only change our perception of reality, but they can also change reality itself. In a remarkable case study, a woman in California had a cancerous tumor, so bad that it was described as resembling "a hand grenade under a thin sheathing of skin."[20] Her doctors, who had suggested she have a mastectomy, sent her to an alternative physician, who assisted her in visualization. One of the exercises involved increasing her body temperature. During this exercise, the temperature of her skin rose by 14 degrees. The woman responded extremely well to this treatment, and upon her return to her primary doctors two weeks later, it was found that the tumor had completely disappeared.[5]

In another study, researchers found that rheumatoid arthritis seemed to be connected to the strength of the individual's psychological defenses. Those patients with weakened psychological defenses were more liable to have rapidly developing cases of the disease, respond poorly to treatment, and become incapacitated.[6]

Maier's research is particularly interested in the knee-jerk reaction of our immune system, which determines whether we become ill as a result of certain stressors. This nonspecific immune response is frequently referred to as the "sickness" response. When activated, it sets in motion a series of physiological and behavioral changes, such as fever, alterations in the liver's metabolism, decreased consumption of food and liquid, and decreased sexual desire. This nonspecific immune response also triggers the classic response to stress commonly referred to as fight-or-flight—the release of stress-fighting hormones, including cortisol.

Maier believes that the sickness pattern is an organized effort on the part of the body, designed to manufacture energy to fight infection and to preserve energy. Maier and his colleagues determined the molecules called proinflammatory cytokines—interleukinl, interleukin 6, and tumor necrosis factor alpha—were signaling the brain.[7]

When Maier inactivated these cytokines or blocked the cerebral receptors that connected them, animals did not show any indication that they were sick following infection. When these cytokines were activated, however, the animals exhibited all of the classic signs of infection, whether they were sick or not.

Interestingly enough, Maier discovered that it is not the cytokines manufactured in the blood that signal to the brain that you are sick.

Remember the blood–brain barrier? The cytokines are too big to get past it. Instead, when infection fighting cells called macrophages attack a bacteria, a cytokine called interleukinl is released into the bloodstream, where it binds to receptors on the paraganglia cells found near the adrenal glands that release the neurotransmitters epinephrine and norepinephrine. These neurotransmitters activate the brain's vagus nerve, which controls the functions of the larynx, stomach, esophagus, heart, lungs, and intestines. This signal triggers the brain to make its own cytokines, setting off the sickness response, which then signals back to the immune system and further activates immune cells. Maier calls this loop from infection-fighting blood cells to cranial nerves to a systemic immune reaction "complete biodirectional immune-to-brain circuitry."[21]

In addition to this chemical brain immune system response, Maier discovered that if animals were stressed by being socially isolated or by being given electrical shock, their brains would produce massive increases in the cytokine interleukinl in the hippocampus.[8] Along with the predicted stress response, the animals exhibited behavioral and physiological changes: a decrease in food and water consumption, fever, increased white blood cell count, and activated macrophages just like those seen in the infection-driven "sickness" response.[9]

The implications of this shared neural loop are that stress and infection sensitize the body's reaction to each other. In other words, an infection primes the circuit so that it has an exaggerated response to later stress and vice versa. According to Maier, "Stress is another form of infection. And the consequences of stress are mediated by the activation of circuits that actually evolved to defend against infection."[10]

For many years, the concept of mind–body interactions has been discounted by traditional medicine. When scientific research demonstrates an example of such a connection, it is often dismissed by the traditional medical community as a placebo effect. Yet the mind–body connection has been proven by the tens of thousands of drug studies that employ the traditionally accepted double-blind, placebo-controlled method.

It is one thing for Deepak Chopra, Adele Davis, Canton Fredericks, myself, or any other alternative medicine practitioners to state their belief in the mind–body connection, but it took a well-respected member of the orthodox medical community to give it mainstream credibility. In 1974, Dr. Herbert Benson and his colleagues pioneered the discovery of the relaxation response, and a year later published the seminal work on the subject, *The Relaxation Response*.[11] Based on studies at Boston's Beth Israel Hospital and Harvard Medical School, Dr. Benson showed that relaxation techniques, such as meditation, have immense physical benefits and are effective in treating such disparate conditions as hypertension, heart disease, and cancer. This book ushered in a new era in the study of the mind–body connection.

In 1993, the field and concept of mind-body medicine were brought into the homes of mainstream America by one of its most respected journalists, when Bill Moyers hosted his PBS television special *Healing and the Mind*. Throughout the series, Moyers explored the uncharted waters of the mind-body connection through a series of interviews with acclaimed experts, as well as ordinary laypeople. The author showed the American public for the first time how the new innovations in the mind–body field were being used to treat stress, chronic disease, and neonatal problems in hospitals throughout America. Moyers also delved into the chemical connection of emotions and their ability to either make us well or make us sick.

Later, experiments conducted by the well-respected Dr. Andrew Weil confirmed that the benefit of a treatment almost always mirrored the expectations of the patient. In one amazing case, reported in his book *Spontaneous Healing*,[12] a woman with advanced lupus and kidney failure was in failing health when she fell in love. Shortly thereafter, her symptoms disappeared. Dr. Weil reported that the remarkable shift in her level of consciousness coincided precisely with the full remission of her disease. The power of her mind, her beliefs, and her attitude was accepted as positively impacting her medical condition.

But this field did not just arrive in the 1970s or 1980s. It merely took that long for it to be accepted by the mainstream. Thirty years ago, the medical establishment laughed at me for stating that simply by changing one's lifestyle, a person's health could be improved. They are not laughing at me today. Virtually every day I see a new report touting the benefits of lifestyle change in combating a wide array of conditions. Just a sampling of the spate of recent reports shows how brain exercise is the key to a healthy mind,[13] that lifestyle plays a significant role in Alzheimer's disease,[14] and that lifestyle is crucial in combating diabetes.[15]

To properly understand the use of mind–body medicine, one must place it in its proper context. Lifestyle changes designed to improve the health of the individual must occur first, for the mind–body techniques are only one of many areas of lifestyle change that synergistically improve health. Recent medical studies confirm that proper diet, exercise, and social support networks are integral pieces of this puzzle.

We all have had the experience of being involved in an extremely stressful situation—an argument with a loved one, the death of a close friend, or being fired from one's job—and shortly thereafter coming down with a cold or just feeling miserable. Up until relatively recently, there was no scientific support establishing a relationship between the two. The thought that feelings could adversely affect physical health was an alien one to the medical community.

But a plethora of scientific evidence has now established a definite link between feelings and physical health. This evidence demonstrates how the brain regulates the immune system, the body's main guardian against infectious diseases, in extremely complex and critical ways by sending a steady barrage of messages to it. As we have seen, however, this is a two-way street, for the brain also receives messages from the immune system.

In all of the cases I've used as illustrations in this chapter, the single constant in successful outcomes was the belief of the individual. This belief was relayed to the brain, to the immune system, or to the nervous system. Once this belief was firmly entrenched, the body and brain went into action and performed miracles.

One of my favorite examples of the power of the mind to control the body is that of the runner Roger Bannister. Until 1954, it was widely believed that humans were incapable of running the mile in under four minutes. It was thought that it was physically impossible for a person to do so. Then Roger Bannister ran the mile in 3:59:4. Less than six weeks after Bannister broke the record, John Landy from Australia lowered the record by another second. And within the next nine years, nearly two hundred people had broken the "impossible" barrier. Now, high school athletes routinely break it. Bannister demonstrated that the barrier was purely psychological. But the significant aspect to this story is that any of those two hundred people could have figured it out on their own. They didn't really need Bannister to show them the fallacy of this belief.

The four-minute mile is a metaphor for life. It is a metaphor for everything that everyone has told you that you could not do. But now you have the knowledge to prove them wrong. Your health is in your hands and in your mind.

PART III

APPENDICES

Appendix I

Purchasing Vitamins, Supplements, and Herbal Remedies

When I am talking with people in my travels, one of the questions they most frequently ask me is, "How can I be sure I am choosing a high-quality supplement?" With the rise in popularity of nutritional supplements, it can be confusing to know how to purchase high-quality vitamins, minerals, and supplements.

Natural health stores or groceries stock most of the vitamins, supplements, and herbs I recommend in this book. Even some mainstream grocery stores carry many of the vitamins and supplements mentioned. If you are able to use the Internet, it is easy to research and purchase supplements and herbal remedies online.

Vitamins and Supplements

When shopping for vitamins and supplements, there are a few important questions you should ask:

- How does the manufacturer select its ingredients?
- What is the specific formula of the vitamin or supplement?
- What is the potency level of the vitamin or supplement?
- Does the manufacturer test for quality control, and if so, how?
- Are the vitamins natural (i.e., from food sources) or do they include added ingredients?

You may wonder whether it is better to choose tablets, capsules, powders, or liquids when purchasing vitamins and supplements. Generally speaking, tablets have a long shelf life, but can contain fillers and stabilizers that may cause allergic reactions. Capsules are generally used for fat-soluble and powdered supplements. The powdered type is most rapidly absorbed and generally contains no additives. The liquid forms may contain coloring agents or sweeteners.

Multivitamins may be useful in combining vitamins and minerals that are more effective when taken together (e.g., a B-complex vitamin). Most multivitamins combine vitamins and minerals in complementary doses. In some of the protocols given earlier in the book, I recommend doses higher than those found in multivitamins. For that reason, with the exception of a B-complex vitamin, I recommend buying vitamins and supplements individually.

Finally, when purchasing supplements, remember these important points:

- Buy from organic sources whenever possible. Avoid artificial ingredients.
- If you have food sensitivities, buy hypoallergenic products. Avoid wheat, yeast, and corn.
- Always examine the expiration date before purchasing.

- If you have any questions or doubts about a product, never hesitate to contact the manufacturer and ask questions. A reputable company will not hesitate to address concerns.

For a more detailed discussion of vitamins and supplements, go to my website: www.garynull.com.

Herbal Remedies

If you are taking herbs, it is essential to take them in proper dosages, because they contain powerful ingredients. For centuries, people have been taking herbs to treat various conditions. When taken in the correct manner, herbs do not have the side effects that traditional medicines may cause. If herbs are used randomly or indiscriminately, however, they may produce unwanted side effects. If you are taking prescription or over-the-counter medications, you should talk with your health care provider before taking any herbal remedies, because some may have adverse interactions with medications. Herbs may be taken in their natural forms of leaves, barks, or roots by brewing them in teas. More commonly, herbs are taken in capsules or tinctures. Herbs can be used in compresses, applied externally with essential oils, or infused in teas, ointments, or salves.

For more information on herbal remedies, including hundreds of scientific studies on the efficacy of herbs for impacting various conditions, along with recommended dosages, go to www.garynull. com.

Reboot Your Brain Meals: Recipes for the Mind

The late comedian Redd Foxx used to joke, "They say you are what you eat. No wonder you look like garbage to me." Truer words were never spoken. You not only literally become what you eat, but what you eat determines how you think, what kind of mood you are in, how you feel, and your emotional stability. Furthermore, it has been proven that what you eat can increase your IQ, enhance your memory, and reverse the aging process.

Through my extensive travels, I have noticed that the vast majority of individuals I meet are nowhere near maximizing their brains' full potential in terms of intelligence, focusing, and memory. Little do they know that with the proper types and amounts of nutrients, they could drastically improve their overall health and brain function.

It is important to consume foods as they were grown in nature. Organic fresh fruits and vegetables, whole grains, legumes, nuts and seeds, and (for those who are not vegetarians) nontoxic animal proteins head the list. Purchase organic foods that have not been exposed to pesticides or other chemical sprays and are not packed with additives.

Eating right does not have to involve a huge effort. Prepare healthy dishes in larger quantities and store them for use throughout the week.

The following recipes were created specifically to promote the health and vitality of your brain. Our brains are under constant assault from a variety of sources: stress, work, home life, improper relationships, free radical damage, electromagnetic radiation, improper nutrition, and so on. To gain the most benefit from my eating plan, you must be consistent in your approach and committed to the health and welfare of your brain. You cannot exercise and eat properly for a month, then take a month off. After all, cell-damaging free radicals never take a day off.

Too many people are literally digging their own graves with their forks. Why not build a temple?

Please note that when soy is mentioned, we mean organic, non-GMO soy only. Also, when wheat is mentioned, please know that you can easily replace it with gluten-free alternatives such as amaranth, quinoa, millet, wild rice, buckwheat, sorghum, and teff, among others.

Recipes

Beverages   340

Main Dishes   376

Desserts   395

Beverages

ALL GREEN
½ cucumber
1 leaf kale
½ bunch parsley
1 small romaine lettuce
3 stalks celery
2 ounces whole aloe vera juice from a bottle

Juice the cucumber, kale, parsley, romaine, and celery, then add the aloe juice.
Serves 1

ANTIOXIDANT PUNCH
1 pineapple, peeled, cored, and cut into 1-inch cubes
4 large limes, peeled and quartered
2 cups unsweetened cranberry juice

1 cup concord grape juice
24 ice cubes
1 large lime, sliced into ½-inch thick half-moons (for garnish)
2 pineapple wedges, sliced into ½-inch thick fans (for garnish)

Separately juice the pineapple and limes. In a large pitcher or punch bowl, combine the pineapple and lime juices with the cranberry juice, grape juice, and ice. Stir together until well combined. Serve garnished with lime and pineapple slices.

ANTIOXIDANT SUPREME
½ honeydew, cubed (do not remove skin)
15 grapes (do not use seedless grapes)
½ cup organic, nonalcoholic red wine (with no sulfites)
2 tbsp aloe vera concentrate

Juice the honeydew and grapes. Blend the juices with the wine and aloe vera concentrate in a container.

APPLE PEAR GINGER ALE
1 large apple, cored and quartered
2 cups sparkling mineral water
1 large pear, cored and quartered
6 ice cubes
1 oz. fresh ginger, sliced into ½-inch pieces

Juice the apple, pear, and ginger. In a large pitcher, combine the apple juice mixture and mineral water. Stir together until well combined. Serve over ice.

APPLE SPROUTS
4 apples, cored and quartered
2 yams, cubed
1 cup alfalfa sprouts

Separately juice the ingredients. Combine the juices and serve immediately.

THE BIG CLEANSE
½ clove organic garlic, peeled
2 cups collard greens, chopped
2 cups organic cauliflower, chopped
½ cup red beet, cubed
1 cup organic chard, chopped
2 large apples, cored and quartered
2 oz. wheatgrass juice

Separately juice the garlic, collard greens, cauliflower, red beet, chard, and apples. Combine the juices and add the wheatgrass juice. Stir well.

(Note: Wheatgrass can be juiced by using a wheatgrass press. You can also make wheatgrass juice by squeezing the grass into clusters with your hand and juicing these hand-squeezed clusters through a traditional fruit and vegetable juicer.)

BLUEBERRY AND PEAR MACADAMIA NUT SHAKE
2 pears (or ½ cup pear juice)
1 banana, mashed
½ cup blueberries
½ cup unsweetened rice milk
½ cup ground or whole white macadamia nuts, unsalted
2 heaping tbsp protein powder
½ tsp pure lemon extract

Juice the pears. In a blender, combine the pear juice with the blueberries, macadamia nuts, mashed banana, rice milk, protein powder, and lemon extract. Blend for 2 minutes, or until smooth. Serve immediately.

BRAIN JUICE

1½ cups organic green beans

½ head organic cabbage, shredded

2 cups organic collard greens, chopped

1 cup organic spinach

2 medium organic peaches, quartered and pitted

3 oranges, peeled and quartered

Separately juice the green beans, cabbage, collard greens, spinach, peaches, and oranges. Combine the juices and serve immediately.

BRAIN POWER

12 lychee nuts (pitted)

2 oranges, quartered

2 mangos, diced and pitted

100 mg ginseng

100 mg ginkgo biloba

Remove the seeds and skin from the lychee nuts. Separately juice the lychee nuts, oranges, and mangos. In a blender or food processor, combine the juices with the herbs and blend until smooth.

CARROT, PINEAPPLE, AND STRAWBERRY JUICE

1 cup of strawberries, halved

4 carrots, sliced

½ pineapple, cubed and peeled

Remove the stems and leaves from the strawberries. Separately juice the strawberries, carrots, and pineapple. Combine the juices and serve immediately.

CHILLING RELAXER

½ pint organic dandelion flowers and stems

2 pints medium organic strawberries

1 medium piece organic cantaloupe (peeled)
2 tbsp organic flax oil
2 oz. organic wheatgrass juice
1 tbsp lecithin

Separately juice the dandelions, strawberries, and cantaloupe. Combine the juices and add the flax oil, wheatgrass juice, and lecithin. Stir well.

(Note: Wheatgrass juice can be made by using a wheatgrass press. You can also make wheatgrass juice by squeezing the grass into clusters with your hand and juicing these hand-squeezed clusters through a traditional fruit and vegetable juicer.)

CHLOROPHYLL BOOST

2 cups organic alfalfa sprouts
2 cups organic spinach, chopped
2 cups organic collard greens, chopped (with ends cut)
5 medium stalks organic asparagus
2 oz. wheatgrass juice
1 apple, cored and quartered (optional)

Separately juice the alfalfa sprouts, spinach, collard greens, and asparagus, and combine with the wheatgrass juice. If you find the greens alone to be too bitter, juice an apple and add the juice to the mixture.

(Note: Wheatgrass juice can be made by using a wheatgrass press. You can also make wheatgrass juice by squeezing the grass into clusters with your hand and juicing these hand-squeezed clusters through a traditional fruit and vegetable juicer.)

CRANBERRY COOLER

4 cups filtered water
2 green tea bags (decaffeinated)

4 large oranges, peeled
2 large limes, peeled
1 large lemon, peeled
1 cup unsweetened cranberry juice
2 cups blueberries
¼ cup honey
1 tsp ground cinnamon
20 ice cubes
1 large lime, sliced into ½-inch thick half-moons (for garnish)

In a small saucepan with lid, combine the water and tea bags, bring to a boil, then simmer, covered, for 8 to 10 minutes, or until fully brewed. Set aside to cool completely. Separately juice the oranges, limes, and lemon. In a blender, combine the juices with the cranberry juice, blueberries, honey, cinnamon, ice cubes, and tea. Blend on high speed for 3 minutes or until well combined. Serve over ice and garnish with lime slices.

CUCUMBER COOLADE
1 large bunch flat-leaf parsley
4 large cucumbers, cut into quarters lengthwise
4 pears, cored and quartered
1 small piece ginger (1-inch square)

Bunch up the parsley and push it through the juicer feed tube, alternating it with the cucumbers, pears, and ginger. Serve immediately.

DEEP-SEA JUICING
1 oz. wakame
1 oz. kombu
1 oz. dulse
2 cups arugula lettuce, chopped

2 cups organic red leaf lettuce, chopped
2 cups organic romaine lettuce, chopped
2 apples, cored and quartered

Cut the wakame, kombu, and dulse into small pieces and chop very finely in a blender or food processor. Separately juice the arugula, red leaf, and romaine lettuces, and the apples. Add the juices to the vegetables in the blender or food processor and blend until well combined. Serve immediately.

DELICIOUS DETOX
½ small watermelon, cubed (do not remove rind)
2 cups frozen cherries (pitted)
2 cups alfalfa sprouts
½ pint blueberries
½ pint raspberries
1 medium organic peach, pitted and quartered

Separately juice the watermelon, cherries, alfalfa sprouts, blueberries, raspberries, and peach. Combine the juices and serve immediately.

DETOX TONIC
1 watermelon, cubed (do not remove rind)
2 grapefruits, peeled and quartered
2 limes, peeled and quartered
8 kiwifruit, peeled
1 lemon, peeled and quartered

Push the watermelon, kiwifruit, grapefruits, limes, and lemon through the juicer feed tube. Serve immediately.

ENZYME ENHANCER
1 medium organic papaya, cubed
½ large organic pineapple, cubed and peeled

6–10 large organic strawberries, halved, with stems and leaves removed

½ medium organic cabbage, chopped

½ small organic kiwi, quartered

Separately juice the papaya, pineapple, strawberries, cabbage, and kiwi. Combine the juices and serve immediately.

EVERGLADES PUNCH

1 honeydew melon, peeled, seeded, and cut into 2-inch pieces (about 8 cups)

4 large oranges, peeled and quartered

4 large limes, peeled and quartered

2 large grapefruits, peeled and quartered

2 large lemons, peeled and quartered

4 mangos, peeled, pitted, and cut into 2-inch pieces

1 cup blueberries

20–40 ice cubes

1 large orange, sliced into ½-inch thick half-moons (for garnish)

Push the melon, oranges, limes, grapefruits, lemons, mangos, and blueberries through the juicer feed tube. Serve over ice and garnish with orange slices.

FATIGUE BUSTER

3 carrots, sliced lengthwise

1 pear, cored and quartered

2 cucumbers, sliced

½ tsp bee propolis

Separately juice the carrots, cucumbers, and pear. Combine the juices and stir in the bee propolis. Serve immediately.

(Note: If you are allergic to bee propolis, replace it with ½ tsp guarana or ginseng powder. The powder can be removed from capsules.)

FLAX CRUNCHER
3 tbsp organic flax seed
1 cup organic puffed rice
1 cup tofu yogurt
½ cup Rice Dream Original

In a grinder, grind the flax seed very finely. In a blender, chop the puffed rice. Add the flax seed, tofu yogurt, and Rice Dream to the chopped puffed rice and blend well.

FOUNTAIN OF YOUTH
1 cup green grapes
1 cup purple grapes
½ cantaloupe, cubed and peeled
2 medium organic zucchini, sliced
1 medium tomato, quartered
2 tbsp vegetarian protein powder

Separately juice the green and purple grapes, cantaloupe, zucchini, and tomato. In a blender, combine the juices with the protein powder and blend well.

FREE RADICAL DELIGHT
1 cup organic grapes
½ medium organic cantaloupe, cubed and peeled
½ cup organic broccoli, chopped
1 cup organic collard greens, chopped (with ends cut)
1 cup organic spinach, chopped (with ends cut)
3 oranges, quartered

Separately juice the grapes, cantaloupe, broccoli, collard greens, spinach, and oranges. Combine the juices and serve immediately.

GARY'S GINGER ALE
organic ginger, 1-inch piece
½ large organic cantaloupe, cubed (do not remove rind)
½ pint organic strawberries, halved and stemmed
1 medium organic orange, quartered (do not remove peel)
4 oz. sparkling water

Separately juice the ginger, cantaloupe, strawberries, and orange.
Combine the juices and add the sparkling water. Serve immediately.

GINGERMINT TEA
8 cups filtered water
4 peppermint tea bags
½ cup freshly squeezed lemon juice
40 ice cubes
1 large lemon, sliced into ½-inch thick half-moons
4 oz. fresh ginger, sliced into ½-inch pieces (for garnish)
1 tbsp plus 1 tsp honey (optional)
fresh mint (optional)

In a small saucepan with a lid, combine the water, tea bags, and
ginger over moderate heat and simmer covered for 8 to 10 minutes,
or until fully brewed. Sir in the honey until well combined and set
aside to cool completely. Combine the tea, lemon juice, and ice
in a large pitcher. Stir together. Serve garnished with lemon slices
and fresh mint.

GREEN POWER PUNCH
2 cups kale, chopped
1 cup broccoli, chopped
2 cups organic parsley, chopped
½ head cauliflower, chopped

1 cup organic spinach, chopped
6 stalks celery
1 medium organic apple, cored and quartered

Separately juice the kale, parsley, spinach, apple, broccoli, cauliflower, and celery. Combine the juices and serve immediately.

HEAD CLEANER
1 small onion, quartered and peeled
3 cloves garlic, peeled
2 stalks celery
1 turnip, halved (do not remove the leaves)
ginger, ½-inch slice
3 tbsp honey

Separately juice the onion, garlic, celery, turnip, and ginger. Combine the juices and add the honey. Stir well.

HOW GREEN IS YOUR JUICE?
2 cups kale, chopped
2 cups spinach, chopped
2 stalks celery
2 tsp Green Stuff powder

Separately juice the kale, spinach, and celery. In a blender, combine the juices with the Green Stuff powder and blend well. Serve immediately.

THE KITCHEN SINK
1 apple, cored and quartered
1 cup spinach, chopped
1 cup kale, chopped
½ cup chard, chopped
½ papaya, cubed

2 cloves garlic, peeled
organic ginger, ½-inch piece
2 tbsp protein powder

Separately juice the apple, spinach, kale, chard, papaya, garlic, and ginger. In a blender, combine the juices and protein powder and mix well.

MELON BOOST
½ medium cantaloupe, peeled and cubed
½ small watermelon (without rind), cubed
1 medium lemon, peeled and quartered
½ tsp vitamin C powder
1 pint raspberries

Separately juice the cantaloupe, watermelon, and lemon. In a blender, combine the juices, vitamin C powder, and raspberries, and mix well.

NUTS AND SEEDS
2½ cups vanilla soy milk
1 pint blueberries
2 frozen bananas, peeled
3 tbsp organic soy butter
3 tbsp organic almond butter
3 tbsp organic cashew butter
3 tbsp organic macadamia butter
3 tbsp organic sunflower butter

In a blender, combine the soy milk, blueberries, and bananas. Add the butters and blend until smooth. Serve immediately.

PURE CITRUS PUNCH
8 large grapefruits, peeled and cubed
12 large oranges, peeled and cubed

8 large limes, peeled and quartered
4 large lemons, peeled and quartered
16–20 ice cubes

Separately juice the grapefruits, oranges, limes, and lemons. Combine the juices and serve over ice.

RELAX YOUR MIND
4 stalks celery
3 carrots, sliced lengthwise
2 apples, cored and quartered
ginger, 1-inch piece
kava kava (1 capsule/25 mg)
chamomile (1 capsule/25 mg)
St. John's wort (1 capsule/100 mg)
valerian (1 capsule/50 mg)
½ tsp nutmeg
½ tsp cinnamon

Separately juice the celery, carrots, apples, and ginger. In a blender, combine the juices, and empty the powder from the capsules into the liquid. Add the nutmeg and cinnamon and mix well.

RUBY RED
1 grapefruit, peeled and quartered
½ cup blueberries
1 pear, cored and quartered
½ cup strawberries
1 tsp lecithin
½ cup ice

In a blender, combine the grapefruit, pear, strawberries, blueberries, and lecithin with ice and blend until smooth.

SLEEP INSURER
ginger, 1-inch piece
½ head cabbage, chopped
½ cup organic basil
2 medium organic bananas
1 cup green beans
valerian root extract
3 stalks organic celery

Separately juice the ginger, basil, green beans, celery, and cabbage. In a blender, combine the juices and bananas. Add 10 to 15 drops liquid valerian root and blend until smooth.

STRONG LUNGS
6 large organic carrots, sliced lengthwise
1 organic apple, cored and quartered
1 organic avocado, peeled, quartered, and pitted
½ large guava fruit, peeled, seeded, and quartered
3 tsp liquid chlorophyll

Separately juice the carrots, apple, avocado, and guava fruit. Combine the juices and add liquid chlorophyll. Stir well.

SUPER VEGETABLE COCKTAIL
1 large bunch flat-leaf parsley (about ½ pound)
2 large tomatoes, cored and quartered
8 large celery stalks
4 large carrots, tops removed and cut into halves lengthwise
4 yellow bell peppers, cored, seeded, and cut into quarters
4 large limes, peeled
sea salt to taste (about ½ tsp)
4 celery stalks (for garnish)
1 large lime, sliced into ½-inch thick half-moons (for garnish)

Separately juice the parsley, then alternate pushing the tomatoes, celery, carrots, peppers, and limes through the juicer tube. Stir in salt until well combined. Serve garnished with celery stalks and lime slices.

VELVETY PECAN MILK

1 cup pecan halves, soaked in 4 cups filtered water for 6 to 8 hours (then discard soaking water, rinse well, and drain)
4 cups filtered water
2 tbsp honey
1 tbsp pure almond flavor
2 tbsp pure vanilla flavor
1 pinch salt

Combine the prepared pecans and 4 cups water in a blender. Blend on medium speed for 30 seconds; increase speed to high, and continue blending for 1 minute.

Transfer the pecan mixture to a cheesecloth-lined sieve and strain into a medium bowl (squeeze or use a spoon to stir and push the milk through while you pour; it will be too rich to strain it through without a bit of mashing). Save the pulp for hot cereal, grain dishes, baked goods, or smoothies.

Rinse and dry the blender, then pour in the strained milk, honey, almond flavor, vanilla flavor, and salt. Blend on high speed until smooth and frothy, about 1 minute. Transfer to a container and refrigerate for 12 hours or until chilled.

VERY BERRY SHAKE

1 cup fresh or frozen blueberries, strawberries and blackberries
1¼ cup soy milk
1 banana
3 tbsp pure maple syrup

1 cup ice cubes

1 tbsp Red Stuff powder

Combine all the ingredients in a blender and blend until smooth.

WISDOM DRINK

3 burdock roots, sliced

2 parsnips, sliced

4 carrots, sliced lengthwise

1 cup parsley greens

1 tbsp blackstrap molasses

Separately juice the burdock, parsnips, carrots, and parsley greens. In a blender, combine the juices and add the molasses. Blend well and serve immediately.

Salads

SPROUT AND VEGGIE SALAD

3 oz. Brussels sprouts

3 oz. lima beans, cooked (chilled)

3 oz. barley, cooked (chilled)

3 oz. soybean sprouts

1½ oz Brazil nuts, chopped

2 tbsp soy oil

1 tsp soy sauce

½ tsp chopped parsley

½ tsp rosemary

½ tsp salt

Steam the Brussels sprouts for 10 minutes. Combine all ingredients and mix well. Serve cool.

Serves 2

MILLET AND GREENS SALAD

3 oz. green pepper, chopped

3 oz. onion, chopped

3 oz collard greens, coarsely chopped

3 oz millet, cooked (chilled)

1½ oz pumpkin seeds

2 tbsp sesame oil

½ tsp thyme

1 tsp tarragon

½ tsp salt

Steam all vegetables for 3 minutes. Combine all ingredients. Mix well. Serve hot or cold.

Serves 2

JAPANESE BUCKWHEAT SALAD

3 cups cooked buckwheat noodles

¼ cup toasted sesame oil

2 tbsp sliced scallions

2 tbsp raisins

2 tbsp sunflower seeds

1 cup broccoli florets, steamed 5 to 6 minutes

1 cup sliced carrots

3–4 tbsp tamari (or soy sauce)

¼ cup gomasio

Combine all the ingredients in a medium bowl and mix well. Serve chilled.

Serves 2

MELLOW RICE SALAD

3 oz. basmati rice, cooked (chilled)

½ oz. pecans, chopped

3 oz. fresh dill, chopped
3 oz. yellow pepper, chopped
1½ tbsp safflower oil
2 tbsp cider vinegar
½ tsp salt

Combine all ingredients.
Serves 1

INDONESIAN SPROUT SALAD
2 cups sunflower sprouts
2 cups bean sprouts
2 cups whole walnuts
½ cup honey
3 cups sliced red cabbage
1 cup diced raw carrots
1 cup sliced onion
½ cup toasted sesame seeds

Coat the walnuts with the honey and place on a lightly greased cookie sheet. Bake in a preheated, 375°F oven for 20 minutes. In a large bowl, toss the sprouts, red cabbage, carrots, onion, and sesame seeds. Then toss the salad with dressing and top with the walnuts before serving.
Serves 2

FABULOUS WILD RICE SALAD
3 cups cooked wild rice
½ cup carrots, sliced
½ cup broccoli florets, steamed 5 to 6 minutes
½ cup fresh parsley, chopped
½ cup zucchini, diced
3 tbsp safflower oil

1 tsp fresh dill, chopped
2 tbsp fresh lemon juice
½ tsp freshly ground black pepper
½ tsp salt

Combine all the ingredients in a medium bowl, mix well, toss, and serve at room temperature.

FOUR-BEAN SALAD
½ cup dry chickpeas
½ cup dry black beans
½ cup dry kidney beans
½ pound fresh string beans, cut into 1-inch pieces
1–2 carrots, grated
3 scallions, sliced
½ green pepper, chopped
1 large celery stalk, diced or chopped
Orange Vinaigrette (see below)

Soak the chickpeas, black beans, and kidney beans in separate pots of water, covered, overnight. Drain. Add unsalted water to each pot and cook the soaked beans, covered, for about an hour, or until tender. Drain, put into separate containers, and refrigerate until chilled. Steam the string beans for 5 minutes, or until just tender. Place in the refrigerator to chill. In a large mixing bowl, combine the chilled beans and the vegetables. Pour the Orange Vinaigrette over the mixture and refrigerate several hours or overnight. Serve on a bed of lettuce topped with some grated, nondairy cheddar cheese, or use this salad to stuff a pita along with the nondairy cheese slices.

Orange Vinaigrette
1 tsp orange zest, minced
16 oz. fresh orange juice

2 tbsp apple cider vinegar

½ sweet onion

2 tbsp of honey

1 garlic clove, finely chopped

1 tsp cumin seed, toasted and ground

1 tsp salt

1 tsp basil

1 tsp fennel

2 tbsp extra virgin olive oil

1 pinch cayenne pepper

2 tbsp apple cider vinegar

1 tbsp kosher salt

Combine all the ingredients in a small bowl and whisk together. Blend until smooth.

GARY'S CHEF'S SALAD WITH CREAMY ITALIAN DRESSING

1 head fresh, young romaine lettuce

1 head butter lettuce (about 1½ pounds)

Creamy Italian Dressing (see page 359)

2 cups Savory Croutons (see below)

1 recipe "Bacon" Bits (see page 358)

4 oz. Vidalia onion, thinly sliced

⅓ cup black olives, pitted

Trim the base of the lettuces and discard any bruised outer leaves. Use the tender inner leaves, keeping the small leaves whole and cutting or tearing the larger outer leaves crosswise into halves or thirds. Wash and dry the greens in a spinner and transfer to a large bowl. Drizzle the dressing onto the salad greens to taste, and gently toss together until well coated. Toss briefly with the croutons, "Bacon" Bits, onion, and olives, and serve immediately.

Savory Croutons
2 cups millet or rice bread, cut into ¾-inch cubes
2 tbsp extra virgin olive oil
1 tbsp grated Parmesan style nondairy cheese
½ tsp dried basil
½ tsp dried marjoram
½ tsp dried oregano
sea salt to taste

Preheat the oven to 425°F. Line an 11×15-inch cookie sheet with parchment paper and set aside. In a medium mixing bowl, toss together the bread, oil, cheese, basil, marjoram, oregano, and salt. Evenly spread the seasoned cubes on the prepared cookie sheet, and bake in the preheated oven for 8 to 10 minutes, or until golden. For uniformity in baking, rotate the sheet from front to back halfway through the baking period. Remove the sheet from the oven and cool the croutons completely.

"Bacon" Bits
1 pound extra firm tofu, crumbled
½ cup extra virgin olive oil
1 large clove garlic, peeled and finely chopped
1 tsp dried marjoram
1 tsp rubbed sage
1 tsp dried basil
½ tsp dried oregano
½ tsp sea salt
freshly ground black pepper to taste (optional)

Preheat the broiler. Line an 11×15-inch cookie sheet with parchment paper and set aside. In a medium mixing bowl, toss together the tofu, oil, garlic, marjoram, sage, basil, oregano, salt, and pepper. Evenly spread the seasoned tofu on the prepared cookie sheet and broil in the preheated oven for 15 minutes, or until golden. For uniformity in broiling, rotate the sheet from front to back halfway through the baking period. Remove the sheet from the oven and cool the bits completely.

Creamy Italian Dressing
1 cup silken tofu
½ cup extra virgin olive oil
½ cup freshly squeezed lemon juice (about 2 large lemons)
½ cup parsley, chopped
2 large cloves garlic, peeled and finely chopped
16 fresh basil leaves
½ tsp sea salt
freshly ground black pepper to taste (optional)

In a blender, combine the tofu, oil, lemon juice, parsley, garlic, basil, salt, and pepper. Blend on medium speed for 3 minutes, or until smooth and creamy. Set aside.

HERBED TOMATO SALAD
1 tsp sea salt
⅛ tsp cayenne pepper
½ tsp freshly ground black pepper
2 tbsp lime juice
2 tbsp fresh dill
½ tsp chopped fresh thyme
3 ripe tomatoes
1 bunch arugula
1 bunch watercress

In a small bowl, combine the salt, cayenne, black pepper, lime juice, dill, and thyme to make a dressing. Cut the tomatoes into thick slices; toss with arugula and watercress. Pour the dressing over the salad and let marinate for 1 hour in the refrigerator. Serve chilled.

INSALATA CAESAR
2 heads fresh, young romaine lettuce (about 1½ pounds)
Creamy Caesar Dressing (see page 361)
2 cups Savory Croutons (see page 358)
4 sheets of julienne strips of sushi nori

Trim the base of the romaine lettuce and discard any bruised outer leaves. Use the tender inner leaves, keeping the small leaves whole and cutting or tearing the larger outer leaves crosswise into halves or thirds. Wash and dry the greens in a spinner and transfer to a large bowl. Drizzle the dressing onto the salad greens to taste, and gently toss together until well coated. Toss briefly with the croutons, top with nori, and serve immediately.

Creamy Caesar Dressing
½ cup extra virgin olive oil
1½ cup water
½ cup tahini
½ cup silken tofu
½ cup freshly squeezed lemon juice (about 1 large lemon)
1 tsp tamari (or soy sauce)
2 tbsp chopped parsley
1 large clove garlic, peeled and finely chopped
½ tsp dried basil
½ tsp paprika
½ tsp sea salt

In a blender, combine the oil, water, tahini, tofu, lemon juice, soy sauce, parsley, garlic, basil, paprika, and salt. Blend on medium speed for 3 minutes, or until smooth and creamy, and set aside.

MIXED BEANS VINAIGRETTE
½ cup cooked lima beans
½ cup canned kidney beans, drained

½ cup green beans, steamed 15 minutes
½ cup chopped yellow bell pepper
½ cup chopped fresh parsley
1–2 tbsp prepared mustard
1–2 tbsp apple cider vinegar
2 tbsp extra virgin olive oil
½ tsp freshly ground black pepper
2 tbsp chopped red onions

Combine all the ingredients in a medium bowl, toss, and serve chilled.

MIXED SPROUT, BEAN, AND NUT SALAD WITH LIME VINAIGRETTE

2 cups sunflower sprouts
2 cups alfalfa sprouts
½ cup radish sprouts
½ cup canned garbanzo beans
½ cup asparagus tips, steamed 8 to 10 minutes
½ cup avocado cubes
½ cup halved seedless grapes
½ cup chopped Brazil nuts
Lime Vinaigrette (see below)

Combine all the ingredients except the Lime Vinaigrette in a large salad bowl and chill for 1 hour. Serve with Lime Vinaigrette.

Lime Vinaigrette
¼ cup lime juice
¼ cup fresh orange juice
¼ cup raw honey
¼ cup orange zest
2 tbsp Dijon mustard
⅛ cup agave
juice from ¼ lemon

1 cup plus 2 tsp light extra virgin olive oil
1 tbsp kosher salt
2 tbsp mint
pinch tarragon seed
pinch white pepper

Place lime juice, orange juice, honey, orange zest, mustard, agave, and lemon juice in a large bowl. While blending ingredients with a whisk in one hand, slowly add the oil. Season with salt, mint, tarragon seed, and white pepper, to taste.

NATURE'S TOTAL SALAD WITH LEMON GARLIC DRESSING
2 heads fresh, young romaine lettuce (about 1½ pounds)
½ pound sunflower sprouts
Lemon Garlic Dressing (see below)
2 ripe Haas avocados, peeled, halved, pitted, and sliced
1 large cucumber, halved, seeded, and thinly sliced
1 cup cooked millet
½ cup unsalted roasted cashews

Trim the base of the lettuces and discard any bruised outer leaves. Use the tender inner leaves, keeping the small leaves whole and cutting or tearing the larger outer leaves crosswise into halves or thirds. Wash and dry the greens and sunflower sprouts in a spinner and transfer to a large bowl. Drizzle the dressing onto the lettuce, add the sprouts, avocados, cucumber, and millet to taste, and gently toss together until well coated. Toss briefly with the cashews and serve immediately.

Lemon Garlic Dressing
½ cup extra virgin olive oil
½ cup freshly squeezed lemon juice (about 2 large lemons)
1 cup parsley, chopped

2 large cloves garlic, peeled and finely chopped

2 tsp sea salt freshly ground black pepper to taste (optional)

In a blender, combine the oil, lemon juice, parsley, garlic, salt, and pepper. Blend on medium speed for 3 minutes, or until emulsified.

PASTA SALAD

4 oz. whole-wheat macaroni, uncooked

1 cup soy cheese

½ tsp dry mustard

2–3 tbsp plain soy yogurt

1 red bell pepper, coarsely chopped

4 scallions, chopped

1 tbsp parsley flakes

1 tsp dill

1 tsp tamari (or soy sauce)

salt and pepper to taste

Cook the macaroni according to the directions on the package. Drain well and chill. In a large mixing bowl, combine the soy cheese, mustard, and soy yogurt. Add the macaroni, toss well, and add the remaining ingredients. Toss again. Serve on a bed of lettuce.

SUCCOTASH SALAD

about 4 quarts filtered water

one 12 oz. package quinoa macaroni

2 large Vidalia onions, peeled and thinly sliced

½ cup extra virgin olive oil

1 small kuri squash, seeded and chopped into ¼-inch pieces (about 2 cups)

½ pound extra firm tofu (crumbled)

10-oz. package frozen lima beans

2 cups fresh corn kernels (about 3 to 4 ears)

one 6 oz. can pitted black olives, sliced

1 large red bell pepper, cored, seeded, and diced
4 large celery stalks, finely chopped
½ cup chopped parsley (curly-leaf preferred)
½ cup freshly squeezed lemon juice
1 tbsp plus 1 tsp sea salt
1 tbsp dried basil
freshly ground black pepper to taste (optional)
sweet relish to taste
paprika to garnish

In a large pot, bring the water to a rolling boil. Stir the macaroni into the water and cook until the pasta is just tender, but not soft, about 4 to 5 minutes. Transfer to a colander, drain, and place in a large mixing bowl to cool. While the pasta is cooling, use a large saucepan to sauté the onions in the oil over moderate heat for 6 to 8 minutes, or until tender. Remove the onions from heat and gently toss into the cooked pasta until well blended. Place the kuri squash pieces on a steamer set into a large pot containing 1 inch of filtered water. Cook, covered, over moderate to high heat until the squash is tender when a fork is inserted into its center, about 8 minutes. Remove the squash from the steamer and gently toss into the macaroni and onion mixture. Add the tofu, lima beans, and corn to the steamer and cook covered for 10 minutes, or until the lima beans are hot. Remove the tofu, lima beans, and corn from the steamer and gently toss into the macaroni mixture. Add the olives, red pepper, celery, parsley, lemon juice, salt, basil, black pepper, and relish to the macaroni and gently toss together until well blended. Serve warm or chilled, garnished with a sprinkling of paprika.

SUPERIOR SPINACH SALAD
3 oz. spinach, coarsely chopped
3 oz. cauliflower florets, cut into bite-size pieces
3 oz. avocado, cut into bite-size pieces
3 oz. marinated artichoke hearts, cut into bite-size pieces

1½ oz. peanuts, chopped

1½ oz. shallots, chopped

1 tbsp sunflower oil

½ tsp oregano

½ tsp sage

½ tsp salt

Combine all ingredients and mix well.

Soups

BLACK BEAN SOUP

3 tbsp olive oil

1 onion, chopped

1 stalk celery, sliced

1½ cups black beans, washed very well

3 cloves garlic

6 cups vegetable stock

1 tsp celery salt, or more to taste

2 tbsp spelt flour

1 lemon, sliced

In a large soup pot, heat the olive oil and sauté the onion and celery until the onion is translucent and the celery is wilted, about 5 minutes. Add the black beans, garlic, and vegetable stock. Bring the mixture to a boil. Cover and simmer for 3 hours, or until the beans are very tender. Add the celery salt and the flour. (If you measure the flour into a sifter and sift it into the soup, you will not have trouble dissolving it.) Remove from heat. Transfer the mixture in batches to a blender and purée. After puréeing each batch, pour the purée into a large bowl. When you have puréed the entire mixture, return it to the pot and cook until it thickens slightly, which will take about 20 to 30 minutes. Some people like a more lemony flavor than others. Garnish the soup with the lemon slices and serve.

CHILLED CANTALOUPE SOUP
1 tsp agar flakes
2 tbsp water
1 cup orange or tangerine juice
1 tbsp lemon juice
2 cups diced cantaloupe
tofu sour cream for garnish

Place agar, water, and ¼ cup of orange juice in a small saucepan. Bring to a boil, reduce heat, and simmer until the agar dissolves, about 10 minutes. Place this mixture in a blender with the remaining orange juice, lemon juice, and cantaloupe pieces. Blend until the mixture is puréed. Chill in the refrigerator for at least 1 hour, preferably longer. Just before serving, return the mixture to the blender for 12 minutes. Serve with a spoonful of tofu sour cream on top.

CHINESE MUSHROOM SOUP
½ cup leeks, chopped
1 scallion, chopped
1 tbsp sesame oil
½ tsp hot sesame oil
1 tbsp tamari (or soy sauce)
2 cloves garlic, sliced
1½ tsp ginger, freshly grated
½ cup firm tofu, diced
½ cup miso paste
5 cups water
½ cup water chestnuts (measured, then chopped)
½ cup bamboo shoots (measured, then chopped)
½ cup dried black mushrooms
½ cup tree ear mushrooms
½ cup shiitake mushrooms (heads only)

1 tsp freshly ground black pepper
1 tbsp nori flakes for garnish

In a large saucepan, sauté the leeks and scallion in the oils over medium high heat for 5 minutes. Add the tamari, garlic, ginger, and tofu, and sauté another 3 minutes. Whisk in the miso paste and water. Add the remaining ingredients, except the nori flakes, reduce the heat to low, and let simmer for 50 minutes. Garnish with the nori flakes.

CINNAMON FRUIT SOUP
1 butternut squash
2 pears
1½ cups unsweetened soy milk
1 tsp pure vanilla extract
½ tsp ground cinnamon
6 orange slices (for garnish)
2 sprigs fresh mint (for garnish)

Separately juice the squash and pears to get ½ cup of squash juice, ¾ cup of squash pulp, and ½ cup of pear juice. In a medium saucepan, combine the juices, pulp, soy milk, vanilla extract, and cinnamon. Bring to a boil over high heat. Reduce the heat to medium-low, and simmer uncovered for 4 to 6 minutes. Serve hot or cold, garnished with the orange slices and mint sprigs, if desired.

COLD STRAWBERRY SOUP
1 pint strawberries, hulled
1 cup fruit juice (orange, papaya, apple, or strawberry)
2 tbsp arrowroot
juice of 1 lemon
honey to taste

½ cup tofu sour cream
tofu sour cream (for garnish)

Place three-quarters of the strawberries and the cup of fruit juice into a blender and purée. Pour the mixture into a saucepan. Dissolve the arrowroot in the lemon juice and pour this mixture into the saucepan, as well. Cook over medium heat until the mixture thickens, about 5 minutes. Remove from heat and sweeten with honey, if desired. Slice the remaining strawberries and fold them, along with the ½ cup of tofu sour cream, into a slightly cooled mixture. Refrigerate 2 to 3 hours, until well chilled. Serve cold with a teaspoonful of tofu sour cream on top.

CREAM OF SWEET POTATO SOUP
2 tbsp unsalted, nondairy butter
3 cloves garlic, minced or pressed
1 large onion, thinly sliced
2 sweet potatoes (about 1 lb.)
2 cups low-sodium vegetable stock
1 bunch fresh watercress
2 cups soy milk
egg substitute (enough to replace 2 egg yolks)

In a large, heavy saucepan, melt the butter. Add the garlic and onion and sauté over medium heat until the garlic turns golden brown. Add the sweet potatoes and stock. Bring to a boil. Then turn the heat down and simmer for 10 minutes, until the sweet potatoes are soft. Wash the watercress well. Save a handful of leaves to be used as a garnish later. Add the rest of the watercress and the milk to the sweet potatoes and simmer for about 10 minutes. Remove from heat. Purée in batches in the blender, and then return to the pot. Heat until the first bubbles appear around the edge, then stir in the egg substitute until the soup thickens.

(Note: This soup can be reheated if not allowed to boil. You may use homemade stock, as long as it has not been made with vegetables that have high sodium content. You might use low-sodium vegetable powder to be sure.)

CREAMY TOMATO SOUP
1 butternut squash
½ tomato
½ cup plus 3 tbsp plain soy yogurt
½ cup chopped tomatoes
2 tsp chopped fresh dill
½ tsp sea salt
¼ tsp pepper
2 tbsp plain yogurt (for garnish)
2 tbsp soy Parmesan cheese (for garnish)
2 sprigs fresh dill (for garnish)

Separately juice the squash and tomato to get ½ cup of squash pulp and ¼ cup of tomato juice. In a medium saucepan, combine the pulp, juice, and soy yogurt. Bring to a simmer over medium-low heat and cook uncovered for 10 to 15 minutes. Add the chopped tomato, 2 tsp dill, salt, and pepper, and remove from the heat. Serve hot or cold, garnished with the yogurt, Parmesan cheese, and dill sprigs, if desired.

PAPAYA NECTAR SOUP
4 small papayas, peeled, seeded, and cut into 2-inch pieces (about 8 cups)
16 large nectarines, pitted and quartered
4 large limes, peeled
⅓ cup lemon flavored nondairy yogurt
fresh mint to garnish

Separately juice papayas, nectarines, and limes. Serve chilled in bowls garnished with a dollop of yogurt and mint leaves.

Breakfast Dishes

TIPS

- Grains cooked in advance may be reheated by steaming.
- Grains are more flavorful when cooked with ½ teaspoon sea salt per cup of dry grain.
- Although unhulled barley is most desirable because it is the whole grain, it has a longer cooking time than "pearled" barley; look for the darker varieties of pearled barley found in health food stores, as they are minimally processed.
- Grade B or C maple syrup is less processed than Grade A, retaining more of its natural minerals.

TROPICAL PARADISE RICE CEREAL

2 cups coconut milk

1 cup pitted fresh or frozen cherries

½ cup chopped pineapple

¼ cup shredded, unsweetened coconut

2 cups cooked sweet rice

½ cup chopped macadamia nuts, toasted (see note below)

2 tbsp almond extract

1 tbsp vanilla extract

In a medium saucepan, combine the coconut milk, banana, cherries, and pineapple. Cook over medium-low heat for 2 to 3 minutes. Add the remaining ingredients, mix well, and cook an additional 2 to 3 minutes. Serve hot.

Serves 2

Note: To toast the nuts, preheat oven to 375°F and place nuts on an ungreased cookie sheet for 10 to 15 minutes or until light brown.

ALMOND CINNAMON MILLET

6 oz. Millet

13 oz. water

1½ oz. almonds, blanched and chopped
1½ oz. brewer's yeast
pinch cinnamon

Cook millet in a saucepan in 13 oz. water. When water comes to a boil, lower heat and cook until water is absorbed. Stir occasionally. Add remaining ingredients. Mix well.
Serves 1

QUINOA PANCAKES
¾ cup quinoa flour
¼ cup rolled oats
½ tsp baking soda
1 tsp baking powder
1 tbsp egg substitute
½ cup fresh extracted apple juice
½ cup soy milk
2 tbsp coconut oil

Mix together quinoa flour, oats, baking soda, baking powder, and egg substitute. Add juice, soy milk, and oil. Pour ¼ cup of batter onto a medium-heat, nonstick skillet. Turn the pancakes as they rice and bubble. Cook for an additional minute. Serve with brown rice syrup or warm molasses.
Serves 2

BLUEBERRY BREAKFAST TREAT
1 cup brown rice, cooked (cooled to room temperature)
½ cup blueberries, cut in half
2 tbsp sunflower seeds
sprinkle of unsweetened, flaked coconut

Combine all ingredients and mix well.

BLUEBERRY BANANA PANCAKES

½ cup spelt flour
½ cup wheat germ
1 tsp baking powder
1 tsp baking soda
dash of ground nutmeg
1 cup plain soy yogurt
½ cup thinly sliced bananas
¾ cup fresh or frozen blueberries
¼ cup oil (sunflower, soy, or safflower)

In a medium mixing bowl, combine the flour, wheat germ, baking powder, baking soda, and nutmeg. Mix well with a fork to remove lumps. Mix in the yogurt, bananas, and blueberries. Heat the oil in a large skillet over medium heat. Pour 3 to 4 tbsp of batter into the oil at a time and cook for 2 to 3 minutes on each side until light brown.

BLUEBERRY BUCKWHEAT-SOY-BANANA PANCAKES

2 tbsp egg substitute
2 tbsp vanilla extract
1 banana, mashed
½ cup rice milk
½ cup spelt flour
½ cup buckwheat flour
½ cup soy flour (optional)
1 tsp baking powder
1 tsp baking soda
4 tbsp raisins
½ cup blueberries
4 tbsp sunflower oil
3 tbsp shredded unsweetened coconut

In a medium mixing bowl, combine the egg substitute, vanilla, banana, and milk, mixing with a fork until well blended. In a separate bowl, combine the flours, baking powder, and baking soda, mixing well. Add the flour mixture to the banana and milk mixture, blending well with a spoon. Stir in the raisins and blueberries. Heat the oil in a large skillet over medium heat. Pour in 2 to 3 tbsp of batter at a time and cook for 35 minutes on each side until light brown. Garnish with coconut.

CREAM OF BARLEY

½ cup silken tofu
2 tbsp chopped walnuts
1 banana, mashed
1 tbsp pure maple syrup
½ cup cooked pearled barley
2 tbsp protein powder

In a saucepan, combine all of the ingredients except the barley and protein powder over low heat, until creamy. Add the barley, stirring until hot. Sprinkle the protein powder on top and serve immediately.

NUTTY BANANA BREAKFAST

6 oz. barley, cooked
3 oz. banana, mashed
1½ oz. walnuts, chopped
2 tbsp agave sweetener

Combine all ingredients and mix well.

NUTTY OATMEAL

6 oz. oatmeal, cooked (cooled to room temperature)
3 oz. pears, cut into bite-size pieces
1½ oz. pecans, chopped
1 tbsp honey

Combine all ingredients. Mix well.

RICE AND STRAWBERRIES
1 cup rice milk
⅛–½ tsp pure vanilla extract
1 tbsp pure maple syrup
½ cup raw cashews
pinch sea salt
½ cup sliced strawberries
1 cup cooked brown rice, hot

In a blender, combine rice milk, vanilla extract, maple syrup, cashews, and salt. Sprinkle strawberries over hot rice. Pour the cashew sauce over all. Serve immediately.

Main Dishes

BAKED RICE PASTA CASSEROLE
3 oz. potato
3 oz. rice pasta, cooked
3 oz. tomato, chopped medium fine
1½ oz. scallions, chopped medium fine
1½ oz. sesame seeds
1½ tbsp sesame oil
¼ tsp thyme
¼ tsp minced garlic
½ tsp salt

Preheat oven to 400°F. Lightly grease 4×8-inch baking pan with sesame oil. Bake potato for 40 minutes. When cooled, cut into ½-inch cubes. Combine all ingredients together. Lower heat to 375°F. Transfer to a baking pan and bake for 15 minutes.
Serves 2

TOFU CAULIFLOWER CASSEROLE
1 head cauliflower
3 tbsp olive oil
½ lb. (about 4 cakes) tofu, pressed and cut into cubes
1 onion, sliced thin
3 cloves garlic, pressed
1½ cups Tahini (sesame seed paste)
1 tbsp tamari (or soy sauce)

Preheat oven to 375°.
Break the cauliflower head into flowerettes and steam until just tender, about 10 minutes. Grease a medium casserole with about 1 tbsp of the olive oil and arrange in it the cauliflower and the tofu. To prepare the sauce, heat the remaining 2 tbsp of oil in a large saucepan. Add the onion and garlic and sauté until golden brown. Add the tahini and tamari, stirring until blended, and cook for an additional 3 to 5 minutes.

Pour the sauce over the cauliflower and tofu and bake for 20 minutes, until heated through.
Serves 3

THE QUINTESSENTIAL MEDITERRANEAN
3 oz. brown rice
3 oz. buckwheat or spelt noodles
3 oz. avocado
3 oz. marinated artichokes
2 tbsp olive oil
2 tsp scallions, chopped
1 tsp parsley, chopped
1 garlic glove, minced
½ tsp basil
½ tsp salt
1 oz. black olives, garnish

In a medium saucepan, cook brown rice in 12 oz. of water for 35 minutes or until done. Cook noodles according to directions on package. Chop the avocado and artichokes into bite-size pieces and place in a medium mixing bowl. Add the remaining ingredients. Toss gently. When the rice and noodles are done, place them on your plates. Top with the avocado mixture, and serve at room temperature.
Serves 2

SQUASH POTATO CASSEROLE
3 oz. sweet potato
3 oz. yellow squash
1 oz. green pepper, chopped
2 tbsp safflower oil
½ tsp thyme
½ tsp basil
½ tsp salt
3 oz. basmati rice, cooked
3 oz. amaranth, cooked

Preheat oven to 400°F. Pierce sweet potato with fork and place in oven for 45 minutes. When potato cools, cut into ½-inch cubes. Lower heat to 375°F. Steam squash and pepper until slightly tender. Lightly grease 4×8-inch casserole pan with safflower oil. Combine all ingredients and mix well. Transfer to casserole pan and place in oven for 15 minutes.
Serves 2

KIDNEY BEAN BONANZA
1½ oz. filberts, chopped
2 tbsp sunflower oil
1 tbsp tarragon
¾ tsp basil
½ tsp salt

⅓ tsp curry

3 oz. brown rice, cooked

3 oz. kidney beans, cooked

1½ oz. cashew pieces

Preheat oven to 375°F. Lightly grease 4×8-inch baking dish with sunflower oil. Place filberts in blender with 2 oz. water, oil, tarragon, basil, salt, and curry. Blend until mixture achieves sauce consistency. Combine brown rice and beans. Transfer to baking dish. Top with filbert sauce. Sprinkle on cashews. Bake, covered, for 15 minutes.
Serves 2

MEXICAN MEDLEY

3 oz. asparagus, cut into ½-inch pieces

3 oz. cauliflower flowerets, cut into bite-size pieces

3 oz. celery, chopped

3 oz. kidney beans, cooked

1½ oz. filberts, chopped medium-fine

2 tbsp sunflower oil

⅔ tsp chopped fresh dill

⅓ tsp chili powder

¼ tsp basil

¼ tsp celery seed

½ tsp minced garlic

½ tsp salt

Steam asparagus and cauliflower for approximately 10 minutes. Combine with celery. Set aside. In a blender, place beans, filberts and remaining ingredients. Purée until smooth. Pour this sauce over the asparagus mixture. Serve at room temperature.
Serves 2

THREE GREEN CURRY CASSEROLE

3 oz. sunflower flour

3 oz. split peas, cooked

2½ tbsp sunflower oil

⅓ tsp curry

¼ tsp minced garlic

¼ tsp salt

¼ tsp thyme

3 oz. spinach, coarsely chopped

3 oz. cauliflower, cut into bite-size pieces

3 oz. brown rice, cooked

3 oz. avocado, sliced

Preheat oven to 375°F. Lightly grease 4×8-inch baking pan with sunflower oil. In a blender, combine sunflower flour, split peas, oil, curry, garlic, salt, thyme and 2 oz. water. Separately, combine spinach, cauliflower, and brown rice. Transfer to a baking pan, add the flour and the beans, cover, and bake for 15 minutes. Place avocado slices on top for garnish.

Serves 2

MAMA'S MAKE-BELIEVE SPAGHETTI

3 oz. spaghetti squash

6 oz. tomato, chopped

3 oz. scallions, chopped

3 oz. green pepper, chopped

1½ oz. onion, chopped

2 tbsp olive oil

¼ tsp basil

1 tsp salt

Preheat oven to 400°F. Cut squash in half; remove the seeds and discard them. Place the squash halves in a baking pan cut side down, with ⅓ inch water. Bake for 40 minutes. Sauté the tomato, scallions, green pepper, and onion in the skillet with olive oil for 5 minutes. Add the basil and salt. Remove the spaghetti from

the squash and combine with the sautéed mixture. Toss gently. Serve hot.
Serves 1

SAVORY STUFFED ARTICHOKES
2 artichokes
4 tbsp orange juice
4 tbsp plus 1 tsp lemon juice
2 cups water
½ cup avocado, chopped
¼ cup fresh tomatoes, chopped
¼ cup black pitted olives, chopped
¼ cup onions, chopped
2 tbsp extra virgin olive oil
½ cup fresh basil, chopped
3 tbsp sesame seeds, toasted
½ cup macadamia nuts, roasted
1 tsp salt
1 sliced lemon (for garnish)

Trim the thorns from the artichoke leaves with a pair of scissors and trim the bottoms so that they will stand upright. In a medium saucepan, simmer the artichokes in the water and lemon juice over medium heat for about 50 to 60 minutes, until the leaves pull out easily. Remove the artichokes from the water and let them cool. Gently pull out the center leaves and scoop out the fuzzy choke with a spoon. Combine the remaining ingredients in a small mixing bowl and stir well. Spoon the stuffing mixture into the centers of the artichokes and garnish with lemon slices.
Serves 4

CAPONATA
2 small eggplants, about ½ lb. each
3 tbsp olive oil

1 large onion, sliced thin
2 cloves garlic, minced
4 stalks celery, chopped
4 tomatoes, peeled and chopped fine
water as needed
4 tbsp pignolia nuts (optional)
2 tbsp capers, drained
2–3 tbsp apple cider vinegar
salt and pepper to taste

Slice the unpeeled eggplants about ¼-inch thick. Arrange on a plate and sprinkle with salt. Set aside for 30 minutes. Drain well and rinse with cold water. Squeeze gently to remove excess moisture and dry on paper towels.

Heat 2 tbsp of the olive oil in a skillet and add the eggplant. Sauté until browned. Remove from pan.

Add the remaining olive oil to the frying pan and sauté the onion and the garlic until the garlic is golden brown. Add the celery, tomatoes and a little bit of water (about 2 to 3 tbsp). Cover and let the mixture steam for 10 minutes. Be sure to stir occasionally.

At this point, add the eggplant as well as the pignolia nuts, capers, and vinegar. Season with salt and pepper to taste, and let simmer for another 10 minutes to let the flavors blend. Be careful not to burn. Serve either hot or cold. The flavor improves if you refrigerate a day or two.
Serves 3

INDIAN EXOTIC RICE
1½ tbsp sesame oil
1 medium onion (preferably Vidalia), chopped
1 small clove garlic, minced
½-inch cinnamon stick or ¼ tsp ground cinnamon
2 whole cloves

½ tsp sea salt

¼ tsp powdered ginger

1 cup jasmine or basmati rice, rinsed once and soaked for
   5 minutes

1¾ cups boiling water

¼ tsp ground turmeric

¼ cup unsweetened coconut milk

¼ cup roasted cashews and pecans

1 tbsp fennel seeds

In a large saucepan, heat the sesame oil over low heat.

Add the onion and garlic and cook until soft, about 10 minutes. Add the cinnamon, cloves, salt, and ginger. Drain the rice and add in the pan. Toss lightly to coat the oil. Add the boiling water to the rice mix. Bring to a full boil. Add the turmeric, coconut milk, nuts, and fennel seed. Reduce the heat and simmer, covered, for 15 minutes. Remove from the heat and leave covered for 5 to 10 minutes before serving.
Serves 2

BRAZILIAN RICE

2 tbsp sunflower oil

3 oz. cauliflower florets, cut into bite-size pieces

2 tbsp fresh chopped parsley

½ tsp soy sauce

½ tsp salt

3 oz. black beans, cooked

3 oz. brown rice, cooked

3 oz. avocado, sliced

Preheat the oven to 350°F. Lightly grease a 4×8-inch baking pan with sunflower oil. Steam the cauliflower about 5 minutes. Combine all the ingredients except for the avocado. Mix well.

Transfer to baking pan and bake for 15 minutes. Garnish with avocado slices.

CHICKPEA HUMMUS WITH TOASTED PITA TRIANGLES
1 sweet onion, chopped
2 cloves garlic, minced
15-oz. can chickpeas (garbanzo beans), drained
½ cup tahini (sesame butter)
½ cup lemon juice
½ tsp pepper
⅛ tsp cayenne pepper
⅓ cup chopped fresh parsley
½ cup water
pita bread
3 tbsp olive oil
garlic powder or garlic salt, to taste

Sauté the onion and garlic in oil until the onion is transparent. Put into a blender or food processor with the chickpeas, tahini, lemon juice, pepper, cayenne pepper, and parsley. Blend until smooth, adding a little water if necessary to achieve desired consistency. Cut the pita bread into triangles, paint lightly with olive oil, and sprinkle with garlic powder or garlic salt. Broil until lightly browned.

GARY'S VEGETABLE PAN
2 tomatoes (yielding ½ cup juice)
1 lb. extra-firm tofu, cut into 1-inch cubes
2 tbsp sunflower oil
½ cup yellow onions, chopped
2 cups frozen peas
1 cup tomatoes, chopped
½ cup plain soy milk
3 tsp apple cider vinegar

½ cup arugula, finely chopped

2 green chili peppers, finely chopped

3 cloves garlic, crushed

2 tsp ginger root, grated

1 tsp ground coriander

1 tsp ground turmeric

½ tsp chili powder

1½ tsp sea salt

Juice the tomatoes to get ½ cup of juice. In a large frying pan, brown the tofu in the oil over high heat. Add the onions. Sauté for 2 to 3 minutes, or until the onions are soft. Reduce the heat to medium-low. Add the ½ cup of tomato juice, peas, chopped tomatoes, soy milk, cider vinegar, arugula, chili peppers, garlic, ginger, coriander, turmeric, chili powder, and sea salt. Simmer, uncovered, for 5 minutes. Serve with a fresh green salad.

GARY'S VEGGIEBALL STEW

1 tsp sea salt

⅛ tsp white pepper

1 tsp Worcestershire sauce

1 tsp grated lemon peel

½ tsp dried thyme

1 tbsp curry powder

1 tsp tamari (or soy sauce)

1 stalk celery, chopped

1 scallion, chopped

2 tbsp egg substitute

1 tbsp Bragg Liquid Aminos

4 oz. seitan, chopped

½ cup spelt flour

1 tbsp extra virgin olive oil

4 cups filtered water

1 cup yellow squash, sliced
1 small turnip, boiled and cubed
1 medium red potato, boiled and shredded
1 cup fresh tomato, peeled, cored, and chopped
1 leek with top sliced off
vegetable broth bouillon cubes, enough for 1 quart
1 tbsp chopped fresh dill

In a medium bowl, combine the salt, pepper, Worcestershire sauce, lemon peel, thyme, curry, tamari, celery, scallion, egg substitute, Bragg Aminos, and chopped seitan. Shape into 1-inch balls and roll in spelt flour. Heat the oil in a skillet and brown the balls, turning gently between a fork and a spoon. Set aside. Save and set aside the drippings. In a large saucepan, with 4 cups water, place the squash, turnip, potato, tomato, leek, and vegetable bouillon cubes. Boil on medium heat for approximately 30 minutes. Add the veggie balls to the soup and heat for 5 to 7 minutes. Sprinkle dill on top.

GOOD SHEPHERD'S PIE
1 large baking potato, peeled and diced
2 tbsp sunflower seed oil
½ cup rice milk
1 tbsp curry powder
½ tsp celery salt
⅛ tbsp freshly ground black pepper
1 tbsp olive oil
1 clove garlic, minced
1 medium onion, chopped
1 scallion, chopped
½ lb. vegetarian meat substitute
1 vegetable bouillon cube
3 oz. tomato paste
¼ tsp sage

1 tbsp spelt flour
1 tsp parsley flakes
1 tsp dried tarragon
½ cup white wine
½ can adzuki beans, cooked
1 pinch paprika

Cook the potato in boiling, salted water. Drain and mash the potato, and add the sunflower seed oil and rice milk. Season with curry powder, celery salt, and pepper. Heat the olive oil and sauté the garlic, onion, and scallion until soft. Add the meat substitute and stir until brown and the flavors are married, about 5 minutes. Crumble the vegetable bouillon and stir it into the onion mixture. Stir in the tomato paste, sage, flour, parsley, and tarragon. Add the wine and continue stirring for a few minutes. Cover and simmer on low for 10 additional minutes. Preheat the oven to 350°F. Lightly coat a soufflé dish or bread pan with oil. Spread the onion mixture on the bottom of the dish. Follow with a layer of cooked adzuki beans, then mashed potatoes, and sprinkle with paprika. Bake for 30 minutes, then brown under broiler for 1 minute and serve.

INDONESIAN KALE

1 cup onions, chopped
3 cups fresh tomatoes, chopped
½ cup extra virgin olive oil
4 cups fresh or frozen kale, chopped
4 cups diced red potatoes, steamed for 15 minutes
4 cloves garlic, sliced
2–3 tbsp curry powder, dissolved in 2 tbsp water
½ tsp ground allspice
½ tsp ground ginger
½ tsp paprika
2 tbsp salt

In a large saucepan, sauté the onions and tomatoes in the oil over medium heat for 15 minutes. Add the remaining ingredients and cook for an additional 5 minutes.

ITALIAN VEGETABLE STEW
2 tbsp olive oil
1 large onion, sliced thin
3 cloves garlic, pressed
1 red pepper, coarsely chopped
1 green pepper, coarsely chopped
2 carrots, sliced thin
1 small zucchini, sliced
½ bunch broccoli, cut into stalks
½ head cauliflower, cut into florets
2 tomatoes, chopped
2 cups red wine
1 tbsp honey
1 tbsp basil
1 tsp oregano
2 tsp parsley flakes
1 tsp tamari (or soy sauce)
1 cup grated soy Parmesan cheese

Heat the oil in a large skillet and add the onion, garlic, red pepper, green pepper, and carrots. Sauté for 5 minutes. Add the zucchini and sauté for 5 minutes longer. Stir in the broccoli, cauliflower, tomatoes, wine, honey, basil, oregano, parsley, and tamari. Cover and simmer for 25 minutes, stirring occasionally. Place in an oiled casserole dish, top with the soy Parmesan cheese, and bake for 20 minutes at 350°F.

MACARONI MARCONI
½ pound quinoa pasta
10 artichoke hearts

3 cloves garlic, minced
2 oz. sundried tomatoes
2 tbsp extra virgin olive oil
1 sprig fresh basil, chopped
15 green olives, pitted and sliced
½ cup grated soy or rice Parmesan (optional)

Cook the pasta according to the package directions. Steam the artichoke hearts until tender. In a skillet, sauté the garlic with the sundried tomatoes in the olive oil, for 3 minutes. Add the basil and olives, and sauté for about 2 minutes more. In a large bowl, toss the mixture with the pasta and Parmesan, and serve.

ORIGINAL BROCCOLI STIR-FRY
1 cup firm tofu
2 cups broccoli florets
2 tbsp hot sesame oil
2 tbsp tamari (or soy sauce)
½ tsp cayenne pepper
1 tsp grated fresh ginger
3 cloves garlic, minced

In a medium saucepan, sauté the tofu and broccoli in the oil for 3 minutes over medium heat. Remove from the pan and place the mixture in a bowl. Combine the remaining ingredients in the saucepan. Cook over medium heat until the mixture simmers, about 1 minute. Add the broccoli mixture and cook, covered, for 2 minutes. Stir well. Serve with short-grain brown rice.

PASTA e FAGIOLI (BEAN SOUP)
3 cloves garlic, diced
½ onion, diced
2 tbsp olive oil

2 8-oz. cans of tomato puree
½ tsp garlic powder
½ tsp oregano
salt and pepper to taste
1 can cannellini beans or white kidney beans
3 cups ditalini pasta or other small noodle, cooked

Sauté the garlic and onion in olive oil. Add the tomato purée, bring to a boil, and add the spices and beans. Cook for 30 minutes over medium-low heat. Add the cooked pasta; if the mixture is too thick, add water to reach the desired consistency.

POTATO CHOWDER
1 lb. golden potatoes, peeled
½ lb. purple potatoes, peeled and cut into ½-inch cubes
2 tbsp extra virgin olive oil
1 medium onion, chopped
2 stalks celery, minced
4 cloves garlic, minced
1 yellow bell pepper, diced
2 scallions, white portion only, chopped
3 cups filtered water
1 cup plain soy milk
½ cup diced carrots (for garnish)
1 bay leaf
1 small jalapeño
1 tsp freshly ground black pepper
1 tsp sea salt
1 tsp dried thyme
1 tsp ground sage
1 tsp dried basil
1 tsp Pick a Pepper or Tabasco Sauce

1 tbsp mustard seeds
1 tbsp fennel seeds
1 tbsp honey
parsley (for garnish)
Hungarian paprika (for garnish)

Steam the potatoes for 10 minutes. In a stockpot, heat the oil over medium heat and sauté the onion, celery, garlic, yellow pepper, and scallions. Add the water, soy milk, carrots, and steamed potatoes to the sautéed vegetables. Add the bay leaf, jalapeño, pepper, salt, thyme, sage, basil, pepper sauce, mustard seeds, fennel seeds, and honey. Stir and simmer for an additional 15 minutes. Garnish with the parsley and Hungarian paprika.

RATATOUILLE
4 tbsp plus ¼ cup extra virgin olive oil
1 small eggplant, peeled and cubed
1 small yellow squash, cubed
½ cup shallots, minced
1 scallion, chopped
2 cloves garlic, pressed
1 small zucchini, cubed
¼ tsp thyme
¼ tsp dried basil
1 small onion, chopped
2 tbsp dulse leaves, minced
½ stalk celery, chopped
½ cup sun-dried tomatoes, reconstituted in ½ cup water
1 tbsp curry powder
sea salt
freshly ground black pepper
½ cup raw sunflower seeds

Heat the olive oil in a large skillet over medium heat. Add the eggplant, yellow squash, shallots, scallion, garlic, and zucchini. Cook, stirring, for 3 minutes. Add the thyme, basil, onion, dulse, and celery, and cook for another 3 minutes. Add the sun-dried tomatoes, curry powder, sea salt, and fresh pepper to taste. Sprinkle with sunflower seeds and serve warm.

SWEET KIDNEY BEAN MASH

1 lb. sweet potatoes or yams, scrubbed well and cut into 2-inch thick slices (about 2 cups)
½ cup extra virgin olive oil
1 8 oz. yellow onion, peeled and finely chopped
2 large celery stalks, finely chopped
3 large cloves garlic, peeled and coarsely chopped
1 pound cooked kidney beans, rinsed and drained
½ cup freshly squeezed lime juice
10 large basil leaves
1 tsp sea salt
1 tsp ground cumin
1 tsp ground chili powder
freshly ground black pepper to taste (optional)
8 slices whole-grain country bread or millet bread, cut into ½-inch thick slices

Place the sweet potato slices in a steamer set into a large pot containing 1 inch of water. Cook, covered, over moderate to high heat until the potatoes are tender when a fork is inserted into their centers, about 15 to 20 minutes. Remove the steamer and run the potatoes under cool water until they can be handled comfortably. Using a small paring knife, remove and discard the peels.

In a medium saucepan, combine the oil, onion, celery, and garlic. Sauté over moderate heat for 5 to 7 minutes, or until the onions are translucent. In a food processor, using a metal blade, combine the sautéed vegetables with the sweet potatoes, beans, lime juice, basil leaves, salt, cumin, chili powder, and black pepper. Process together until smooth and creamy, for about 2 minutes. Set aside.

Lightly toast the bread on both sides. Spread the bread slices with the sweet mash and serve warm.

TANTALIZING TEMPEH DINNER
2 tbsp soy oil
½ oz. dulse, dry
3 oz. chickpeas, cooked
3 oz. soybean sprouts
3 oz. broccoli florets, cut intobite-size pieces
3 oz. tempeh, cut into ½-inch cubes
1 tsp fresh chives, chopped
1 tsp onion, minced
½ tsp salt

Preheat oven to 350°F. Lightly grease a 4×8-inch baking pan with the soy oil. Soak and rinse the dulse 2 or 3 times in cold water. Combine with the chickpeas, soybean sprouts, broccoli, tempeh, chives, onion, and salt, and mix well. Transfer to a baking pan and bake for 20 minutes.

TEX-MEX TOFU SCRAMBLER
½ cup sunflower seeds
6 tbsp extra virgin olive oil
4 1-oz. slices tempeh
½ cup lecithin granules (optional)
1 tbsp onion powder
1 tbsp dry mustard
1 tbsp dried basil

1 tbsp ground turmeric

1 tbsp ground cumin

1 tbsp celery salt

1 tbsp sea salt

1 lb. soft tofu, well-drained, chopped, and crumbled

1 cup mushrooms, sliced

3 tbsp tamari (or soy sauce)

1 Vidalia onion, peeled and finely chopped

4 large cloves garlic, peeled and finely chopped

1 yellow bell pepper, cored, seeded, and finely chopped

½ cup zucchini, finely chopped

1 tomato, cored and finely chopped

1 ripe Haas avocado, peeled, halved, pitted, and finely chopped

1 tbsp balsamic vinegar

½ cup fresh cilantro, finely chopped

freshly ground black pepper to taste (for garnish)

2 large limes, sliced into 1-inch thick wedges (for garnish)

In a large cast-iron frying pan, over moderate to low heat, roast the sunflower seeds until golden and transfer to a small dish. Set aside. Preheat the broiler and brush the frying pan with 2 tbsp oil. Evenly space the tempeh in the pan and broil for 5 minutes, or until golden. Remove the pan from the oven, transfer the tempeh to a paper towel–lined plate, and set aside. In a small mixing bowl, combine the lecithin, onion powder, mustard, basil, turmeric, cumin, celery salt, and sea salt. Stir together until well combined and set aside. In a large mixing bowl, toss together 2 tbsp of the oil with the tofu and the spice mixture until well combined. Set aside. In the frying pan, combine the remaining 2 tbsp oil with the mushrooms and tamari. Toss together until well mixed and broil for 5 minutes, or until the mushrooms are golden. Remove the pan from the oven and toss in the prepared tofu, onion, garlic, yellow pepper, zucchini, tomato, avocado, vinegar, cilantro, and black pepper until well combined. Return to the broiler and broil, mixing occasionally, until golden, for about 10 minutes. Serve hot, garnished with the tempeh, sunflower seeds, and lime, accompanied by whole-grain toast.

Desserts

STRAWBERRY SUNSHINE

6 oz. brown rice, cooked (cooled to room temperature)
3 oz. strawberries, halved
1½ oz. sunflower seeds
1½ oz. figs, chopped
sprinkle of coconut, shredded and unsweetened

Combine all ingredients. Mix well.
Serves 1

SUNNY RICE PUDDING

3 oz. mango
3 oz. brown rice, cooked
5 tsp carob powder
1½ oz. sunflower seeds
1 oz. date sugar
1 tsp vanilla
1½ oz. dates
2 heaping tsp egg substitute

Combine all ingredients and purée until smooth. Transfer to saucepan and cook over medium heat for 5 minutes, stirring frequently. Chill in the refrigerator for 45 minutes.
Serves 2

KIWI PUDDING

5 oz. strawberries
2 oz. kiwi

3 oz. millet, cooked
4 oz. maple syrup
6 oz. coconut milk
2 heaping tsp egg substitute
1 tsp vanilla
1 tsp fresh mint
1 tsp lemon juice
pinch cinnamon
1½ oz. slivered almonds

Place all ingredients except the almonds in a blender. Purée until smooth. Transfer to a saucepan and set over medium heat for 5 minutes, stirring constantly. Chill for 45 minutes in the refrigerator. Top with almonds when chilled.
Serves 3

PEACH JULEP PUDDING
6 oz. peaches, sliced
3 oz. barley, cooked
8 oz. peach juice
4 oz. barley malt
1½ oz. walnuts
1 tsp vanilla
2 tsp fresh mint
1 tsp lemon juice

Place all ingredients in a blender. Puree until smooth. Transfer to a saucepan and set over medium heat for 5 minutes, stirring frequently. Chill for 45 minutes in the refrigerator.
Serves 2

BLACKBERRY NECTARINE FRUIT SALAD
1 large cantaloupe, peeled, seeded, and cut into 1-inch pieces
   (about 4 cups)

8 large nectarines, pitted and sliced (about 4 cups)
4 cups blackberries
1 tbsp freshly squeezed lemon juice
3 tbsp freshly squeezed lime juice
2 tbsp powdered brown rice syrup (optional)

In a large bowl, combine the cantaloupe, nectarines, and blackberries. Drizzle the juices onto the fruit and gently toss together until well coated. Spoon into small bowls, sprinkle on the powder, and serve.

CAROB POWER BROWNIES
½ cup sunflower seeds
1½ cups brown rice flour
½ cup carob powder
½ tbsp baking powder
½ tbsp ground nutmeg
½ tbsp sea salt
½ cup extra virgin olive oil
5 large bananas, peeled and coarsely chopped (about 2 ½ cups)
1 cup apple juice
1 cup apricot juice
1 tbsp honey
1½ tsp pure banana flavor
1 cup walnuts, coarsely chopped
1 cup oat bran
½ cup plus 2 tbsp rice bran
½ cup dairy-free carob chips

Preheat the oven to 350°F. Line two 12-well muffin tins with paper baking cups and set aside. Using a small food processor or coffee grinder, process the sunflower seeds until powder-fine. Transfer to a mixing bowl and set aside. To make the brownies, in a large mixing bowl, sift together the flour, carob powder, baking powder, nutmeg, and salt. Whisk together until well mixed. Set aside. In a food processor, using the metal blade, combine the oil and bananas. Process until creamy, about 1 minute. Pour in the apple juice, apricot juice, honey, and banana flavor. Process until well blended. With a rubber spatula, gradually add the wet ingredients to the dry, making sure they are well blended before each addition. Scrape off any excess batter from the side of the bowl. Stir in the walnuts, oat bran, rice bran, and chips until well mixed. Spoon the batter into the prepared muffin tins (the wells will be half full). Bake in the middle level of the preheated oven for 35 to 40 minutes. For uniformity in baking, rotate the tin from front to back halfway through the baking period. The brownies are done when a tester inserted in the center comes out clean. Remove the brownies from the oven and let cool completely, about 15 to 20 minutes. Serve with a glass of rice milk, soy milk, or nut milk.

CHERRY GRAPE KANTEN

6 cups pineapple juice

½ cup plus 2 tbsp agar flakes (available at your local health food store)

8 medium ripe peaches, peeled, pitted, and sliced (about 3 cups)

½ large pineapple, peeled, cored, and cut into 1-inch pieces (about 2 cups)

2 cups seedless green grapes

2 12-oz. packages frozen pitted cherries

2 tbsp freshly squeezed lemon juice

In a medium saucepan, bring the pineapple juice to a boil over high heat. Reduce heat to moderate and stir in the agar. Simmer, uncovered, stirring occasionally, for 10 minutes, or until the agar is completely dissolved. In a large mixing bowl, toss the peaches, pineapple, grapes, and cherries together with the lemon juice until well combined. Transfer to a 7×11-inch baking dish and pour in the pineapple juice mixture. Let cool for 15 minutes, then refrigerate for 30 to 45 minutes, or until congealed. Spoon into small bowls and serve.

COLD CHERRY SOUP
2 cups cherries, pitted and stemmed
1 lemon, peeled and quartered
1 cup strawberries, hulled
1 cup blueberries
½ cup agar
cinnamon, to taste
1 orange, peeled and in wedges

Juice the cherries and lemon. In a blender, blend the cherry juice together with the strawberries, blueberries, and agar. Serve in a bowl with cinnamon garnish and orange wedges.

HEAVENLY ROASTED NUTS
1 cup walnuts
1 tbsp honey
1 tsp extra virgin olive oil
1 tsp freshly squeezed lemon juice

Preheat oven to 350°F. Line an 11×15-inch cookie sheet with parchment paper and set aside. In a medium mixing bowl, toss together the nuts, honey, oil, and lemon juice until well combined. Evenly spread the nuts on the prepared sheet. Bake on the middle rack of the preheated oven for 8 to 10 minutes, or until the nuts are golden. Remove the sheet from the oven and slide the parchment paper to a wire rack until the nuts are completely cool (about 10 minutes). Serve alone, or use the nuts as a topping for cereal, salads, nondairy yogurt, or nondairy frozen dessert.

Appendix III

Testimonials

Depression

I was dissatisfied with my body. My energy was low, and I was very overweight. My acquaintances and friends were depressing me to the point of irritability. I had a fear of public speaking and did not know where to turn for guidance. I joined Gary's health support group. I lost sixteen pounds without dieting. My increasing energy made me feel young again. I need less sleep and find I am not distracted with other people's petty, unimportant issues. My toxic relationships were dismissed. My self-esteem replaced them. I learned to be the real me, healthy and vital.

—Alexandra M.

Mental Fatigue

I was concerned about my health. My blood pressure and cholesterol were elevated. I had a stressful life due to being mentally fatigued and could not control these feelings. I suffered an acid reflux condition that I assumed was caused by my job. My body was falling apart. I detoxed and carefully followed Gary's protocol. I felt stronger each week and released stress each day. My blood pressure is now normal, my digestion is improved, and I lost fifteen pounds. I do aerobics at home in the morning, yoga during evening hours, bike, walk, and run. My uncluttered environment and journal writing give me a new constructive outlet.

—Alice

Brain Allergies

I had many allergies and frequent upper-respiratory infections. My life was unmanageable, and my stress was overwhelming. My blood pressure and cholesterol were elevated. I heard about Gary Null's support groups and detoxification. I needed to change and decided to enter a group as soon as one was formed. That was the beginning of the best part of my life. My energy built, my headaches stopped, and my cholesterol and blood pressure lowered. I have a new body from exercising, using weights, doing chi gong, and deep breathing. I feel calm, more patient, and less irritable. I love my food and progressive life.

—Bob

Depression

I weighed 210 pounds, smoked three packs of cigarettes a day, drank alcohol, felt depressed, and had knee pains and upper-respiratory infections. One day I looked at the very aged man in the mirror and was shocked. Today I follow Gary Null's protocol. I drink purified water, use supplements, and feel terrific. I haven't had a cold in five years; no more upper-respiratory infections. I follow an organic, vegan diet and do not take vaccines. My neighbors tell me I look forty-five years old. They admire my changes. I appreciate my healthy lifestyle. I am confident and pleased with my life, and I am no longer depressed.

—Job

Brain Trauma

In 1989 I attended a Gary Null retreat. I learned the benefits of vegetarianism, juicing, supplements, and meditation. In 1994 I became disabled because of carbon monoxide poisoning. I am still in the process of recovery. I no longer work. I cannot see computer screens. Surgery for two detached retinas affected my eyesight. My blood pressure was extremely high. My heartbeat accelerated to a dangerous level. I took several pharmaceutical drugs to control these conditions. A few years later, seizures began with Alzheimer's-like symptoms. Abnormally severe edema in my legs incapacitated me. I was in a coma for sixty days. Nursing home care was considered. My health took an upward turn on the Gary Null protocol. Juicing, stress management, and homework opened me to my potentials and purpose in life. I discovered the best of what works and realized I was not doing anything worthwhile. Today I no longer need a compressor for leg edema. My leg size decreased 30 percent. I sleep less, lost twenty-three pounds, and exercise with hand weights. I recently received a Bowflex to build my upper body. My blood pressure is lower. My brain speed seems to be faster.

—Michael

Migraine

I was labeled disabled for four years. Migraine headaches caused me to be bedridden, and I used pain medication for a spinal disc injury. I was swollen after eating my usual meat, wheat, sugar, coffee, and dairy. My cholesterol was high. Candida plagued my body. I threw up after meals and was stressed by anxiety attacks. One day, after reading one of Gary's books, I saw him on PBS. I joined a support group in 1994. I attended classes open to change, and after two weeks on the protocol being vegan, organic, and never returning to toxic foods, the change began. I exercise in a rehab center for my back problem. Probiotics and sensible eating eliminated throwing up. I am a vegetarian cook and intend to study vegetarian meal preparation. My back pain is sporadic and not as acute. I am still in recovery but use no medication. I never looked at life as I do now.

—Barbara

Memory Loss

I was bedridden for two weeks with Epstein Barr disease and could not walk more than three minutes at a time. I lost some of my memory. I returned to work but only put in five hours a day, and went to bed as soon as I returned home. Stair climbing was difficult. My physician could do no more and suggested I do independent research. A homeopathic examination revealed food sensitivities. The day I watched Gary on PBS changed my life. I donated to the station and soon joined a support group. Today I carefully follow the protocol. I gave up chocolate without difficulty. At first the new food choices were difficult to accept, but today I am vegan and feel 1,000 percent better. I work seven hours a day and exercise after work. I walk one and a half hours and am training to race walk in the New York Marathon. I still need eight hours of sleep, possibly because of Epstein Barr, but my waking hours are productive. With a clear mind, good memory, energy, and concentration, I plan future occupations in art and volunteer work.

—Cathy T.

Insomnia

I could not sleep well and was tired all day long. I wanted to be healthy and change my work. I decided to join a support group. I heard members of Gary's groups speak of their successes. I intended to change my work and life. I was overweight. My hair and nails were weak. I had a swollen knee because of three automobile accidents. I suffered with skin eruptions. The group had a wonderful effect. I became friends with several people and spoke to them during the week. We motivated each other. Today I am twenty-five pounds thinner. My hair and nails grow rapidly. The swelling in my knee has lessened. I no longer have skin eruptions. My energy is high all day long because I sleep well. I have also actualized a new career.

—Eileen

Anxiety

I used to feel no one understood my problem and fear of isolation. I was reticent about meeting with a group of people to improve my life, but I did and felt that the group enhanced my progress. I stayed on the protocol and lost ten pounds. I now feel joy and happiness; I feel really good about myself. I can now easily help other people. Praying and listening to my inner voice brought good results. The protocol cleaned my body and mind.

—Kenneth L.

Brain Trauma

Brain surgery left me with numb fingers and cold extremities. I had flu-like symptoms, a constant "frog" in my throat, fatigue in the morning, tinnitus, dizziness, constipation, and a general lack of motivation that interfered with my work performance. I was angry and soon went on disability. The first time Gary Null spoke about support groups on his show, I listened but did nothing. At that stage I could not really help myself. Feeling totally locked in, I pulled up some inner courage and went to the first meeting. I began the protocol. In a short amount of time, it was evident the protocol was working. I began to feel better; the pains and other symptoms lessened. As I continued and listened to the lectures, which were quite penetrating and motivating, I noticed all the symptoms I once had were gone. Today I am a functioning, healthy woman.

—Yvonne

Depression

I was prescribed Prozac for Multi-menopausal Syndrome by my gynecologist. I gained weight and lost energy. My hair and nails were weak. I had difficulty sleeping and felt depressed. I thought I followed a sensible eating plan. I did not connect food and aging. I began the detox protocol carefully and followed it diligently. I wanted to reverse my aging and clean my system out. I lost weight and am keeping it off. I have good energy. My hair and nails are growing to pre-menopausal thickness and strength. I discontinued the Prozac when I began the protocol and am not depressed. I sleep well, look well, and get healthier each day.

—Maria R.

Memory Loss

At age seventy-five, we were not happy with symptoms of getting old. We both had memory difficulties. We did not like to be homebodies and wanted this part of our lives to be active. There is so much to experience and learn. We rejoined a support group and feel we have reversed aging. We follow the protocol and noticed we have increased brain power. It is sad watching our friends fail physically. They are closed to the ideas of detoxification and diet changes. We are the only couple in our group not taking medications. We study piano and are writing a book. This is a wonderful time of life.

—Wilma and Myron

Headaches

My blood pressure was a bit high, and I did get headaches. I was curious about this thing called a detox protocol. I did not feel unhealthy, but I decided to attend a group and see if it would impact in any way. I came to each meeting and listened and learned. I lost weight without dieting. My waistline is smaller. My blood pressure is normal. I need less sleep, and my headaches are gone. The protocol and the science behind it are valid. It was a wonderful experience.

—Bob

Depression

I was depressed and overweight, and uncomfortable with the extra pounds. I held anger in and did not discuss, understand, or share my feelings with anyone. I was afraid to take risks, such as asking for a raise. Being timid and angry was not a good place to be. I knew and trusted Gary Null, so I joined a group to see if I could be happy and make changes. I am on the protocol and love it. My depression lifted as my health increased. I exercise without fear of injury. I lost twenty pounds, and my energy is high. I cope, do not hold anger in, and speak my mind. I spoke up at work and got a raise.

—Maria T.

Memory Loss

My memory has significantly improved. I can now connect the names and faces of my friends. I am calmer and more relaxed. My energy level has gone up. I can get through the day without feeling drowsy.

—Joyce C

Depression/Anxiety

I am much more relaxed, I am more able to handle stress, and I need less sleep. My vision is clearer, my hair has gone back to its original color, and I feel twenty years younger. My meditation is now much deeper and richer, and I have less anger and depression. I feel sexy (at fifty-nine!), and I'm thinking about companionship. People who haven't seen me in a while blurt out, "My God, what have you done to yourself? You look fabulous!" I lost sixteen pounds and went down two sizes in clothing, and my abdomen went from forty-four inches to thirty-nine inches. Most days I do twenty to thirty stretching exercises, and I am now willing to challenge my values and beliefs.

—Molly

Headaches

I feel energetic, attractive, and strong. The changes I was able to make during this protocol were more marked than any changes I have been able to make in several years. I followed the protocol closely, and I no longer get headaches, whereas before I usually got at least one severe headache a month. I lost twelve pounds and several inches from my hips and waist. My blood pressure dropped to 102/60. My self-confidence and energy level rose to a new high. I received many comments on my shiny hair, and people commented on how nice my skin was. I feel more confident, positive, clearheaded, and able to focus on other life goals. I feel like a different person: stronger, happier, and enthusiastic.

—Elaine

Depression

Mentally, I am more clear-thinking, making decisions regarding my life and business more quickly, as opposed to laboring over them. I have no depression, but a general feeling of grounding and balance. Affirmations work.

—Liz

Headaches

I am migraine-free. My circulation has improved in my fingers and toes, and I have lots of energy. My sleep has improved, and I wake up energized.

—Jayne

Memory Loss

I had heard about Gary Null from a friend who had been listening to his daily radio program in New York. I decided to go to his office, where he had mentioned there would be a support group. I was showing signs of Alzheimer's that were getting worse and worse. I was overweight, and I had blotches of skin discoloration all over my body. I thought Gary's protocol was too harsh to try, so I decided not to go on it. After a few months, however, when my condition got worse, I went back to his office and immediately began the program.

I had not exercised for quite some time. Now, every day, I would set aside time to walk. My bowel habits became more regular, and suddenly I was remembering things that I used to forget. I could easily recall the names of friends I would run into on the street, whereas before I would have difficulty doing so. I feel that Gary's protocol has given me my life back, for it doesn't matter how good of shape your body is in if your mind is forgetful.

—Rita

Depression

I feel a balance, peacefulness, quietness, and contentment. My depression is gone. This is new for me; I feel joyful. I am now walking two to three miles, four or five times per week. I feel lighter, see the world in a more positive way, and feel content and happier. People are telling me how great I look.

—Louise

Memory Loss

I am now in my early forties, and I feel great! I feel better than I did in my twenties. I am generally sharper, with better memory, and I am experiencing greater mental stability. I have much greater focus and discipline about my daily life and my long-term life goals. I exercise, meditate, eat right, and take supplements daily. My dry skin on my feet cleared up, my thinning hair improved, and my allergies are gone. I have not had any colds or flu since beginning the program. I need less sleep and wake up refreshed and ready for a wonderful day. The dietary changes expanded my food choices. In place of meat, dairy, sugar, and wheat items, I found a whole new world of grains, beans, legumes, fruits, and vegetables to eat. I enjoy exercising but never made time for it on a regular basis, and now I do. In summary, I have achieved that which I set out to do: I am healthier in body, mind, and spirit. I look forward to waking up each day with good health, happiness, and fulfillment.

—Pat

Depression

I feel more worthy of living and of being alive. At the start of the program, I didn't care! My depression has diminished noticeably. Life is no longer happening to me. I am involved. I'm not as timid, and I cry less. I am more in control of my emotions. I am happier.

—Jennie

Brain Allergies

As a child my food sensitivities were treated with antibiotics and medications to no avail. I was weak in every aspect of my being, and pale with dark circles under my eyes. Within two weeks on Gary Null's allergy protocol, I felt remarkably better. Nine months later, I find I can tolerate most all foods. My thinking is clear, and my moodiness, depression, lethargy, and poor complexion have reversed. I feel vital, healthy, and alive. I anticipate studying Oriental Medicine, and I continue research on internal energy.

—Peter

Brain Trauma

In February 1997, I had brain surgery due to a tuberculum sellae meningioma that was wrapped around my pituitary gland and destroyed my optic nerve. I was diagnosed with hypothyroidism. My craniotomy surgery lasted twenty hours. I was in intensive care three days. I was weak and could not walk or even brush my teeth. I joined a support group eight months after surgery and began the protocol. I came into the Gary Null Running and Walking Club two months later and soon discontinued steroids, seizure pills, Synthroid, laxatives, and antacids. I no longer discuss my illness, but speak of my health. I am naturally positive in thought, behavior, and speech. My physician does not understand my physical, emotional, and mental recovery in so short a time. I feel great and push forward without an attitude of handicap.

—Frank E.

Parkinson's Disease

My doctors had given up on me. They didn't tell me that, but I could see it in their eyes and hear it in their voices. They told me that I had Parkinson's and that there was no cure for it. They told me that Janet Reno and Muhammad Ali had forms of it, and they were leading productive lives. This may sound strange, but the thing I feared the most about my condition was being unable to stop my shaking. This may sound selfish, but it is true. I visited Gary in his office on Seventy-Second Street and Broadway, where he had me go to get my blood work done. Then he designed a program for me that changed my life. At first, I did not think I could go through with it. Now, I know I can. Although my shaking has not completely gone away, it has lessened a great deal. My wife is amazed at my progress, and I look forward to living the rest of my life knowing that one day, I will not be shaking at all.

—Joseph

Memory Loss

I was overjoyed to come into a Reversing the Aging support group. My memory was getting worse; I left my car keys in the trunk lock, and my car was stolen. I was not organic, but had been juicing and using supplements for a year before beginning the protocol.

Once I used organic produce and juice, I began to feel stronger. I did not get sore throats since I began taking vitamin C at night. I decided to work less. A short time later, I dated a man for the first time since my divorce eight years earlier. I felt happy and prayed for the return of my car. A short time later, I spotted it while taking a long walk on an alternative trail. This increased my spiritual belief. I am building a cohesive relationship between my boyfriend, son, and myself. I sleep better, exercise, and work on an eating plan to prevent overeating.

—Virginia C.

Alzheimer's Disease

I am speaking for my wife, who gave me permission to do so. She is a little shy about these things, but she wants everyone to know her results. Two years ago, she and I attended a lecture by Dr. Null. What he said gave us hope that my wife's Alzheimer's could be improved. We joined one of Gary's support groups, and it has changed our lives. Alzheimer's runs in my wife's family. So, when she began forgetting things, we both suspected she had fallen victim to this dreaded disease. Her condition soon worsened, and her doctors could not give her anything to improve her condition. In Gary's support group, we completely changed our diets and began exercising. My wife said she could feel something like electricity in her brain that improved her memory and bettered her overall mood. People mistakenly believe that only one spouse gets a disease like Alzheimer's. This is not true. For when she got it, it affected me, as well. Though she is not totally cured, she is a changed person. As a result, I, too, am a changed person.

—Egbert

Mental Fatigue

I had a "fuzzy" toxic head. I also had a lack of focus. The intensive focus on body, mind, spirit became clear in manifestation. I feel I have more focus and motivation and a new sense of who I am. My awareness is heightened. I believe I am moving toward divine health.

—Faye Marie L.

Headaches

I was diagnosed with a small melanoma in my right eye. I am legally blind in my left eye. The cancer options were horrendous: removing the eye, doing radiation, or leaving it with the chance it would metastasize to my liver. I often had migraine headaches, chronic lower back pain, prostate problems, a rotator cuff injury in my right shoulder, and arthritis in a toe. I was overweight. It was time to change strategies and rid myself of these conditions. Gary's words were powerful. I had to become my own authority. Since beginning the protocol, the cancer has not grown for eight months. Migraine headaches virtually disappeared about two months after changing my diet. I lost thirty-five pounds, and my back has improved. Saw palmetto and other herbs did not relieve my prostate problem in the past, but they are quite effective now. My body is receptive to healing. The other minor conditions have improved. Although my energy level varies, I feel more energetic and younger in a body that knows how to heal itself

—Eugene

Headaches

I suffered with bothersome tension-type headaches that sometimes became debilitating migraines. Since joining the group, I am eating a primarily vegetarian diet. I eliminated caffeine and sugar. I can state that I no longer have tension head aches. I feel very fortunate.

I see changes in my physical health and awareness around me. Understanding my life energies further empowered me with insight and understanding.

—Natalie K.

Parkinson's Disease

I am a Parkinson's patient. I had hypertension, B-simplex outbreaks, and arthritis and skin problems. I became aware of the importance of nutrition and studied various theories, but my physical problems continued. Parkinson's symptoms caused me shame in public. I could not write, and I typed with two fingers. My hands trembled when I put food in my mouth. I was prescribed medications, but past experiences were unpleasant, so I refused them. I began Gary's detoxification protocol and learned the specifics of diet and organics, the biochemical necessity of green juices and grasses, and the importance of attitude and beliefs. Things began to look up. I uncluttered my life of people and objects, and I now honor myself and share my knowledge with others. I am alert without past negative influences. These are my happiest and proudest times. I am seventy now, and I intend to live another twenty years.

—Thomas

Appendix IV

Endnotes

Chapter 1

1. E. Gould, A. J. Reeves, F. Mazyar, P. Tanapat, C. G. Gross, and E. Fuchs, "Hippocampal Neurogenesis in Adult Old-World Primates," *Neurobiology* 96 (1999): 5263–67.
2. Agency for Toxic Substances and Disease Registry, "2003 CERCLA Priority List of Hazardous Substances," www.atsdr.cdc.gov/clist.html.
3. John Carpi, "Stress: It's Worse than You Think," *Psychology Today* (1996).
4. J. Douglas Bremner, *Does Stress Damage the Brain? Understanding Trauma-Related Disorders from a Neurological Perspective* (New York: W. W. Norton & Co., 2002).
5. "New Studies of Human Brain Show Stress May Shrink Neurons," Stanford News Service press release, August 14, 1996, http://news.stanford.edu/pr/96/960814shrnkgbrain.html.
6. Robert Sapolsky, *Why Zebras Don't Get Ulcers: An Updated Guide to Stress, Stress-Related Diseases, and Coping* (New York: W. H. Freeman, 1998).
7. American Psychiatric Association, "Code 292.00, Nicotine Withdrawal," *Diagnostic and Statistical Manual of Mental Disorders*, 4th ed., revised (Washington, DC: American Psychiatric Association, 1994).
8. Joel Fuhrman, interview on *The Gary Null Show* on VoiceAmerica, November 11, 2004. Joel Fuhrman, MD, is a board-certified family physician.

Chapter 2

1. J. Madeleine Nash, "Fertile Minds," *Time*, February 3, 1997.
2. Stephen Nohlgren, "Challenging, Nurturing the Brain Keeps It Healthy," *St. Petersburg Times*, March 13, 2005.
3. Lawrence C. Katz, *Keep Your Brain Alive* (New York: Workman Publishing, 1998).
4. J. Weuve, J. H. Kang, J. E. Manson, M. B. Breteler, J. Ware, and F. Grodstein, "Physical Activity, Including Walking, and Cognitive Function in Older Women," *Journal of the American Medical Association (JAMA)*, 292 (2004), 1454–61.
5. N. Scarmeas, G. Levy, M.X. Tang, et al., "Influence of Leisure Activity on the Incidence of Alzheimer's Disease," *Neurology* 57 (2001), 2236–42.
6. K. Yaffe, D. Barnes, M. Nevitt, L. Lui, and K. Covinsky, "A Prospective Study of Physical Activity and Cognitive Decline in Elderly Women: Women Who Walk," *Archives of Internal Medicine* 161 (2001), 1703–08.
7. AARP, "Let's Dance to Health," www.aarp.org/health/fimess/get_motivated/ lets_dance_to_health.html.
8. Yaffe et al., "A Prospective Study of Physical Activity."
9. Ursula Lehr, "Longevity: A Challenge for the Individual and the Society" (speech presented at Colegio de Medicos de Madrid, May 18, 2000), www.segg.es/segg/html/socios/formacioncontinuada/ casos_clinicas/lehr.htm.
10. Marc Kaufman, "Meditation Gives Brain a Charge, Study Finds," *Washington Post*, January 3, 2005, wwwwashingtonpost.com/wpdyn/ articles/2430062005Jan2.html.
11. Ibid.
12. P. C. Bickford et al., "Diets High in Antioxidants Can Reverse Age-Related Declines in Cerebellar Beta-Adrenergic Receptor Functions and Motor Learning" (paper presented at the AGE Annual Meeting, Seattle, 1999); and L. Buee, "Cerebrovascular Aging," *Therapie* 54 (1999), 155–65.
14. A. M. al-Awadhi and C. D. Dunn, "Effects of Fish-Oil Constituents and Plasma Lipids on Fibrinolysis in Vitro," *British Journal of Biomedical Science* 57 (2000), 273–80.
15. "Fish Oil Holds Promise in Alzheimer's Fight," U.S. Department of Veterans Affairs press release, May 29, 2005, www.sciencedaily.com.
16. S. M. Loriaux, J. B. Deijen, J. F. Oriebeke, and J. H. De Swart, "The Effects of Nicotinic Acid and Xanthinol Nicotinate on Human

Memory in Different Categories of Age: A Double-Blind Study," *Psychopharmacology* 87 (1985), 390–95.

17. J. E. Alpert and M. Fava, "Nutrition and Depression: The Role of Folate," *Nutrition Review* 55 (1997), 145–49.

18. Marc Kaufman, "Meditation Gives Brain a Charge, Study Finds," *The Washington Post*, January 3, 2005.

19. J. Areart-Treichel, "Nutrient Combo Boosts Memory—At Least in Rats," *Psychiatric News* 37 (2002), 58.

20. Ibid.

21. R. P. Ostrowski, "Effect of Coenzyme Q10 (coQ10) on Superoxide Dismutase Activity in ET1 and ET3 Experimental Models of Cerebral Ischemia in the Rat," *Folia Neuropathology* 37 (1999), 247–51.

22. M. E. Rhodes, P.K. Li, J. F Flood, and D. A. Johnson, "Enhancement of Hippocampal Acetyicholine Release by the Neurosteroid Dehydroepiandrosterone Sulfate: An in Vivo Microdialysis Study," *Brain Research* 733 (1996), 284–86.

23. T. Maurice et al., "Dehydroepiandrosterone Sulfate Attenuates Dizocilpine-Induced Learning Impairment in Mice via Sigma 1 Receptors," *Behavioral Brain Research* 83, (1997),159-64.

24. H. D. Danenboerg et al., "Dehydroepiandrosterone (DHEA) IncreasesProduction and Release of Alzheimer's Amyloid Precursor Protein," *Life Science* 59 (1996), 1651–57.

25. H. Nagasawa, K. Kogure, K. Kawashima, et al., "Effects of Codergocrine Mesylate (Hydergine) in Multi-infarct Dementia as Evaluated by Positron Emission Tomography," *Tohoku Journal of Experimental Medicine* 162 (1990), 225–33.

26. M. Ditch, F. J. Kelly, and O. Resnick, "An Ergot Preparation (Hydergine) in the Treatment of Cerebrovascular Disorders in the Geriatric Patient: Double-Blind Study," *Journal of the American Geriatric Society* 19 (1971), 208–17.

27. H. Emmenegger and W. Meier-Ruge, "The Actions of Hydergine on the Brain: A Histochemical, Circulatory and Neurophysical Study," *Pharmacology* 1(1968), 65–78.

28. P. M. Kidd, "A Review of Nutrients and Botanicals in the Integrative Management of Cognitive Dysfunction," *Alternative Medicine Review* 4 (1999), 144–61.

29. P. J. Deiwaide et al., "Double-Blind Randomized Controlled Study of Phosphatidylserine in Senile Demented Patients," *Acta Neurological Scandinavica* 73 (1986), 136–40.

30. D. Bagchi, R. L. Krohn, M. Bagchi, et al., "Oxygen Free Radical Scavenging Abilities of Vitamins C and E, and a Grape Seed

Proanthocyanidin Extract in Vitro," *Research Communications in Molecular Pathology and Pharmacology* 95 (1997), 179–89.

31. P. Jones and D. Takai, "The Role of DNA Methylation in Mammalian Epigenesis," *Science* (2001), 1068–70.

Chapter 3

1. "Depression in Elderly," HealthyPlace.com, www.healthyplace.com/communities/depression/elderly.asp.
2. Ricki Lewis, "Evening Out the Ups and Downs of Manic-Depressive Illness," *FDA Consumer Magazine*, June 1996.
3. Ronald M. Podell, *Contagious Emotions: Staying Well When Your Loved One Is Depressed* (New York: Pocket Books, 1993).
4. Lewis Harrison, Interview on *The Gary Null Show* on VoiceAmerica, November 30, 2004.
5. Ibid.
6. T. L. Brink, J. A. Yesavage, O. Lum, P. Heersema, M. B. Adey, and T. L.Rose, "Screening Tests for Geriatric Depression," *Clinical Gerontologist* 1(1982), 37–44; see also J. A. Yesavage, T. L. Brink, T. L. Rose, O. Lum, V. Huang, M. B. Adey, and V. O. Leirer, "Development and Validation of a Geriatric Depression Scale: A Preliminary Report," *Journal of Psychiatric Research* 17 (1983), 37–49; and J. I. Sheikh, J. A. Yesavage, J. O. Brooks III, L. F. Friedman, P. Gratzinger, R. D. Hill, A. Zadeik, and T. Crook, "Proposed Factor Structure of the Geriatric Depression Scale," *International Psychogeriatrics* 3(1991), 23–28.
7. R. C. Casper, "Nutrients, Neurodevelopment, and Mood," *Current Psychiatry Report* 6 (2004), 425–29.
8. J. E. Alpert and M. Fava, "Nutrition and Depression: The Role of Folate," *Nutrition Review* 55 (1977), 145–49.
9. D. Frizel et al., "Plasma Magnesium and Calcium in Depression," *British Journal of Psychiatry* 115 (1969), 1275–77.
10. H. Beckman, M. A. Strauss, and E. Ludolph, "DL-Phenylalanine in Depressed Patients: An Open Study," *Journal of Neural Transmission* 41 (1977), 123–34.
11. K. D. Hansgen, J. Vesper, and M. Ploch, "Multicenter Double-Blind Study Examining the Antidepressant Effectiveness of the Hypericum Extract LI 160," *Journal of Geriatric Psychiatry and Neurology* 7, (1994), 15–18.
12. H. Schubet and P. Halam, "Depressive Episode Primarily Unresponsive to Therapy in Elderly Patients: Efficacy of Ginkgo Biloba Extract (EGb

761) in Combination with Antidepressants," *Geriatric Forschung* 3 (1993), 45–53.

13. Michael J. Norden, *Beyond Prozac: Brain-Toxic Lifestyles, Natural Antidotes & New-Generation Antidepressants* (New York: ReganBooks, 1995).

Chapter 4

1. Richard Restak, Interview on *The Gary Null Show* on VoiceAmerica, November 24, 2004. Richard Restak, MD, is a preeminent neuropsychiatrist and author of several books, including *The New Brain: How the Modern Age Is Rewiring Your Mind* (New York: Rodale, 2003).

2. *The Gary Null Show* on VoiceAmerica, November 24, 2004. Data taken from W. E. Narrow, D. S. Rae, and D. A. Regier, "NIMH Epidemiology Note: Prevalence of Anxiety Disorders. Population Estimates Based on U.S. Census Estimated Residential Population Age 18 to 54 on July 1, 1998." Unpublished.

3. "Anxiety: Should You Let It Worry You?" PDRHealth.com, www.pdrhealth.com.

4. "Anxiety Disorders," in *Merck Manual of Geriatrics*, 3rd ed., (Whitehouse Station, NJ: Merck Research Laboratories, Division of Merck & Co., Inc., 2000).

5. L. N. Robins and D. A. Regier, eds., *Psychiatric Disorders in America: the Epidemiologic Catchment-Area Study* (New York: The Free Press, 1991).

6. L. N. Robins and D. A. Regier, eds., *Psychiatric Disorders in America: the Epidemiologic Catchment-Area Study* (New York: The Free Press, 1991).

7. Anxiety Disorders Association of America website, www.adaa.org, adapted from A. J. Land and M. B. Stein, "Anxiety Disorders: How to Recognize and Treat the Medical Symptoms of Emotional Illness," *Geriatrics* 56 (2001), 24–27, 31–34.

8. Norman Brown, "Do You Suffer High Anxiety? Research Reveals More about How Stress Affects Body and Mind. Here Is the Rundown on Causes and Therapies," *VFW Magazine*, January 2003.

9. Ibid.

10. D. S. Charney, G. R. Heninger, and P. I. Jatlow, "Increased Axiogenic Effects of Caffeine in Panic Disorders," *Archives of General Psychiatry* 42 (1985), 233–43.

11. J. P. Boulenger, T. W. Uhde, E. A. Wolff III, and R. M. Post, "Increased Sensitivity to Caffeine in Patients with Panic Disorders: Preliminary Evidence," *Archives of General Psychiatry* 41 (1984), 1067–71.

12. M. Y. Geng, H. Saito, and N. Nishiyama, "Protective Effects of Pyridoxal Phosphate against Glucose Deprivation-Induced Damage in Cultured Hippocampal Neurons," *Journal of Neurochemistry* 68 (1997), 25000–6.

13. R. A. Akhundov, V. V. Rozhanets, T. A. Voronina, and A. V. Vaidman, "Mechanism of the Tranquilizing Action of Electron Structural Analogs of Nicotinamide," *Biull Eksp Biol Med.* 101 (1986), 329–31.

14. A. Palatnik, K. Frolov, M. Fux, and J. Benjamin, "Double-Blind, Controlled, Crossover Trial of Inositol versus Fluvoxamine for the Treatment of Panic Disorder," *Journal of Clinical Psychopharmacology* 21 (2001), pp. 335–39.

15. K. D. Hansgen, J. Vesper, and M. Ploch, "Multicenter Double-Blind Study Examining the Antidepressant Effectiveness of the Hypericum Extract LI 160,"*Journal of Geriatric Psychiatry and Neurology* 7, (1994), 15–18.

16. T. Field, "Massage Therapy Effects," *American Psychologist* 53 (1998), 1270–81.

17. Stephanie Marohn, interview on *The Gary Null Show* on VoiceAmerica, November 22, 2004. Stephanie Marohn is a writer and editor of books on psychospirituality and alternative thought.

Chapter 5

1. Paul Scheele, interview on *The Gary Null Show* on VoiceAmerica, November 29, 2004. Paul Scheele is the founder of Learning Strategies Corporation.

2. Ibid.

3. Dharma Singh Khalsa, interview on *The Gary Null Show* on VoiceAmerica, November 26, 2004. Dr. Singh Khalsa is president and medical director of the Alzheimer's Prevention Foundation International in Tucson, Arizona.

4. "Staying Sharp, Memory Loss and Aging," 2004 AARP Foundation and the Dana Alliance for Brain Initiatives.

5. T. D. Smith, M. M. Adams, M. Gallagher, J. H. Morrison, and P. R. Rapp, "Circuit-Specific Alterations in Hippocampal Synaptophysin Immunoreactivity Predict Spatial Learning Impairment in Aged Rats," *Journal of Neuroscience* 20 (2000), 6578-93.

6. A. D. Mooradian, "Effect of Aging on the Blood-Brain barrier," *Neurobiology of Aging* 9 (1988), 31–39.
7. Gary Null, *Healing the Brain Naturally*, DVD, directed/performed by Gary Null (2011; New York City: Gary Null & Associates, 2011.)
8. Elisa Lottor and Nancy Bruning, *Female and Forgetful: A Six-Step Program to Help Restore Your Memory and Sharpen Your Mind* (New York: Warner Books, 2002).
9. C. Decarle, B. L. Miller, G. E. Swan, et al., "Predictors of Brain Morphology for the Men of the NHLBI Twin Study," *Stroke* 30 (1999), 529–36.
10. J. S. Rhodes, H. van Praag, S. Jeffrey, I. Girard, G. S. Mitchell, T. Garland Jr., and F. H. Gage, "Exercise Increases Hhippocampal Neurogenesis to High Levels but Does Not Improve Spatial Learning in Mice Bred for Increased Voluntary Wheel Running," *Behavioral Neuroscience* 117 (2003), 1006–16.
11. Gary Null with Dharma Singh Khalsa, "Improving Memory Function," November 26, 2004.
12. R. G. Thompson, C. J. Moulin, S. Hayre, and R. W. Jones, "Music Enhances Category Fluency in Healthy Older Adults and Alzheimer's Disease Patients," *Experimental Aging Research* 31 (2005), 91–99.
13. B. Draganski, C. Gaser V. Busch, G. Schuierer, U. Bogdahn, and A. May, "Neuroplasticity: Changes in Grey Matter Induced by Training," *Nature* 427 (2005), 311–12.
14. M. C. Morris, D. A. Evans, J. L. Bienias, C. C. Tangney, and R. S. Wilson, "Vitamin E and Cognitive Decline in Older Persons," *Archives of Neurology* 59 (2002), 1125–32.
15. Ibid.
16. M. S. Morris, P. F. Jacques, I. H. Rosenberg, and J. Selhub, "National Health and Nutrition Examination Survey: Hyperhomocysteinemia Associated with Poor Recall in the Third National Health and Nutrition Examination Survey," *American Journal of Clinical Nutrition* 73 (2001), 927–33.
17. H. P. Volz, U. Hehnke, and W. Hauke, "Improvement in Quality of Life in the Elderly: Results of a Placebo-Controlled Study on the Efficacy and Tolerability of Lecithin Fluid in Patients with Impaired Cognitive Functions," *MMW Fortschr Medicine* 146 (2004), 99–106.
18. P. M. Kidd, "A Review of Nutrients and Botanicals in the Integrative Management of Cognitive Dysfunction," *Alternative Medicine Review* 4 (1999), 144–61.

Chapter 6

1. S. Kaplan, "The Restorative Benefits of Nature: Toward an IntegrativeFramework," *Special Issue: Green Psychology, Journal of Environmental Psychology* 15 (1995), 169–82.
2. Edward O. Wilson, *Biophilia: The Human Bond with Other Species* (Cambridge: Harvard University Press, 1986).
3. Annual Meeting of the Society of Psychophysiological Research in Montreal, Canada, October 1981.
4. A. Watanabe et al., "Effects of Creatine on Mental Fatigue and Cerebral Hemoglobin Oxygenation," *Euroscience Research* 42 (2002), 279-85.
5. V. Darbinyan, A. Kteyan, A. Panossian, E. Gabrielian, U. Wikman, and H. Wagner, "Rhodiola Rosea in Stress-Induced Fatigue: A Double-Blind Crossover Study of a Standardized Extract SHR5 with a Repeated Low-Dose Regimen on the Mental Performance of Healthy Physicians during Night Duty," *Phytomedicine* 7 (2000), 365–71.
6. A. A. Spasov, G. K. Wikman, V. B. Mandriko I. A. Mironova, and V. V. Neumoin, "A Double-Blind, Placebo-Controlled Pilot Study of the Stimulating and Adaptogenic Effect of Rhodiola Rosea SHR5 Extract on the Fatigue of Students Caused by Stress during an Examination Period with a Repeated Low-Dose regimen," *Phytomedicine* 7 (2000), 85–89.

Chapter 7

1. E. Mohr, T. Mendis, and J. D. Grimes, "Late Cognitive Changes in Parkinson's Disease with an Emphasis on Dementia," *Advances in Neurology* 65 (1995), 97–113.
2. Joan Stephenson, "Exposure to Home Pesticides Linked to Parkinson's Disease," *JAMA* 283 (2000), 3055–56.
3. P. C. Holland, J. S. Han, and M. Gallagher, "Lesions of the Arnygdala Central Nucleus Alter Performance on a Selective Attention Task," *Journal of Neuroscience* 20 (2000), 6701–06.
4. From the website of the National Parkinson's Foundation.
5. D. E. Riley, "Secondary Parkinsonism," in *Parkinson's Disease and Movement Disorders*, 3rd ed., edited by J. Jankovic and E. Tolosa (New York: LW&W, 1998), 317–28.
6. A. J. Hughes, S. E. Daniel, L. Kilford, and A. J. Lees, "Accuracy of Clinical Diagnosis of Idiopathic Parkinson's Disease: AClinicopathological

Study of 100 Cases," *Journal of Neurology, Neurosurgery, and Psychiatry* 55 (1992), 181–84.

7. A. I. Tröster, J. A. Fields, and W. C. Koller, "Parkinson's Disease and Parkinsonism," in *Textbook of Geriatric Neuropsychiatry*, 2nd ed., edited by C. E. Coffey and J. L. Cummings (Washington, DC: American Psychiatric Press, 2000), 559–600.

8. J. R. Chacon, E. Duran, J. A. Duran, et al., "Usefulness of Olanzopine inthe Levodopa-Induced Psychosis in Patients with Parkinson's Disease," *Neurologia* 17 (2002), 7-11.

9. C. W. Olanow, P. Jenner, N. Tatton, and W. Tatton, "Neurodegeneration and Parkinson's Disease," in *Parkinson's Disease and Movement Disorders*, 3rd ed., edited by J. Jankovic and E. Tolosa (New York: LW&W, 1998), s26–s33.

10. S. Fahn, "An Open Trial of High-Dosage Antioxidants in Early Parkinson's Disease," *American Journal of Clinical Nutrition* 53 (1991), 3805–3825.

11. W. Hellenbrand, H. Boeing, B. P. Robra, et al., "Diet and Parkinson's Disease: A Possible Role for the Past Intake of Specific Nutrients. Results from a Self-Administered Food-Frequency Questionnaire in a Case-Control Study," *Neurology* 47 (1996), 644–50.

12. M. Ebadi, J. F. Rodriguez-Sierra, and N. S. Norton, "Glutathione and Metallothionein in Neurodegeneration: Neuroprotection of Parkinson's Disease," *NEL* 18 (1998), 111–22.

13. "Jefferson Researchers Show Melatonin's Potential Benefits in Preventing Parkinson's Damage," Thomas Jefferson Medical College press release, October 24, 1999, www.mult-sclerosis.org/news/Octl999/MelatoninParkinsons.html.

14. D. Bagchi, R. L. Krohn, M. Bagchi, et al., "Oxygen Free Radical Scavenging Abilities of Vitamins C and E, and a Grape Seed Proanthocyanidin Extract in Vitro," *Research Communications in Molecular Pathology and Pharmacology* 95 (1997), 179–89.

Chapter 8

1. "Latest Facts & Figures Report," Alzheimer's Association (accessed January 2, 2013), www.alz.org/alzheimers_disease_facts_and_figures.asp.

2. Adapted from the Alzheimer's Information Site, www.alzinfo.org.

3. Ibid.

4. Adapted from the Administration on Aging's website, www.aoa.gov/ALZ/Public/alzcarefam/disease_info/questions_to_ask_pf.asp.

5. Alzheimer's Association International Conference on Prevention of Dementia, June 18–21, 2005, Washington, DC, www.alz.org/preventionconference/pc2005/.
6. "Exercise Slows Development of Alzheimer's-Like Brain Changes in Mice, New Study Finds," NIH News, April 25, 2005.
7. J. Verghese, R. B. Lipton, M. J. Katz, C. B. Hall, C. A. Derby, G. Kuslansky, A. F. Ambrose, M. Sliwinski, and H. Buschke, "Leisure Activities and the Risk of Dementia in the Elderly," New England Journal of Medicine 348 (2003), 2508–16.
8. P. E. Newman, "Could Diet Be One of the Causal Factors of Alzheimer's Disease?" Medical Hypotheses 39 (1992), 123–26.
9. S. Yehuda and S. Rabinovitz, et al., "Essential Fatty Acids Preparation (SR3) Improves Alzheimer's Patients' Quality of Life," International Journal of Neuroscience 87 (1996), 141–49.
10. M. Sano, C. Ernesto, et al., "A Controlled Trial of Selegiline, Alphatocopherol, or Both as Treatment for Alzheimer's Disease: The Alzheimer's Disease Cooperative Study," New England Journal of Medicine 336 (1997), 1216–22.
11. P. M. Kidd, "A Review of Nutrients and Botanicals in the Integrative Management of Cognitive Dysfunction," Alternative Medicine Review 4 (1999), 144–61.
12. P. L. Le Bars, M. M. Katz, N. Berman, et al., "A Placebo-Controlled, Double-Blind, Randomized Trial of an Extract of Ginkgo Biloba for Dementia," JAMA 278 16 (1997), 1327–32.
13. Q. Wang, K. Iwasaki, T. Suzuki, H. Arai, Y. Ikarashi, T. Yabe, K. Toriizuka, T. Hanawa, H. Yamada, and H. Sasaki, "Potentiation of Brain Acetylcholine Neurons by KamiUntanTo (KUT) in Aged Mice: Implications for a Possible Antidementia Drug," Phytomedicine 7 (2000), 253–58.
14. H. Arai, T. Suzuki, H. Sasaki, T. Hanawa, K. Toriizuka, and H. Yamada, "A New Interventional Strategy for Alzheimer's Disease by Japanese Herbal Medicine," Nippon Ronen Igakleai Zasshi 37 (2000), 212–15.
15. S. S. Xu, Z. X. Goa, Z. Weng, et al., "Efficacy of Tablet HuperzineA onMemory, Cognition and Behavior in Alzheimer's Disease," Chung k Uo Yao LiHsueh Pao 16 (1995), 391–95.

Chapter 9

1. J. P. Boulenger, T. W. Uhde, E. A. Wolff III, and R. M. Post, "Increased Sensitivity to Caffeine in Patients with Panic Disorders: Preliminary Evidence," Archives of General Psychiatry 41 (1984), 1067–71.

2. A. Mauskop and B. M. Altura, "Role of Magnesium in the Pathogenesis and Treatment of Migraines," *Clinical Neuroscience* 5 (1998), 24–27.
3. A. Peikert et al., "Prophylaxis of Migraine with Oral Magnesium: Results from a Prospective Multicenter, Placebo-Controlled and Double-Blind Randomized Study," *Cephalagia* 16 (1996), 257–63.
4. B. Claustrat, J. Brun, M. Geoffriau, R. Zaidan, C. Mallo, and G. Chazot, "Nocturnal Plasma Melatonin Profile and Melatonin Kinetics during Infusion in Status Migrainosus," *Cephalagia* 17 (1997), 511–17.
5. T. Field, "Massage Therapy Effects," *American Psychologist* 53 (1998), 1270–81.

Chapter 10

1. Scott Shepherd, "Head Trauma," August 20, 2004, www.emedicine.com.
2. S. Moochhala and J. Lu, "Potential Use of Stem Cell Therapy for Traumatic Brain Injury," Defence Medical & Environmental Research Institute, 117510. DSO National Laboratories, Singapore.
3. J. H. Bower, D. M. Maraganore, and B. J. Peterson, "Head Trauma Preceding PD," *Neurology* 60 (2003), 1610–15.
4. D. Shoumitro, I. Lyons, M. Koutzoukis, I. Au, and G. McCarthy, "Rate of Psychiatric Illness 1 Year after Traumatic Brain Injury," *American Journal of Psychiatry* 156 (1999), 374–78.
5. James M. Connor, Andrea A. Chiba, and Mark H. Tuszynski, "The Basal Forebrain Cholinergic System Is Essential for Cortical Plasticity and Functional Recovery Following Brain Injury," *Neuron* 46 (2005), 173–79.
6. F. Yang, G. P. Lim, A. N. Begum, O. J. Ubeda, M. R. Simmons, S. S. Ambegaokar, P. P. Chen, R. Kayed, C. O. Glabe, S. A. Frautschy, and G. M. Cole, "Curcumin Inhibits Formation of A Oligomers and Fibrils and Binds Plaques and Reduces Amyloid in Vivo," *Journal of Biological Chemistry* 280 (2005), 5892–5901.
7. Joie Gunei, "The Curry Cure," *UCLA Daily Brain Online*, January 14, 2005.
8. P. J. O'Connor, N. P. Pronk, A. Tan, and R. R. Whitebird, "Characteristics of Adults Who Use Prayer as an Alternative Therapy," *American Journal of Health Promotion* 19 (2005), 369–75.

9. R. F. Palmer, D. Katerndahl, and J. Morgan-Kidd, "A Randomized Trial of the Effects of Remote Intercessory Prayer: Interactions with Personal Beliefs on Problem-Specific Outcomes and Functional Status," *Journal of Alternative and Complementary Medicine* 10 (2004), 438–48.

Chapter 12

1. K. D. Hansgen, J. Vesper, and M. Ploch, "Multicenter Double-Blind Study Examining the Antidepressant Effectiveness of the Hypericum Extract LI 160," *Journal of Geriatric Psychiatry and Neurology* 7, (1994), 15–18.
2. T. Field, "Massage Therapy Effects," *American Psychologist* 53 (1998), 1270–81

Chapter 13

1. D. S. Knopman, S. T. DeKosk, J. L. Cummings, et al., "Practice Parameter: Diagnosis of Dementia (an Evidence-Based Review). Report of the Quality Standards Subcommittee of the American Academy of Neurology." *Neurology* 56 (2001), 1143–53.
2. Adapted from the Administration on Aging's website, www.aoa.gov/ALZ/Public/alzcarefam/diseasejnfo/questions_to_ask_pf.asp.
3. Alzheimer's Association International Conference on Prevention of Dementia, June 18–21, 2005, Washington, DC, www.alz.org/preventionconference/pc20057.
4. "Exercise Slows Development of Alzheimer's-Like Brain Changes in Mice, New Study Finds," *NIH News*, April 25, 2005.
5. J. Verghese, R. B. Lipton, M. J. Katz, C. B. Hall, C. A. Derby, G. Kuslansky, A. F. Ambrose, M. Sliwinski, and H. Buschke, "Leisure Activities and the Risk of Dementia in the Elderly," *New England Journal of Medicine* 348 (2003), 2508– 16.
6. R. A. Whitmer, E. P. Gunderson, E. Barrett-Connor, C. P. Quesenberry, and K. Yaffe, "Obesity in Middle Age and Future Risk of Dementia: A 27-Year Longitudinal Population-Based Study," B.7M, doi: 10.1 136/bmj.384446.466238 .EO (published April 29, 2005).
7. M. Sano, C. Ernesto, et al., "A Controlled Trial of Selegiline, Alphatocopherol, or Both as Treatment for Alzheimer's Disease: The Alzheimer's Disease Cooperative Study," *New England Journal of Medicine* 336 (1997), 1216–22.

8. P. M. Kidd, "A Review of Nutrients and Botanicals in the Integrative Management of Cognitive Dysfunction," *Alternative Medicine Review* 4 (1999), 144–61.

9. P. L. Le Bars, M. M. Katz, N. Berman, et al., "A Placebo-Controlled, Double-Blind, Randomized Trial of an Extract of Ginkgo Biloba for Dementia," *JAMA* 278, no. 16 (1997), 1327–32.

10. Q. Wang, K. Iwasaki, T. Suzuki, H. Arai, Y. Ikarashi, T. Yabe, K. Toriizuka, T. Hanawa, H. Yamada, and H. Sasaki, "Potentiation of Brain Acetylcholine Neurons by Kami Untan To (KUT) in Aged Mice: Implications for a Possible Antidementia Drug," *Phytomedicine* 7 (2000), 253–58.

11. H. Arai, T. Suzuki, H. Sasaki, T. Hanawa, K. Toriizuka, and H. Yamada, "A New Interventional Strategy for Alzheimer's Disease by Japanese Herbal Medicine," *Nippon Ronen Igakleai Zasshi* 37 (2000), 212–15.

12. S. S. Xu, Z. X. Goa, Z. Weng, et al., "Efficacy of Tablet Huperzine A on Memory, Cognition and Behavior in Alzheimer's Disease," *Chung k Uo Yao LiHsueh Pao* 16 (1995), 391–95.

Chapter 15

1. C. B. Pert and S. H. Snyder "Opiate Receptor: Demonstration in Nervous Tissue," *Science* 179 (1973), 1011–14.

2. Irving Kirsch and Guy Sapirstein, "Listening to Prozac but Hearing Placebo: A Meta-Analysis of Antidepressant Medication," *Prevention and Treatment* 1 (1998), article 0002a.

3. S. F. Maier and L. R. Watkins, "Cytokines for Psychologists: Implications of Bidirectional Immune-to-Brain Communication for Understanding Behavior, Mood, and Cognition," *Psychological Review* 105 (1998), 83–107.

4. S. E. Hammack, K. J. Richey, L. R. Watkins, and S. F. Maier, "The Role of Corticotropin Releasing Hormone in the Dorsal Raphe Nucleus in Mediating the Behavioral Consequences of Uncontrollable Stress," *Journal of Neuroscience* 22 (2002), 1020–26.

5. Marc Barasch, "Welcome to the Mind-Body Revolution," *Psychology Today* (1996).

6. Soloman, G. E., "The Emerging Field of Psychoneuroimmunology," *Advances* 2(1985), 6–19.

7. Maier and Watkins, S.F Maier and L.R. Watkins, "Cytokines for psychologists: Implications of bidirectional immune-to-brain

communication for understanding behavior, mood, and cognition." *Psychological Review*, Vol 105(1), Jan 1998, 83-107.

8. K. A. O'Connor, J. D. Johnson, M. K. Hansen, Frank J. L. Wieseler, E. Maksimova, L. R. Watkins, and S. F Maier, "Peripheral and Central Proinflammatory Cytokine Response to a Severe Acute Stressor," *Brain Research* 991 (2003), 123–32.

9. Ibid.

10. Beth Azar, "A New Take on Psychoneuroimmunology," *Monitor on Psychology* 32 (2001).

11. Herbert Benson, *The Relaxation Response* (New York: Avon Books, 1975); and Herbert Benson, *Beyond the Relaxation Response* (New York: Berkley Books, 1985).

12. Andrew Weil, *Spontaneous Healing* (New York: Ballantine Books, 1996).

13. Lauran Neergaard, "Brain Exercise Is Key to Healthy Mind," AssociatedPress, June 20, 2005.

14. Kathy Facklemann, "Lifestyle Link to Alzheimer's Strengthens," *USA Today*, June 19, 2005.

15. David M. Nathan and Linda Delahanty, "Better Waysto Beat Diabetes," *Newsweek*, June 9, 2005.

Index